FOUNDATIONS OF NURSING PRACTICE

Second Edition

Foundations of
Nursing
Practice

MAKING THE DIFFERENCE

EDITED BY

RICHARD HOGSTON AND
PENELOPE M. SIMPSON

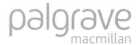

First edition 1999
Reprinted three times
Second edition 2002

Published by
PALGRAVE MACMILLAN
Houndmills, Basingstoke, Hampshire RG21 6XS and
175 Fifth Avenue, New York, N.Y. 10010
Companies and representatives throughout the world

PALGRAVE MACMILLAN is the global academic imprint of the Palgrave Macmillan division of St. Martin's Press, LLC and of Palgrave Macmillan Ltd. Macmillan® is a registered trademark in the United States, United Kingdom and other countries. Palgrave is a registered trademark in the European Union and other countries.

ISBN 0–333–98592–3 paperback

This book is printed on paper suitable for recycling and made from fully managed and sustained forest sources.

A catalogue record for this book is available from the British Library.

A catalog record for this book is available from the Library of Congress.

10 9 8 7 6 5 4 3
11 10 09 08 07 06 05 04 03

Editing and origination by Aardvark Editorial, Mendham, Suffolk

Printed and bound in Great Britain by
Bath Press, Bath

Contents

List of Figures

List of Tables

List of Charts

Notes on Contributors

SID CARTER MSc, BA, RN(LD), PGCEA, AdvCert (Human Sexuality) is a Lecturer (Clinical) in Learning Disabilities at the European Institute of Health and Medical Sciences, University of Surrey. His clinical work centres on the empowerment of people with cognitive impairments. Sid's research interests include the skills of professionals working with people with learning disabilities, and the psychophysiology of emotion as it relates to learning.

NADIA CHAMBERS MA, PGDipEd, BSc(Hons), ENB HA, RGN has just taken up the post of Consultant Nurse Elderly Care at Southampton General Hospital, having been a Senior Lecturer at the University of Portsmouth heading up Clinical Governance and Clinical Leadership Education at the School of Postgraduate Medicine. Her clinical practice focus is tissue viability, especially in elderly care. Her recent research includes an illuminative evaluation of continuing education in the principles of wound care, collaborative action research into nurses' self-efficacy in wound care and a study of how, why and when primary health-care nurses involve patients in the nursing management of chronic leg ulcers. Nadia is a member of the Tissue Viability Society and has presented work at the Fifth and Sixth International European Wound Management Association Conferences and the First International Conference for Evidence-based Nursing.

MOLLY COURTENAY PhD, MSc, BSc, CertEd, RGN, RNT has a nursing background in general medical and intensive care settings. She has worked as a lecturer in several academic institutions and currently holds a Senior Lecturer post at Buckinghamshire Chiltern University College. In 1996, she completed a PhD on infection control, and she has more recently undertaken research examining the use of larva therapy in the management of wounds. Molly is also involved in nurse prescribing practice and publication.

IAN DOUGLAS RGN, DPSN, RCNT, RNT, BA(Hons), MSc is a Senior Lecturer at South Bank University. His area of speciality is accident and emergency nursing, his current research interest lying in the epidemiological distribution of accidents related to accident and emergency services. He has for many years had an interest in and association with reflective practice development.

DEBRA ELLIOTT MSc, BSc(Hons), RNT, CertEd(FE), CertHE, RGN is Senior Nurse for Acute Medicine in Portsmouth, prior to this being Ward Manager of the Emergency Medical Unit at Southampton General Hospital. She also spent 5 years as a Senior Lecturer at the School of Health Studies, University of Portsmouth, seconded by the Queen Alexandra's Royal Naval Nursing Service, in which she served for 10 years. Debra has extensive clinical experience gained in the NHS and the Services in the areas of intensive care, coronary care and acute and emergency medicine, her main research interest and published work to date being related to resuscitation, particularly advanced life support.

ANITA J. GREEN MA, BA(Hons), RCNT, RGN, RMN is a Lecturer (Clinical) in the European Institute of Health and Medical Sciences, University of Surrey. She has worked in both acute mental health and drug and alcohol services, and is currently working with the staff of the Drug and Alcohol Services of Sussex Weald and Downs NHS Trust. Anita's research interest focuses on clients' experiences of the drug and alcohol service, in particular methadone prescribing. She has a consultancy relationship with the Drug and Alcohol Services and a nursing college in St Petersburg, Russia, and is currently completing an evaluation of that project.

RICHARD HOGSTON MSc(Nurs), PGDipEd, BA(Hons), RN is Director of The School of Nursing, Social Work and Applied Health Studies at the University of Hull, having been Nursing Officer for Education and Training at the NHS Executive. Previous to that, Richard was Principal Lecturer/Subject Leader for Nursing Studies at the School of Health Studies, University of Portsmouth, where his main teaching and research interests concentrated upon quality and management together with expertise in curriculum development.

MELANIE JASPER MSc, BNurs, BA, RN, RM, RHV, NDNCert, PGCEA is a Principal Lecturer working primarily in the Centre for Health Research in the School of Health and Social Care, University of Portsmouth. She is Course Leader for the MSc in Nursing Studies and focuses her teaching on the area of critical nursing theory and research methodology. She has a particular interest in the development of reflective writing in professional development, and in the use of portfolio construction in lifelong learning.

JANET McCRAY MSc, BSc(Hons), RNT, RN(LD), CertEd is currently a Principal Lecturer in Primary Care and Disabilities in the School of Health and Social Care, University of Portsmouth. While working in practice, Janet had a wide range of experiences supporting people with learning disabilities, largely in the community setting. She has more recently developed educational programmes that enhance interprofessional working, in particular between nurses and social workers. Janet now works in the field of primary care and disability studies.

BARBARA MARJORAM TD, MA, RN, CertEd is Deputy Head of Pre Registration Education at the School of Nursing and Midwifery, University of Southampton. She combines over a quarter of a century of clinical and teaching experience. Her previous publications have been related to the use of information technology in nursing and nursing practice.

SUSAN MOORE MSc, MBA, PGDipEd, BA(Hons), DipN(Lond), CertGer, RMN, RGN is Head of Department, Mental Health and Disability Nursing, St Bartholomew School of Nursing and Midwifery, City University. She was formerly Ward Manager of an assessment and treatment unit within the Department of Psychiatry of Old Age, Oxford Mental Healthcare NHS Trust. She has been a nurse for 24 years, during which she has been a manager, teacher and clinician. Her abiding interest lies in working with older people with mental health problems, including the sociology and social policy applied to this speciality.

SOMDUTH PARBOTEEAH MSc, SRN, RCNT, RNT, CertEd, DipN(Lond) is Senior Lecturer in Adult Nursing at De Montfort University and is involved in teaching life sciences and essential nursing skills. His research interests include the use of knowledge maps as a heuristic device for integrating theory and practice.

PHIL RUSSELL MSc, MA, BA(Hons), DipNE, RNT, RN is a Senior Lecturer at the School of Health and Social Care, University of Portsmouth. He is a nurse and practising counsellor with a particular interest in bereavement and palliative care. Phil teaches counselling, health psychology and interpersonal skills to a wide range of health-care professionals.

RUTH SADIK MSc, BA(Hons) Health Studies, RNT, RCNT, RSCN, RGN, CertEd(FE) currently teaches applied physiology relating to respiratory disorders in both children and adults. She is Senior Lecturer in Child Health and Programme Leader at the School of Nursing and Midwifery, Chester College of Higher Education.

PENELOPE M. SIMPSON MSc, DipEd, CertEd, DN(Lond), RCNT, RN is a Lecturer in the School of Nursing and Midwifery, University of Southampton and has been a nurse for more than 30 years. She currently teaches foundation nursing skills and therapeutic interventions. Her published work includes the nutritional impact of alcohol on elderly people, surgical nursing and client profiles in nursing.

CATHERINE THROWER MSc, BSc(Hons), DipNE, RNT, RN, RM gained an honours degree in Psychology from Portsmouth Polytechnic and an MSc in Health Psychology from City University, London. She worked in nurse education from 1989 until 2001, when she took a clinical post. Her clinical experience has been predominately in care of the older adult, her area of speciality being dementia care.

GRAHAM WATKINSON MA(Ed), RN, RNT, CertEd, MIHPE has worked operationally in acute care as manager, teacher and clinician specialising in intensive and coronary care nursing. His main research interests include promoting health within higher education, and the bereavement and loss aspects of organ donation. Graham lectures in Health Promotion and is adviser to the University of Portsmouth.

Acknowledgements

Many thanks to Richard Hogston, who started the whole project, to the authors, publishers and all at Aardvark for their patience, to the many student reviewers of all the chapters, and especially to my husband, David, for his support and forbearance throughout.

PENELOPE M. SIMPSON

Every effort has been made to trace all the copyright holders, but if any have been inadvertently overlooked the publishers will be pleased to make the necessary arrangements at the first opportunity.

Introduction

This text is designed to be used as a study guide to support many aspects of your learning throughout the common foundation programme. Each chapter has been written by an enthusiastic subject specialist, and we hope that their passionate interest will be infectious. The chapters are not meant to be read in any particular order but to be tackled when they feel relevant to your progress and experience. Their interactive style is intended to make you think, various activities enlivening the text and enabling you to apply your knowledge in practice settings. Constant reference is made to complementary texts, current evidence and further reading. Objectives give you an idea of what you can achieve by working through each chapter, and a running glossary within the chapters will enhance your vocabulary and understanding. Cross-referencing within and between chapters increases the coherence of the text. Client case studies draw on all four branches of nursing and feature a range of settings to encourage you to reflect on your reading and its application to clients. At the end of the chapters, there are review questions to enable you to check your knowledge gain.

Each of the chapters discusses a particular topic. In Chapter 1, the five stages of the problem-solving approach to care known as the nursing process will be used to help you to focus on the example of the client in pain. You will be enabled to map your own concept of health and, through Chapter 2 on health promotion, identify the concept of health gain. Nurses tend to deal with uniquely vulnerable clients, and nursing can carry risks to nurses, so Chapter 3 will identify some of the many safeguards, legal and otherwise, available to protect you and your clients. Eating and drinking, normal enough activities, can pose particular problems for clients, so you will be encouraged in Chapter 4 to look at your own knowledge and habits, aiming to help clients to achieve optimum nourishment for their changing needs. Logically, elimination follows, and Chapter 5 will help to dispel some taboos and myths, with a healthy emphasis on achieving and attaining relative normality across the life span. Chapter 6, on respiration and circulation, will explore the nurse's role in assessing and implementing the care of clients with difficulties of breathing and maintenance of the circulation. Body image and sexuality may be markedly affected by problems of diminished health, this being an area that demands sensitive and thoughtful care, as outlined in Chapter 7. Other body systems, their purpose and functioning, and what can go wrong will be explored in Chapter 8, covering the musculoskeletal system, the skin, lever systems and movement. Nursing covers the life span from cradle to grave. Loss and changes in health status can make clients question or confirm their beliefs, particularly when life is limited, so Chapter 9 will examine spirituality, dying and death. The role of the nurse and his or her professional responsibilities, including account-ability, will be clearly explained in Chapter 10, on wound care. Working in a team is a key part of nursing, and social behaviour and professional interactions will enhance your skill in therapeutic and other communication; this topic is covered in Chapter 11. Knowing yourself better, the subject of Chapter 12, will enable you to give of yourself to clients and colleagues without being dimin-ished. The image of nursing that you started out with is likely to be much changed as you progress in your career, and reflective practice, explained in Chapter 13, will be one tool to help you with this. As nursing takes place in a political arena, nurses should also be political, Chapter 14 encouraging you to understand the climate in which current developments were conceived. Inter-professional practice, Chapter 15, will be a clear focus for the future, as will challenges to professional practice, outlined in Chapter 16; these will enable you to look forward to the next part of your programme.

We hope you enjoy this new edition, finding it stimulating and thought-provoking, and we wish you well in your nursing career.

RICHARD HOGSTON

Chapter

Managing Nursing Care

1

Contents

Learning outcomes

The purpose of this chapter is to explore how nurses manage care; it will take you through a five-stage problem-solving approach known as the nursing process. At the end of the chapter, you should be able to:

- Define the stages of the nursing process

- Undertake a nursing assessment

- Identify nursing diagnoses from the assessment data

- Devise and implement a plan of care

- Evaluate your actions

- Consider the link between evaluation and quality of care.

Throughout the chapter, a working example using a client who is experiencing pain will be used to demonstrate how each of the stages of the nursing process is applied. The chapter also provides an opportunity for you to undertake some exercises that will assist you with your care-planning skills.

■ What is the Nursing Process?

nursing process

a five-stage problem-solving framework enabling the nurse to plan individualised care for a client

The **nursing process** is a problem-solving framework that enables the nurse to plan care for a client on an individual basis. The nursing process is not undertaken once only, because the client's needs frequently change and the nurse must respond appropriately. It is thus a cyclical process consisting of the five stages shown in Figure 1.1. The nursing process originated in the USA and was formally introduced into the UK in 1977 when the then General Nursing Council introduced its revision of the nursing syllabus. It was an attempt to move nursing away from its traditional 'task-orientated' approach to a more scientific and individualised one.

The nurse is an autonomous practitioner whose responsibilities are now governed by the Nursing and Midwifery Council (NMC) *Code of Professional Conduct* (NMC, 2002). This requires nurses to be accountable for the care that they prescribe and deliver with the nursing process, enabling them to document their actions in a logical and rational manner. Today, one's ability to use the nursing process is central to *Making a Difference* (DoH, 1999), *Fitness for Practice* (UKCC, 1999) and therefore *The NHS Plan* (DoH, 2000) and is governed by the learning outcomes of preregistration courses as outlined by the statutory body, the NMC, and embedded in parliamentary statute. This states that conditional to registration is the ability to:

> Undertake and document a comprehensive, systematic and accurate nursing assessment of the physical, psychological, social, and spiritual needs of patients, clients and communities

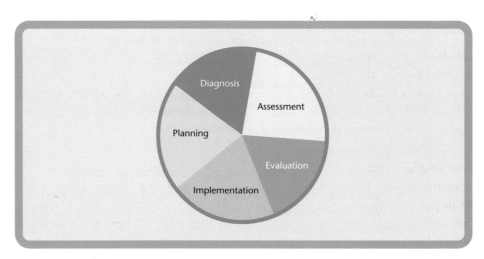

Figure 1.1 ● The nursing process

Provide a rationale for the nursing care delivered which takes account of social, cultural, spiritual, legal, political and economic influences

Evaluate and document the outcomes of nursing and other interventions

(DoH, 2000a)

The Nursing and Midwifery Council (NMC) replaced the United Kingdom Central Council for Nursing, Midwifery and Health Visiting (UKCC) and the four National Boards in April 2002. It is likely that the new Nursing and Midwifery Council will retain the standards and codes published by the UKCC until such time as they are revised.

Failure to keep a record of nursing care or to use the nursing process can lead to a breakdown in the quality of care that is provided. The Clothier Report (DoH, 1994), which was published following the inquiry into Beverley Allitt (the nurse who was convicted of the murder of children in a hospital in Grantham, Lincolnshire), noted how:

Despite the availability of a nurse with responsibility for quality management, there were no explicit nursing standards set for ward four. In addition the nursing records were of poor quality and showed little understanding of the nursing process.

The Commission for Health Improvement (CHI) is now responsible for clinical governance reviews in NHS Acute Trusts. In its guidance (CHI, 2001), it states that 'clinical governace is to ensure patients receive the highest quality of NHS care possible including a patient centred approach and a commitment to quality'. Thus, the importance of understanding and using a systematic approach (such as the nursing process) to the provision of nursing care cannnot be overestimated.

There has been some debate within the profession over the number of stages needed in the nursing process, some suggesting four and others five. With a four-stage approach, the nurse does not have time to reflect on the assessment data that have been collected and instead moves from assessment to planning. The five-stage process enables the nurse to identify the client's nursing diagnosis in order to plan the appropriate care.

The nursing process should not be seen as a linear process: it is a dynamic and ongoing cyclical process (Figure 1.1). Assessment, for example, is not a 'one-off' activity but a continuous one. Take the example of the individual who is in pain – it is not enough to make a pain assessment that may warrant an intervention; the nurse then needs to make a reassessment after having evaluated whether the pain-relieving intervention has been successful.

The nursing process is a problem-solving activity. Problem-solving approaches to decision-making are not unique to nursing. The medical profession uses a specific format based upon an assessment of the body's systems. A number of questions are asked in a systematic manner to enable the doctor to make a diagnosis based upon the information that has been collected. Problem-solving approaches are also taken outside the health-care field. Car mechanics undertake a sequence of activities in order to diagnose what is wrong with your car when you tell them that there is a squeak or a rattle.

Stage 1: Assessment

Sources of assessment data

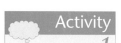

Activity 1

Think about the client and other sources that you may be able to consult to assist you when conducting a comprehensive assessment. Write them down in a list.

Before beginning to consider what sort of information you might need to collect, we need to look at the skills that are necessary to ensure that the data analysed are comprehensive. Assessment is not an easy process as it includes collecting information from a variety of sources. The quality of the assessment will, however, depend on one's ability to put together all the sources at one's disposal. Spend a few minutes on Activity 1.

The sources that you have listed in Activity 1 have probably included the following:

- Your client
- Relatives, friends and significant others
- Current and previous nursing records
- The records of other health professionals such as doctors and physiotherapists
- Statements and information from the police, ambulance personnel, witnesses at an accident scene and others.

Your client

The first and most important source for data collection is obviously the individual whom you are assessing. It will not, however, always be possible to obtain all the information you require, for a number of reasons, so you will also need to consult other people.

Relatives, friends and significant others

If you are assessing a baby, most of the verbal information you require will be obtained from his or her parent(s) or guardian(s). With a child, you will need to qualify some of your information through the same source. In the case of an adult who is unconscious or is having difficulty breathing, you will again need to obtain data from friends, relatives, ambulance personnel, the police and so on. The same applies if the client has difficulty understanding as a result of dementia or severe learning disabilities.

Nursing, medical and other records

It will not always be possible to have immediate access to existing records, especially in an emergency or with a first consultation, but these sources hold valuable information that you need to analyse. They provide details that may assist and prompt you. If the client has been admitted to a hospital, you may have a letter from the GP, district nurse, health visitor or community psychiatric nurse. Similarly, on discharge from hospital, you will provide discharge information if community-based professionals need to be involved. Telephone calls to these professionals, visits and case conferences may also feature.

Skills

Having considered some of the sources at your disposal, we now need to think about what other factors have a bearing on a successful assessment. Spend a few minutes on Activity 2.

As we are beginning to see, the process of assessment is a complex one. Although we have identified some of the sources of information, the quality of the information collected depends upon a number of other factors. In your list from Activity 2, you may have included:

- Listening
- Observing
- The use of verbal and non-verbal communication and open and closed questions
- Physical examination
- Measurements.

Listening

One of the most important features of an assessment interview is the nurse's ability to listen to the client. This means giving the client time to answer questions. You will appreciate from your own life experience that when you are asked a question, you want time to think and then answer without interruption. A premature interruption may lead to clients withholding information or not feeling that you are really interested in what they have to say. Although it is important for you to focus on the information you require and not digress, the

> **Activity**
> **2**
>
> Spend a little while thinking about what sorts of skill you need in order to conduct your assessment. Write them down in list form.

> **CONNECTIONS**
>
> *In Chapter 11 you will find a detailed examination of how the nurse can most effectively use some of these skills. You may wish to consult this before reading on.*

fact that Mrs Jones has been admitted as an emergency and is meant to be on the school run in an hour will be the only thing of interest to her until you are able to contact someone who can collect her children.

Observation

CONNECTIONS

Chapter 6 explains some causes of cyanosis and identifies the difference between central and peripheral cyanosis.

Observation can in itself provide the nurse with a great deal of information. The bluish tinge (cyanosis) seen around the mouths, nailbeds and faces of some breathless patients may be indicative of respiratory distress and will be an indication of how little oxygen is circulating in their blood. A yellowish tinge to the skin (jaundice) may be indicative of biliary disease. Similarly, facial and other body expressions may give you an indication of pain.

Open and closed questioning

closed questions

those designed to elicit a simple 'yes' or 'no' answer

open questions

those in which clients can express their answers in as many words as they choose

Both these methods of communication need to be used when collecting information. The use of **closed questions** allows the client who is, for example, breathless, anxious, in pain or depressed to answer with a simple 'yes' or 'no'. **Open questions**, however, will allow you to provide your clients with a full opportunity to tell you the history of their illness or pain.

Physical examination

CONNECTIONS

Chapter 8 briefly outlines the structure and function of the skin. Chapter 10 classifies wounds and has a section on wound assessment.

The physical examination of clients allows you to observe and make a judgement about their symptoms. You will be able to determine the integrity (state) of the skin, which is an important consideration in an immobile client. Physical damage such as wounds can be seen, as can even the small puncture marks left by an intravenous drug abuser. Skin that feels very warm and moist to the touch may be a sign of pyrexia.

Measurements

CONNECTIONS

Chapter 6 explores blood pressure and explains how to take an arterial blood pressure reading.

Measurements come in many forms, for example the taking of a blood pressure, pulse or temperature. Also included here is the use of other assessment tools such as a nutritional analysis, a pressure sore risk calculator (for example Norton or Waterlow) or a pain chart.

Data collection

As we have seen, nurses must, in order to be able to plan care for their clients, be able to gather information that will enable them to make informed decisions.

But what information do nurses need to gather, what questions should they ask and how much do they need to know? The answer is determined on an individual basis, the nurse collecting both subjective and objective information. Before looking in detail at what information should be collected, undertake Activity 3.

From the activity, in addition to name, age and date of birth, you may have collected some of the following information:

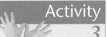

Activity 3

Select a friend or relative and ask them if you can spend about 20 minutes undertaking a health assessment.

Now take a blank piece of paper and collect the information that you feel is important when making some decisions about your chosen person's health status.

Physical health information
- Current and past health problems
- Nutritional and dietary information
- Patterns of activity and rest
- Stamina
- Physical parameters
- Factors affecting health (cigarettes, alcohol and so on)
- Dental, hearing, vision and so on
- Elimination patterns
- Sexual history.

Psychological information
- How does the client react to stress, challenge and so on?
- What are the person's hopes, expectations, demands?
- Communication
- Values and beliefs.

Social health information
- What is the person's lifestyle?
- Employment/unemployment details
- Family or other responsibilities
- Leisure
- Exercise
- Social environment/networks.

How did you decide what you needed to ask, how did you decide to word the questions, and did you collect everything to enable you to feel that you had conducted a thorough assessment?

Framework for assessment

One way of organising the information that you need to collect is by using a nursing framework. The 'activities of living' framework devised by Roper et al.

Chart 1.1 ● The activities of living

- Maintaining a safe environment
- Breathing
- Eliminating
- Controlling body temperature
- Working and playing
- Sleeping

- Communicating
- Eating and drinking
- Personal cleansing and dressing
- Mobilising
- Expressing sexuality
- Dying

(2000) uses a list of the client's activities of living (Chart 1.1) as a framework for assessment, the nurse systematically collecting the physical, psychological, socio-cultural and economic aspects of these activities.

Breathing, one of the activities of living, will now be used as a framework to demonstrate the type of information that the nurse needs to collect during an assessment. At any given time during the assessment process, it may be necessary to concentrate more on one activity than another.

Breathing

CONNECTIONS

Chapter 6 provides methods of respiratory assessment.

The information that the nurse needs to collect about this and any other activity of living depends on the answers to certain trigger questions. You may, for example, start off by asking your client whether she has any problems with breathing. Even though the answer may be 'no', you would, as a professional, need to investigate further. The client whom you are assessing may not feel that she has a problem with breathing, but consider the following questions:

1. 'Do you smoke?' The answer here may be 'yes' even though the client has said she has no problems with breathing. Indeed, she may still feel that she does not have any problems. This is, however, a trigger for further questioning.
2. 'Do you suffer from any breathlessness?' The answer at the outset may again be 'no', but if you ask about running up the stairs or running for a bus, the client may admit that, yes she does then, but this is because she does not usually do any exercise.
3. Taking this one step further allows the nurse to extract even more information about the status of the client's breathing: 'Do you cough?' The answer may be 'no', but when prompted the client may admit to coughing for a little while in the morning, although this clears rapidly and she thinks nothing of it.

If the client is a normal healthy young adult, the nurse may at this stage still perceive that the client does not actually have a problem with breathing in the short term even though she is partaking in health-damaging behaviour. In the long term, however, the consequences are obvious. At this stage in the assessment process, it may be sufficient to make a note of the information gathered so far; when it comes to planning care, the action that will be prescribed will then include health education about smoking. This will be expanded in the section on planning and implementation below.

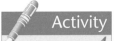

Activity

4

Read the client profiles in Casebox 1.1 on the next page. Choose one of the profiles and, for any two of the activities of living, write down the information that you would need to collect during a nursing assessment.

Summary and worked example

This section has introduced you to the nursing process and looked in some detail at assessment. The activities should have enabled you to experience some of the issues that you need to consider when undertaking a nursing assessment. We have examined the skills that the nurse needs to use when assessing clients, and we have been introduced to one assessment framework that may assist the nurse during the process. By way of a summary of the information that needs to be gained when undertaking an assessment, the following section takes pain as an example and outlines the questions and methods that can be employed when assessing a client's pain. This will be revisited as we consider the other four stages of the nursing process later in the chapter. Having read this summary, you may like to return to the client profile that you chose and identify the information you feel would be important for your chosen profile. Alternatively, you might like to take the opportunity to participate in the assessment process during your practice placements in the common foundation programme.

▪ Pain Assessment

The assessment of pain is a complex activity that involves a consideration of the physical, psychological and cultural aspects of the individual. Because pain is a subjective experience, the nurse needs to be able to summarise the information gained against some objective criteria. This is essential for diagnosis and for evaluating the effectiveness of interventions. Only the person experiencing the pain knows its nature, intensity, location and what it means to them. One of the most seminal, widely used and accepted definitions of pain was put forward by McCaffery (1979), who suggests that pain is 'whatever the experiencing person says it is and exists whenever he says it does'.

CONNECTIONS

Chapter 6 deals with pain arising from circulatory problems.

Assessments of the patient's pain experience

To begin with, it is essential to identify the characteristics of the client's pain. This means that the nurse should consider:

- *The type of pain:* is it crampy, stabbing, sharp? How the client describes the pain may help in diagnosing its cause. Myocardial (heart) pain is often described as stabbing, but biliary pain as cramping or aching
- *Its intensity:* is it mild, severe or excruciating? Pain assessment scales are helpful here. The nurse can ask the patient to rate the pain on a scale of 0 to 10, zero being no pain and 10 intolerable pain. With children, a range of pictures showing a child changing from happy to sad can be used. Colour 'mood' charts, with a series of colours from black through grey to yellow and orange, have also been used and are very useful for clients who have difficulty grasping numbers or articulating exactly what their pain is like
- *The onset:* was it sudden or gradual? Find out when it started and in what circumstances. What makes it worse? What makes it better? What was the patient doing immediately before it happened?
- *Its duration:* is it persistent, constant or intermittent?
- *Changes in the site:* there may be tenderness, swelling, discolouration, firmness or rigidity. With appendicitis, a classic sign is the movement of pain

Casebox 1.1

Joan Harris is a 69-year-old lady who tripped and fell over a protruding pavement slab this morning while out shopping. She has been admitted to the orthopaedic ward of her local NHS Trust hospital suffering from a fractured neck of femur. Mrs Harris is pale and is anxious about who will look after her cat while she is in hospital. She is complaining of severe pain in her hip and knee, and has grazes and cuts to her lower leg.

Amanda Cohen is 29 years old and has profound learning disabilities. She lives in staffed residential accommodation with two other young women. For 2 weeks, Amanda has been showing signs of distress – hitting her face, lifting her jumper and crying. It was at first thought that this might be because of premenstrual tension. After a while, however, someone thought to arrange a dental inspection under anaesthetic: the dentist found a particularly nasty dental abscess. (Adapted from NHSE, 1993)

Andrew Holly is 5 years old and has been admitted to the accident and emergency department of the local NHS Trust hospital. He is complaining of a very sore and painful arm, is very withdrawn and is sobbing. He is accompanied by his mother, his 2-year-old sister and their newborn baby brother.

Alison Simpson, 21 years old, lives in a hostel for people with mental health problems. She has no close family, having left home at 18. She finds it difficult to develop relationships and is suspicious of people who try to befriend her. Alison is very withdrawn and has on two occasions attempted to take her own life through an unsuccessful paracetamol overdose. She was found this morning slumped in a corner, covered in blood and complaining of extreme pain in her left hand. On the floor nearby was a razor blade, and on examination she had severe lacerations to her left forearm.

Chart 1.2 ● Common symptoms of disease that influence the response to pain

- Anorexia
- Diarrhoea
- Dyspnoea
- Immobility
- Dryness of the mouth
- Malaise and lassitude
- Nausea and vomiting
- Inflammation
- Anxiety and fear
- Constipation
- Cough
- Oedema
- Depression

from the umbilicus to the right iliac fossa. In a myocardial infarction (a heart attack), pain classically radiates down the arm, and with biliary pain it can radiate to the shoulder
- *Its location:* ask the patient to be as specific as possible, for example indicating the site by pointing
- *Any associated symptoms:* Chart 1.2 shows some of the common symptoms of disease that can influence the response to pain
- *Signs* such as redness, swelling or heat.

Summary

Table 1.1 provides a summary of some of the issues to consider when assessing pain. In essence, this section demonstrates how much detail the nurse needs to collect when making a full assessment of the client's pain. Consider your own experiences of pain, both personally and from clients you have nursed in clinical practice, and reflect on how comprehensive the assessment was then.

Table 1.1 Assessment of pain

Initial sympathetic responses to pain of low-to-moderate intensity	Parasympathetic responses to intense or chronic pain	Verbal responses	Muscular and postural responses
Increased blood pressure	Decreased blood pressure	Crying	Increased muscle tone
Increased heart rate	Decreased heart rate	Gasping	Immobilisation of the affected area
Increased respiratory rate	Weak pulse	Screaming	
Decreased salivation and gastrointestinal activity	Increased gastrointestinal activity	Silence	Rubbing movements
Dilated pupils	Nausea and vomiting		Rocking movements
Increased perspiration	Weakness		Drawing up of the knees
Pallor	Decreased alertness		Pacing the floor
Cool, clammy skin	Shock		Thrashing and restlessness
Dry lips and mouth			Facial grimaces
			Removal of the offending object

Stage 2: Nursing Diagnosis

nursing diagnosis

the second stage of the nursing process, often described as a 'nursing problem', for which the nurse can independently prescribe care

The second stage of the nursing process is making a **nursing diagnosis**. This enables the nurse to translate the information gained during the assessment and identify the nursing problems. In order to avoid confusion, it is worth noting that 'diagnosis' is not a concept unique to medicine: car mechanics diagnose mechanical problems, teachers diagnose learning difficulties, and consequently nurses diagnose nursing problems.

The language of nursing diagnosis originated in North America in the 1970s in an effort to move the art, science and theoretical basis of nursing forward. The benefits in a clinical setting have been positively described by Mills et al. (1997) and Hogston (1997).

Nursing diagnosis is a critical step in the nursing process, depends on an accurate and comprehensive nursing assessment and forms the basis of nursing care-planning. Nursing diagnosis is the end-product of nursing assessment, a clear statement of the patient's problems as ascertained from the nursing assessment increasingly being referred to as a nursing diagnosis (Roper et al., 2000). Gordon (1987), for example, suggests that a nursing diagnosis 'Describes actual or potential problems that nurses, by virtue of their education and experience, are capable and licensed to treat'. More recently, Weber (1991) stated that a nursing diagnosis is 'A statement that describes the actual or potential health problems of a client based on a complete holistic assessment. The problem/s must be at least partially resolved through nursing interventions.' Furthermore, the International Council of Nurses has, for the purposes of the International Classification for Nursing Practice, defined a nursing diagnosis as 'a label given by a nurse to the decision about a phenomenon which is the focus of nursing intervention' (ICN, 1999). A visit to the website at www.icn.ch is recommended for more detailed information.

Chart 1.3 ● Key components of a nursing diagnosis

A nursing diagnosis:

- is a statement of a client's problem
- refers to a health problem
- is based on objective and subjective assessment data
- is a statement of nursing judgement
- is a short concise statement
- consists of a two-part statement
- is a condition for which a nurse can independently prescribe care
- can be validated with the client

Source: Adapted from Shoemaker (1984), Bellack and Edlund (1992) and Iyer et al. (1995).

This provides a reasoned argument for defining patients' problems as nursing diagnoses and was the definition adopted by Hogston (1997) in an article published on nursing diagnosis in the UK. In summary, the key components of what constitutes a nursing diagnosis are outlined in Chart 1.3.

Making a nursing diagnosis

Nursing diagnoses can be actual or potential. Actual diagnoses are those which are evident from the assessment, for example pain caused by a fractured neck of femur. Potential diagnoses, on the other hand, are those which could or will arise as a consequence of the actual diagnoses. For example, an individual who is normally active but is confined to bed is at risk of becoming constipated or developing a pressure sore. In this instance, two potential diagnoses arise:

- a potential risk of constipation as a result of enforced bedrest
- a potential risk of pressure sore development from enforced bedrest.

▦ Stage 3: Planning Nursing Care

There are two steps to the planning stage:

- Setting goals
- Identifying actions.

A **goal** is a statement of what the nurse expects the client to achieve and is sometimes referred to as an objective. In other words, goals are the intended outcomes and can be short term or long term. Goals are client centred and must be realistic, being stated in objective and measurable language. They help both nurse and client to define how the nursing diagnosis will be addressed. Goals serve as the standard by which the nurse can evaluate the effectiveness of the nursing actions.

When writing goals, they need to conform to the MACROS criteria; they should be:

- **M**easurable and observable so that the outcome can be evaluated
- **A**chievable and time limited
- **C**lient centred
- **R**ealistic
- **O**utcome written
- **S**hort.

Activity 5

Return to the two activities of living that you assessed during Activity 4. Try to identify one actual and one potential nursing diagnosis. Use the guidelines in Chart 1.3 to ensure that your diagnoses meet the criteria.

CONNECTIONS

Chapter 5 considers the causes, diagnosis and treatment of constipation.

goal
the intended outcome of a nursing intervention, sometimes referred to as an objective

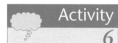

Activity

6

For the diagnoses that you identified during Activity 4, try to identify one short-term and one long-term goal for your chosen client. Remember to ensure that they meet the MACROS criteria.

Using the example of pain, the short-term goal will be that the client will state that he is comfortable and pain free within 20 minutes. The long-term goal, however, is that the client will state within 12 hours that he feels in control of his pain. (It is important to remember to take account of the non-verbal clues discussed earlier – is the client really pain free?) With the move to shorter hospital stays and the emphasis on care in the community, it may not always be necessary to formulate both long- and short-term goals for all problems. It is, however, always better to have a number of short-term goals that are reached so that new goals can be set rather than having a long-term goal that takes weeks to achieve. With Mrs Harris (see Casebox 1.1 above), who will have surgery for her hip, this will be a series of goals that progress her towards full mobility following her operation, for example: 'Mrs Harris will walk one way to the toilet unaided by [enter date]. Mrs Harris will be able to climb one set of stairs by [enter date].' This avoids a long-term goal that reads 'Mrs Harris will be fully mobile by [enter date].'

Action planning

The next stage is to plan the nursing care that will ensure that clients achieve their goals. This is where the nurse prescribes nursing actions that can then be implemented and evaluated. In 'care-planning' language, these are the nursing actions – the prescribed interventions that are put into effect in order to solve the problem and reach the goal. It is against these actions that the nurse may, when evaluating care, have to make some adjustments if the actions have not been effective. In today's NHS, when we are seeing a decreasing number of registered nurses against an increase in those of bank and agency nurses and unqualified health-care support workers, documenting the prescribed nursing care ensures a degree of continuity. In this way, the care plan can be seen as the diary of the client's nursing care. When planning nursing care, use the REEPIG criteria, which will ensure that your plan of care is:

● *Realistic:* it is important that the care can be given within the available resources, otherwise it will not be achievable
● *Explicit:* ensure that statements are qualified. If you suggest that a dressing needs changing, state exactly when. This will ensure that there is no room for misinterpretation
● *Evidence based:* nursing is a research-based profession. When planning nursing care, the research findings that underpin the rationale for care must be considered
● *Prioritised:* start with the most pressing diagnosis. Given that time is of the essence, the first priority may be, for example, to plan care for the client's pain

- *Involved:* the plan of care should involve not only the client, so that he or she is aware of why such care is needed, but also the other members of the health-care team who have a stake in helping the client back to health, for example physiotherapists and dietitians
- *Goal centred:* ensure that the care planned meets the set goals.

Returning now to the example of pain, the nurse needs to make decisions about what sorts of intervention will most effectively relieve Mrs Harris's pain. This involves not only decisions about prescribed medications, but also other considerations such as how often the pain assessment tool should be used and what alternative non-pharmacological methods, such as comfort through pillows, the use of skin traction for the leg and distraction therapy, can be implemented. The nursing care plan for Mrs Harris may therefore detail the following nursing actions:

> ### Activity 7
> Return to the client for whom you chose to identify nursing diagnoses and goals. Consider what nursing care you would need to plan in order to achieve those goals.

> ### CONNECTIONS
> *Chapter 8 examines the development of pressure sores and methods of prevention.*

- Give the prescribed analgesic and monitor its effects. Record them on the pain chart
- Apply skin traction
- Nurse on a bed equipped with a pressure-reduction mattress
- Ensure 2-hourly changes of position by attaching a trapeze pole to the bed, and encourage Mrs Harris to change her position regularly
- Ensure that Mrs Harris has a supply of chosen reading/writing materials and access to the television and radio.

Stage 4: Implementation

Implementation is the 'doing' phase of the nursing process. This is where the nurse puts into action the nursing care that will be delivered and addresses each of the diagnoses and their goals. The nurse will undertake the instructions written in the care plan in order to assist the client in reaching these goal(s). This will involve a process of teaching and helping clients to make decisions about their health. It also involves deciding upon the most appropriate method for

Chart 1.4 ● Other members of the health-care team

- Physiotherapist
- Community psychiatric nurse
- Speech therapist
- Health visitor
- District nurse
- Podiatrist
- Social worker
- Occupational therapist
- Dietitian
- Key worker
- School nurse
- GP

providing nursing care, and the liaison and involvement of other health professionals. Look at the list of health professionals in Chart 1.4. Do you know what their primary roles and functions are and when you might need to involve them?

■ Managing Nursing Care in the Clinical Environment

A number of different approaches to the delivery of nursing care are available to nurses. These include task allocation, patient allocation, team nursing, primary nursing, the key worker and caseload management. The benefits or otherwise of each of these methods need to be considered in the light of the skill mix of available staff (that is, the number and grade of qualified and unqualified staff) and what it is that the nursing team wants to achieve. It is difficult to evaluate the right approach without considering the benefits or drawbacks of each of these methods. The published reports of clinical governance reviews by the CHI (see above) will also consider the management and organisation of nursing care.

Task allocation

task allocation

the provision of nursing care that centres on a range of tasks allocated to nurses/support workers

Task allocation (also known as functional nursing) is a highly ritualistic method of organising care that centres on nurses and support workers being assigned tasks. With this system, one nurse will be assigned to undertake the observations of temperature, pulse, blood pressure and respiration. Another nurse undertakes all the dressings, whereas another takes care of the drugs. This is a very fragmented method of providing nursing care that will ensure that the client receives aspects of care from a multiplicity of nurses and support workers, akin to a production line process. The emphasis on tasks naturally removes the notion of individualised client care and is as such incompatible with the nursing process.

Client allocation

client allocation

individualised care provided by a named nurse, often assisted by a support worker

One step removed from task allocation is **client allocation**. Here, total care for a number of clients is undertaken by one nurse, often assisted by a support worker. Although this system means that there is an emphasis on total client care being delivered by an individual nurse for a designated period of time, continuity of care may become compromised if the same clients are not cared for on a regular basis by the same nurse. With this system, extra attention needs to be paid to the detail in the nursing care plan because of the number of nurses who may have contact with a client.

Team nursing

Team nursing occurs where a designated group of clients is cared for by a team of two or more nurses (at least one of whom is a registered nurse) who accept collective responsibility for the assessment, planning, implementation and evaluation of the clients' care. Although each team will be headed by a team leader, each registered nurse is accountable for his or her actions in accordance with the Code of Conduct (NMC, 2002). This is important to remember in an effort to counteract any criticism surrounding who is ultimately responsible under a system of collective responsibility.

team nursing
care provided by a team of nurses/support workers led by a 'team leader'

There is a plethora of literature available on team nursing, although much of it compares team nursing with primary nursing and is now rather dated. The literature suggests that many nurses who have striven towards a system of primary nursing have used team nursing as a 'stepping stone' (Wilson, 1991). The seminal research undertaken by Chavigny and Lewis (1984) set out to compare primary and team methods of care delivery and to estimate their effect on both quality and cost. The research found that team nursing tended to promote more client contact than did primary nursing, that clients' satisfaction was high but that there were no significant differences in cost or quality. In contrast, the research conducted by Reed (1988) concluded that, compared with team nursing, primary nursing afforded an increase in the quality of care and increased job satisfaction for nurses.

Walsh and Ford (1989) have described how team nursing and client allocation evolved as the successor to task allocation on the premise that being cared for by a team rather than an array of nurses led to more holistic care. They suggested that team nursing really resembles a small-scale version of task allocation, especially if there is a lack of continuity between shifts when the same team may not be on duty, leading to fragmentation of care. Consequently, there has to be a commitment to ensure that tasks are not assigned to each team member.

Team nursing has received a positive press from student nurses. Lidbetter's (1990) small-scale study describes how students working in a hospital ward practising team nursing spent more time working alongside a qualified nurse and rated their skill acquisition and their evaluation of the effectiveness of client care higher than did those from a ward practising primary nursing. Students were also, as a learning experience, afforded the opportunity to assume the role of team leader, under supervision.

Primary nursing

Primary nursing has been described as a professional patient-centred practice (Manley, 1990). In this approach, the primary nurse accepts full responsibility

primary nursing
care provided on an individual basis by a named nurse who, in its purest form, holds 24 hour accountability for the package of care

and accountability for his or her clients during their stay. In its purest form, the implication is that the primary nurse has 24 hour responsibility 7 days a week (Manthey, 1992). In reality, a team of associate nurses continues to provide nursing care under the direction of the primary nurse and in his or her absence. Again, accountability and autonomy rest with the individual registered nurse under the Code of Conduct (NMC, 2002). There is a great deal of literature on the efficacy of primary nursing, some of the discussion centring on the difference between primary nursing and the named nurse approach. For a full and lively debate on the issue, the reader is referred to the chapter on primary nursing in *New Rituals for Old* by Ford and Walsh (1994).

Person-centred planning

Popular in the field of learning disabilities, a person-centred approach to planning care is advocated in the White Paper *Valuing People* (DoH, 2001a). Person-centred planning starts with the individual, is seen as 'a mechanism for reflecting the needs and preferences of a person with learning disability and covers issues such as housing, education employment and leisure' (DoH, 2001a). At the time of writing, central guidance is to be published and readers are referred to the White Paper and the Department of Health website (www.doh.gov.uk/learning disabilities) for further information.

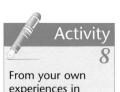

Activity

8

From your own experiences in clinical practice, what method(s) of care organisation have you experienced? Write down two positive aspects and then consider whether one of the other methods described above would have been suitable and why.

Caseload management

This is the most popular method of organising nursing care in the community setting. It revolves around the designated named nurse with extended qualifications in health visiting/district nursing who acts as the caseload manager. Caseloads are normally organised either geographically or by GP attachment, each caseload manager leading a team of qualified nurses and health-care support workers. Continuity of care is maintained because the teams are organised to ensure that a member of the team is available every day of the week; as such, it is less affected by the demands of the shift system. Each registered nurse is accountable for his or her own actions (NMC, 2002), the caseload manager being responsible for ensuring that the skill mix and resources are adequate.

■ Stage 5: Evaluation

At the beginning of this chapter, it was noted that the stages of the nursing process need to be seen as ongoing rather than as once-only activities. This means that the final stage, evaluation, is in reality the end of the beginning and where the process in essence restarts. One of the key components of quality nursing practice is the nurse's ability to make a clinical judgement based upon a sound knowledge base. Evaluation is about reviewing the effectiveness of the care that has been given, and it serves two purposes. First, the nurse is able to ascertain whether the desired outcomes for the client have been achieved. Second, evaluation acts as an opportunity to review the entire process and determine whether the assessment was accurate and complete, the diagnosis correct, the goals realistic and achievable, and the prescribed actions appropriate. The nursing process provides nurses with a tool by which client outcomes are regularly monitored, and can be seen as a vehicle for improving the quality of nursing care and ultimately benefiting the client (Fitzpatrick et al., 1992).

Increased health-care costs require managers throughout the professions to reduce expenditure and seek the most cost-effective options. The population at large are also more informed about health-care matters and are arguably less passive recipients of health care, demanding a detailed and open explanation for their care (Hogston, 1997). It is therefore the responsibility of each nurse to ensure that the prescribed care takes account of these issues. Given that nursing records are legal documents that could be used in a court of law, extreme care and accuracy are essential when completing the care plan to which the registered nurse puts her signature.

In order to raise standards of care, and in keeping with the clincial governance agenda, the government has published benchmarks in eight fundamental aspects of care (DoH, 2001b), one of which focuses on record-keeping. Readers should familiarise themselves with this particular benchmark. It is important to note that the document stresses that the 'eight aspects are by no means an exhaustive account of every fundamental aspect of care, but it represents those elements identified by patients and professionals as crucial to the quality of a patient's care experience' (DoH, 2001b; www.doh.gov.uk/essenceofcare).

Methods of evaluating nursing care

Having discussed the importance of evaluation and the place it has in maintaining quality, it is important to consider some of the methods that nurses can use. First of all, undertake Activity 9.

Your list from Activity 9 may have included some of the following:

- Nursing handover
- Reflection
- Patient satisfaction or complaint
- Reviewing the nursing care plan.

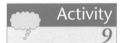

Activity
9

How do you think that nursing care is evaluated? You may have witnessed some methods in your own clinical placements; write them down as a list. If you have not, try to think generally about how you evaluate any service you have received – buying a meal or an item from a shop, for example.

Nursing handover

You may have had experience of a nursing handover, which is where a team of nurses hand over information about the nursing care of clients to another group of nurses, usually at the end of a shift, for example from day care to night care. Using the nursing care plan as the focus, nurses share information about the clients and their planned care. This serves as a valuable forum for evaluating care through a discussion of its effectiveness. The variety of experiences and professional expertise held by a number of nurses allows a sharing of that information. The importance of nursing handover was stated by the Audit Commission (1992) as being critical for maintaining continuity of client care.

Reflection

CONNECTIONS

Chapter 13 reviews types of reflection, thoughtful practice and reflection in practice settings.

The role of reflection in quality and evaluation has been discussed in some detail in the literature, and Chapter 13 discusses the concept in more detail. Reflection can, however, be both formal and informal. You probably reflect on your experiences both socially with other friends who are nurses and more formally in lecturer-led tutorials. This leads to an analysis of your actions and some of the ways in which you could have done things differently or which you would want to repeat. The use of critical incident analysis, for example, enables nurses to evaluate a given situation or event; this is a tool that is used by qualified nurses in their personal portfolios, which must be kept in order for the nurses to be eligible for triennial re-registration (see Chapter 13).

Patient satisfaction

The appreciation that is sometimes offered by clients through, for example, a letter is an indicator of how satisfied individuals have been with their nursing care. In contrast, a letter of complaint may lead to an investigation into the reasons why a client has not been satisfied with the care received. Although the number of letters of complaint appears to be on the increase, this is probably the result of a culture comprising a more informed public. In many ways, such letters lead to an analysis of what went wrong; this may not necessarily be a result of poor nursing care but of other environmental factors. Hopefully, however, such publicity allows those who have control over resources to evaluate the priorities.

Health-care providers are now required to publish statistics on indicators of quality ranging from, for example, how long clients have to wait in accident and emergency departments to the number of clients who receive a visit from the community nurse within the 2 hour appointment time. In the same vein, letters and cards of satisfaction should be closely monitored.

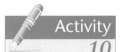

Activity
10
Review the assessment, nursing diagnosis, goal(s), planned care and method of implementation for your chosen client and then write an evaluation statement. Remember to ask the questions outlined in the text.

Reviewing the nursing care plan

This is where the nurse evaluates the effectiveness of the care that has been given against the set goals and writes an evaluation statement. When evaluating care, it is useful to ask yourself a series of questions about each of the stages of the nursing process, which will provide you with answers about your plan of care:

● Have the short-term goals been met?
● If the answer is 'yes', has the diagnosis been resolved? If so, it no longer needs to be addressed
● If the answer is 'no', why have the goals not been met? Did they meet the MACROS criteria?
● Was the planned care realistic? Did it meet the REEPIG criteria?
● Has a new diagnosis arisen or a potential diagnosis become an actual one?
● Was the method of care delivery appropriate?
● Was there effective communication within and between the nursing staff and other members of the multidisciplinary team?
● How satisfied was the client with the care?

Finally, take a look at the completed care plan for Mrs Harris outlined in Figure 1.2 and compare it with your own completed care plan.

Nursing diagnosis:	Pain due to fractured neck of femur.
Goal: Short term:	Mrs Harris states that she is comfortable with a pain scale rating below 2 within 15 minutes.
Goal: Long term:	Mrs Harris feels that she is in control of her pain and that it is no longer a major concern for her within 24 hours.
Nursing actions:	Give the prescribed analgesic and monitor its effects.
	Apply skin traction.
	Nurse on a bed equipped with a pressure-relieving mattress.
	Ensure 2-hourly changes of position by attaching a trapeze pole to the bed, and encourage Mrs Harris to change her position regularly.
	Ensure that Mrs Harris has a supply of chosen reading/writing materials and access to the television and radio.
Evaluation:	Mrs Harris states that she is comfortable and her pain scale rating remains below 2.

Figure 1.2 ● Worked example of a care plan for Mrs Harris

■ Information Technology and Care-planning

The input of information technology to health care is having a significant impact on the NHS as advanced computerised information systems record and evaluate everything from finance to personal records. From your own experiences, you may already have seen laptop/palm-top and office-based computers that can record client details and an analysis of nurses' workload. As the NHS network expands, all health-care workers are able to access electronic records, email and increasingly the World Wide Web. This will provide nurses with rapid access to client data such as previous nursing records. There are also currently a number of care-planning computer packages used by different NHS Trusts.

Computerised care-planning offers the nurse a number of advantages. It is quick, because there are a number of templates for common nursing diagnoses. Although these are sometimes criticised for moving towards a more communal rather than an individualised approach to nursing care, each of the templates has a menu of options that can be tailored to the individual client. The ability to raise at the push of a button a client's previous records is also an advantage and generally allows a more rapid search than does a paper-based system.

Computerised care-planning is, however, only as effective as the person who operates the system and generates the care plan. The skills of assessment, identifying nursing diagnoses and goal-setting, and the required nursing actions, can only be effective if the nurse has a sound knowledge base and uses the skills outlined within this chapter. The profession should, and indeed does, welcome the move to more electronic-based systems, if only because the approach is fast and usually efficient. The government has published its strategy through the NHS Information Authority (2002); a visit to its interactive website at www.nhsia.nhs.uk is recommended in order to appreciate the rapid advances in this area.

■ Chapter Summary

This chapter has introduced you to a systematic method for delivering nursing care through the framework known as the nursing process. You have been introduced to the five basic stages of assessment, diagnosis, planning, implementation and evaluation. Using the vehicle of structured activities, you have been offered the opportunity to develop a care plan for a chosen client.

At this stage, you may feel that the nursing process is a complex activity that demands a great deal of thought and practice, but your skills and experiences will continue to grow and develop as your professional career continues. Working through a structured chapter such as this is no substitute for practice and experience, but the principles of care-planning and the issues you need to consider are offered as the basis of accountable nursing practice. You may, for example, have been surprised at how complex and comprehensive the process of assessment is. The depth of material that you needed to collate when undertaking your assessment may have led you to reflect on the importance of probing and accurate questioning. As you progress in your chosen professional career, you will find that your ability to plan care will become greater. The important point to remember is that the whole practice and process of nursing is ever changing, new strategies, treatments and knowledge arriving almost daily. New research informs nursing practice and must be incorporated into one's professional repertoire. The process of nursing, like the process of learning, is an ongoing rather than a once-only activity.

● **Test Yourself!**

1. Name the stages of the nursing process.

2. Give two reasons for using the nursing process.

3. What sort of information needs to be collected during a nursing assessment?

4. How many types of nursing diagnosis are there?

5. What are the two stages of the planning phase?

6. What criteria should goals conform to?

7. How can the nursing care plan be evaluated?

References

Audit Commission (1992) *Making Time for Patients: A Handbook for Ward Sisters*. HMSO, London.

Bellack, J.P. and Edlund, B.J. (1992) *Nursing Assessment and Diagnosis*, 2nd edn. Jones & Bartlett, London.

Chavigny, K. and Lewis, A. (1984) Team or primary nursing care? *Nursing Outlook* **32**(6): 322–7.

CHI (Commission for Health Improvement) (2001) *A Guide to Clinical Governance Reviews in NHS Acute Trusts*. CHI, London.

DoH (Department of Health) (1994) *The Allitt Inquiry. Independent Inquiry Relating to Deaths and Injuries on the Children's Ward at Grantham and Kesteven Hospital During the Period February–April 1991* (Clothier Report). HMSO, London.

DoH (Department of Health) (1999) *Making a Difference: Strengthening the Nursing, Midwifery and Health Visiting Contribution to Health and Healthcare.* DoH, London.

DoH (Department of Health) (2000a) *Nurses, Midwives and Health Visitors (Training) Ammendment Rules Approval Order 2000.* Stationery Office, London.

DoH (Department of Health) (2000b) *The NHS Plan.* Stationery Office, London.

DoH (Department of Health) (2001a) *Valuing People: A New Stratgy for Learning Disability for the 21st Century.* Stationery Office, London.

DoH (Department of Health) (2001b) *Essence of Care: Patient-focused Benchmarking for Health Care Practitioners.* DoH, London.

Fitzpatrick, J.M., While, A.E. and Roberts, J.D. (1992) The role of the nurse in high quality patient care: a review of the literature. *Journal of Advanced Nursing* **17**: 1210–19.

Ford, P. and Walsh, M. (1994) *New Rituals for Old: Nursing Through the Looking Glass.* Butterworth Heinemann, Oxford.

Gordon, M. (1987) *Nursing Diagnosis: Process and Application,* 2nd edn. McGraw-Hill, New York.

Hogston, R. (1997) Nursing diagnosis: a position paper. *Journal of Advanced Nursing* **26**: 496–500.

ICN (International Council of Nurses) (1999) *International Classification for Nursing Practice.* ICN, Geneva.

Iyer, P.W., Taptich, B.J. and Bernocchi-losey, D. (1995) *Nursing Process and Nursing Diagnosis,* 3rd edn. W.B. Saunders, Philadelphia.

Lidbetter, J. (1990) A better way to learn? *Nursing Times* **86**(29): 61–4.

McCaffery, M. (1979) *Nursing Management of the Patient with Pain.* J.B. Lippincott, Philadelphia.

Manley, K. (1990) Intensive care nursing. *Nursing Times* **86**(19): 67–9.

Manthey, M. (1992) *The Practice of Primary Nursing.* King's Fund, London.

Mills, C., Howie, A. and Mone, F. (1997) Nursing diagnosis: use and potential in critical care. *Nursing in Critical Care* **2**(1): 11–16.

NHSE (National Health Service Executive) (1993) *Learning Disabilities.* DoH, London.

NHS Information Authority (2002) *Information for Health.* information@nhsia.nhs.uk

NMC (Nursing and Midwifery Council) (2002) Code of Professional Conduct. NMC, London. www.nmc-uk.org/cms/content/publications.

Reed, S.E. (1988) A comparison of nurse-related behaviour, philosophy of care and job satisfaction in team and primary nursing. *Journal of Advanced Nursing* **13**: 383–95.

Roper, N., Logan, W., and Tierney. A. (2000) *The Roper-Logan-Tierney Model of Nursing: Based on Activities of Living.* Churchill Livingstone, Edinburgh.

Shoemaker, J. (1984) Essential features of a nursing diagnosis. In Kim, M.J., McFarland, G. and Mclane, A. (eds) *Classification of Nursing Diagnoses.* C.V. Mosby, St Louis.

UKCC (United Kingdom Central Council for Nursing, Midwifery and Health Visiting) (1999) *Fitness for Practice*. UKCC, London.

Walsh, M. and Ford, P. (1989) *Nursing Rituals: Research and Rational Actions*. Butterworth Heinemann, Oxford.

Weber, G.J. (1991) Nursing diagnosis: a comparison of text book approaches. *Nurse Educator* **16**(2): 22–7.

Wilson, J. (1991) Step by painful step. *Nursing Times* **18**(87): 42–4.

2

Promoting Health

Contents

Learning outcomes

This chapter will provide the reader with a broad introduction to health and health promotion. It is intended to stimulate thought and challenge areas of life that are often taken for granted, promoting discussion and reflection. At the end of this chapter, you should be able to:

- Express what health means to you

- Identify contemporary challenges to health

- Recognise that health promotion is a wide concept that includes health education

- Define the key *Our Healthier Nation* targets

- Discuss the role of the nurse as a health promoter

- Evaluate health.

Throughout the chapter, exercises are given to provide an opportunity for you to explore the notion of health in a holistic way.

In July 2000 the government set out its plan to invest in and reform the delivery of health care to create a modern and dependable NHS following years of under-funding (DoH, 2000a). Emphasis was placed on the imperative that nurses, midwives and health visitors should 'take a lead in the way local health services are organised and in the way that they are run'. Through collaboration and partnership, the overarching outcome of improving the general health and life expectancy of the whole population can, it is felt, be achieved. It is inappropriate to attempt to condense, and therefore gloss over in one chapter, material that only a whole text on health promotion can properly cover. Further reading is therefore essential in gaining a good grasp of the many facets of this topic. To this end, a list of suggested texts can be found at the end of this chapter.

■ What is Health?

Before we can examine health promotion, and its integral function within contemporary nursing, we need to define just what health is. Most people know what it is like to experience health on a day-to-day basis, but when you ask someone what it is like to be healthy, or perhaps the less personal question 'What is health?', you inevitably get an answer or definition that seeks to explain what *ill-health* is. It seems easier to turn the question around by asking what it is like not to be healthy and then to speculate that the reverse is health. Unfortunately, if you do this you fall into the trap of oversimplification, which this chapter will seek to clarify.

Health is a slippery concept to grasp in comparison with ill-health, which seems so solid and tangible. The following examples have all been drawn from real-life situations. To maintain confidentiality, clients' names have been changed. Try to justify whether these people are healthy.

Example 1

Jill, a student nurse, was on a short placement to a special school for children with health problems. It cared for and educated a whole range of children whose needs were different from those who passed through what can be called the normal state education system. Many children were playing in the school playground when a 6-year-old girl named Samantha caught Jill's attention. Bending down to listen to the child's breathless voice, Jill picked Samantha up and sat her on her knee. She had seen the child playing joyfully a few moments earlier as though she had not a care in the world. After a few minutes of conversation, Samantha stated that she needed a heart transplant. 'There is nothing wrong with my heart', she pointed out. 'The loving part works just fine, it's the pumping part that has a problem.' In the medical sense, this child was clearly very sick, yet having watched her at play and talked with her, Jill was taken aback by the composed, almost matter-of-fact way in which the child had come to terms with a life-threatening illness. Indeed, she had a very positive outlook on her potentially negative condition.

Example 2

Annie, who is 42 years old, has been married to Jim for 20 years. Unfortunately, shortly after they were married, Annie had a road traffic accident, which resulted in her being hospitalised and undergoing an exploratory laparotomy for abdominal pain. During the surgery, the surgeon discovered that Annie had an ovarian cancer that had been **asymptomatic** until the accident. The diseased organ was successfully removed, and there were no other signs of injury. Was Annie healthy before her accident? It appears not, but as far as Annie was concerned, she certainly was.

asymptomatic

without symptoms

Example 3

This final example concerns two people and the intimate relationship that they share. Rachel, a 21-year-old married woman, had been looking forward to the birth of her first child. Her pregnancy had been relatively straightforward as far as she was concerned, with some morning sickness during the first trimester (third) of pregnancy. A routine ultrasound scan had demonstrated that all was progressing well, and there were no specific concerns for either mother or child. When Sam was born at full term (40 weeks) weighing over 3.6 kg (8 lb), Rachel went through an unexpectedly difficult labour, the prime reason being that Sam had a larger than normal head. A diagnosis of **hydrocephalus** was made. This condition resulted in Sam having many epileptic fits during the first few months of his life. Rachel coped very well with Sam, but during his first Christmas, Sam's fits became more severe, progressing to **status epilepticus**. The consequence was that Sam sustained some brain damage due to a prolonged period of **apnoea**. He is now not expected ever to walk or indeed feed himself. Would you consider Rachel to be healthy in her present circumstances, looking forward to perhaps many years caring for her son? What about Sam and the potential he has for development? How does he fit into your definition of health? Or perhaps he doesn't.

hydrocephalus

an excess of cerebrospinal fluid inside the skull ('water on the brain')

status epilepticus

an almost continuous succession of epileptic attacks

apnoea

cessation of breathing

A consideration of these three very different examples, involving four individuals, will demonstrate that health takes on many different forms. You may, of course, argue that these examples all involve a great deviation from the 'normal', whatever that is. Is someone who has a headache healthy? Is a hangover the residue of having had a great time or is it a transitory unhealthy state?

Some Concepts of Health

Enabling people to achieve better health is a fundamental part of good nursing practice, whether in the community or in an acute hospital setting. Whether involved in primary prevention, secondary health care, tertiary rehabilitation or palliative care, a nurse who thinks critically about those whom he or she seeks to help may be able to promote their health and alleviate their suffering. At a superficial level, this seems obvious, so why is it so difficult to achieve continually in practice with all clients and patients? Perhaps we need to be more critical and define what we mean by health. First of all, consider your own definition of health, as in Activity 1.

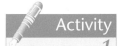

Activity 1

What does being healthy mean to you (as a daughter/son, wife/husband, parent, member of a student group or community, and so on)? Write your answer on a separate sheet of paper. You may wish to review/revise this over time and file it within your portfolio.

Many experts agree that it is difficult to define precisely what health is, although over 50 years ago the World Health Organization (WHO, 1947) put forward a definition that many writers have used as a substructure to build upon:

> A state of complete physical, mental and social well-being and not merely the absence of disease and infirmity.

This definition is very exclusive in that it excludes so many people from ever achieving or hoping to achieve this elusive state of perfection. Is health the same as well-being? Could Sam (see above) aspire to this? Dubos (1979) states that:

> Health and disease cannot be defined merely in terms of anatomical, physiological, or mental attributes. The real measure is the ability of the individual to function in a manner acceptable to himself and to the group of which he is part.

Pike and Forster (1995) complement Dubos' statement by arguing that it is important to take into account people's own perceptions and views on health and that different people will see and express these in different ways. Furthermore, Seedhouse (1986), in his book of the same title, describes health as the 'foundations for achievement'. The idea that health is a particular, precisely determined, fully informed 'structure' to which each individual can strive is, he argues, absurd. It is as nonsensical as the supposition that there can be a faultless person.

Seedhouse (1997) has developed these ideas further into what he calls the foundations theory of health promotion. Fundamental to this is the extent to

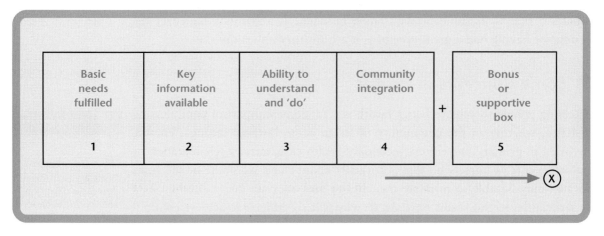

Figure 2.1 ● The foundations theory of health promotion (adapted from Seedhouse, 1997)

which a person's autonomy reflects his or her health status. As long as the foundations for health are complete in the context for that individual, he or she may be in a position to attain optimal health. A simplified version of this theory is included in Figure 2.1, but readers are strongly advised to consult the original text.

According to the foundations theory, a person will have a high level of health providing he or she can stand upon the four central boxes (with support from the fifth when, and as, required). Movement towards X will require additional provision or maintenance. Consequently, if any of these boxes is damaged or missing, only a lower level of health can be achieved.

Check back to Activity 1 and review your statement about what health means to you. You may wish to revise this.

Challenges to Health

Our health is in a dynamic state of continuity and change, constantly being challenged, stressed, abused and even enhanced by our genetic make-up and lifestyle, and by our wider ecological environment. It is truly amazing that, for the majority of people, their health seems to be in a stable state most of the time. In these first few years of a new millennium, our ideas about health and illness are changing. Conquered infectious diseases of the past are ridiculing modern antibiotic therapy through developed resistance. Each time it is informed of a case of necrotising fasciitis, or when antibiotic-resistant bacteria, for example methicillin-resistant *Staphylococcus aureus* (MRSA), close down yet another hospital ward, the media propagates the notion that 'superbugs' with flesh-eating powers lurk within our hospitals. According to Emmerson et al. (1996), however, there is no evidence of an increase in infection rate from MRSA since 1980.

Other organisms that were previously routinely killed by simple hygiene methods are now reasserting their influence, perhaps because of our complacency. Yet it only takes a few *Escherichia coli* bacteria in the wrong place at the wrong time to cause acute, even life-threatening, illness. During the winter of 1996/97, *E. coli* 0157 food poisoning occurred in North Lanarkshire, resulting in the deaths of 18 elderly people and close to 400 reported cases of infection. The source of the outbreak was strongly associated with cooked meat products sold by a local butcher. Food hygiene can thus be seen to be an important aspect of caring for sick and vulnerable people to ensure safety in practice.

> **CONNECTIONS**
>
> *Chapter 3 reviews the essentials of food hygiene.*

Health may be affected in a more insidious way as a result of intensive farming methods, perhaps where animals are fed contaminated or the wrong types of food, resulting in, for example, the foot and mouth disease crisis of 2001 or the bovine spongiform encephalitis (BSE) epidemic. The number of confirmed BSE cases has fallen from over 23,000 in 1994 to around 1,300 in 2000. Since its establishment on 1 April 2000, the Food Standards Agency has been fully involved in the protection of public health, with responsibility for BSE controls relating to the food chain (Department for Environment, Food and Rural Affairs, 2001).

BSE is considered by some 'experts' to be transmissible to man, resulting in Creutzfeldt–Jakob disease (CJD). The causative virus in BSE and CJD is a 'slow virus', an agent inducing slow, degenerative encephalopathy (cerebral dysfunction characterised by disorientation and excitability of the central nervous system). In humans this progressive dementia is usually fatal within 6 months. The Department of Health (DoH) publishes monthly updates on the number of deaths and probable cases of CJD in the UK (http://www.doh. gov.uk/cjd).

New-variant CJD (nvCJD), the hitherto unrecognised variant of CJD discovered by the National CJD Surveillance Unit and reported in the *Lancet* on 6 April 1996, has been shown to account for 110 definite or probable cases up to 2 April 2002 (DoH, 2002). Precisely defining the number of cases is difficult because of the complexities of data collection and the different varieties of CJD, and the results of the few post mortem examinations currently being carried out in the elderly following dementia-related illness may mean that the figure of 109 is an underestimate (MAFF and FSA, 2001). No test is currently available to detect those who may be infected with vCJD at the preclinical stage. Sporadic cases appear to occur spontaneously with no identifiable cause and, according to DoH statistics (2002), account for 85 per cent of all cases. In contrast, **iatrogenic** infection appears to have occurred accidentally as the result of medical interven-

iatrogenic

arising as a result of diagnosis or treatment

tion, for example from contaminated neurosurgical instruments, dural grafts and treatment with human growth hormone.

Challenges to health may occur in a crude cyclical fashion, whereby diseases pose no real threat until safeguards are removed or 'fail-safe' conditions are disrupted, often through complacency or neglect. This may be true for tuberculosis, which could be said to be revisiting the UK (even though it was never completely eradicated). An opportunistic infection, tuberculosis seems to be almost endemic where the most vulnerable are at risk because of poor or inadequate housing and diet. Those who live as part of society's underclass in a state of relative poverty fall victim to it. This heterogeneous group consists of the disempowered, the frail, the young, the elderly, the single parents with no real chance of escaping welfare under the present system and the long-term unemployed. There seems to be a sense of hopelessness within some communities, which squeezes health and vitality out of the everyday lives of the disenfranchised.

◼ The Goldfish Bowl Society

The goldfish bowl society (Figure 2.2) is an oversimplification that attempts to illustrate how equal access to basic 'essentials' such as nutritious food and warm, dry housing is not available to all. Tuberculosis kills, albeit slowly. Yet if you have a healthy immune system and are adequately nourished and housed, your body will rebuff these disease-causing **pathogens**. The vicious cycle of ill-health, unemployment and poverty is self-reinforcing and must be broken.

pathogens

disease-causing organisms

◼ Promoting Health

Promoting health and preventing ill-health can, even from the few illustrations given above, be seen as a complex business. The BSE problem involves the interests of commercial organisations and agriculture, as well as having a political element, with potential global repercussions. The jobs and livelihoods of some farmers and those within the beef and livestock industry are at stake. There is, of course, the possibility of widespread trans-species infection. Tuberculosis has its roots in poverty, involving the homeless and the vulnerable. *Escherichia coli* food poisoning, like so many other bacterial infections, is preventable if scrupulous hygiene standards and thorough food preparation are implemented.

Some key aspects of health promotion are thus beginning to emerge: organisational, social, individual and environmental. Kelly et al. (1993) argue very forcibly that health cannot be effectively promoted unless these four aspects are combined in an integrated approach. Their main objection is that many health-promoting activities focus lower than these four levels without the key element of integration.

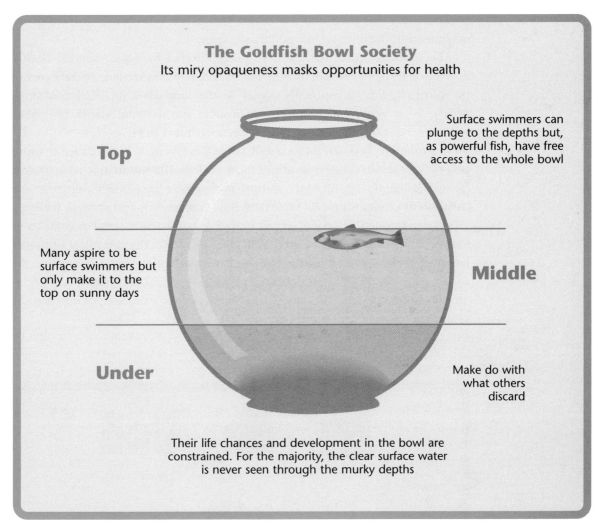

Figure 2.2 ● The goldfish bowl society

Two further aspects of health promotion are the political and the spiritual. This is not to say that these aspects have to be overtly integrated to achieve health, but unless they are accounted for in a thoughtful manner, intolerance and non-receptiveness will result in at worst failure and at best partial success. Thus, nurses need not only carefully consider the client's political values and spiritual beliefs, but also be aware of their own. Nurses and others involved in the promotion of health should take a more critical stance. Seedhouse (1997) views health promotion as an 'endeavour to help individuals, ...ultimately as a task for governments'. It is they who can ensure that everyone's chances for health are maximised throughout an individual's life span.

The spiritual aspect of health is rarely referred to within general health-promotion texts, but within nursing this aspect may be a most important part of the client's health. It especially comes to the fore when an individual crisis occurs, be it acute or chronic, or indeed in the terminal stages of life. A schematic representation of all these aspects is shown in Figure 2.3.

According to Petersen and Lupton (1996), everyone is being called upon to play their part in creating a healthier, more ecologically sustainable environment through attention to 'lifestyle' and an involvement in various collective and collaborative endeavours. All these concerns, expectations and projects are being articulated through an area of expert knowledge and action that has come to be known as 'the new public health'. This takes as its foci the categories of 'population' and the 'environment', conceived in their widest sense to include the social, environmental, organisational, political, spiritual and individual. Let us attempt to examine each of these six key components; there will, of necessity, be some overlap and integration.

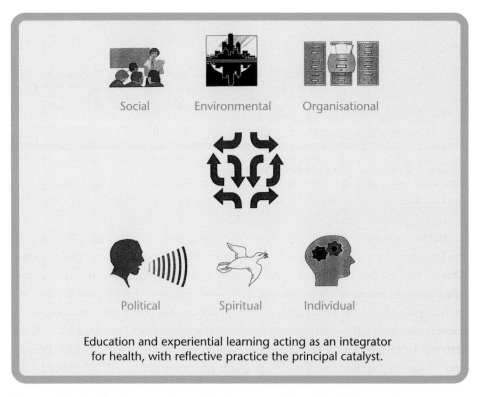

Figure 2.3 ● The integration of six aspects of health within nursing

Social health

The social group into which we are born, or subsequently move, may have an influence on our health for better or for worse. It may shape, constrain or indeed enable health to be realised. Factors such as class, gender, ethnicity and age may sway an individual's genetic predisposition. Biology, lifestyle behaviour and the environment all influence health. Much research has focused on the growing links between social class and health inequalities. The Black Report (DHSS, 1980) provided a modern benchmark of the relationship between mortality, morbidity and social class. The major findings of the report were that:

1. Throughout the life span, those in the lower social classes had higher death rates than those above them.
2. At birth, children born into a lower social class were of a lower weight, often because of poor maternal diet.
3. The ill-effects of major diseases were more profound in the lower social classes than in those at the top of the social scale.

The economy of the late 1990s and this new millennium adds a different slant worthy of mention. The middle classes are now feeling the effect of financial stress that may affect their health and well-being. International competition for work results in the 'downsizing' of companies and the further casualisation of labour. Middle and senior management are now experiencing what once lay within the realm of the working classes: short-term contracts and insecurity. A job for life is becoming a thing of the past, today's emphasis being on flexibility and diversity. But not everyone can cope with managing the enormity of this type of change, often resulting in strains within seemingly secure families.

As Graham (1987) suggests, the social and material circumstances in which people live are strongly linked to their individual behaviour. The continual existence of widespread inequalities in health some 50 years after the foundation of the NHS is an indication of its inability to tackle inequalities. The NHS is geared to respond to present need, dealing with illness; that is what it is good at. In the very near future, it will have to shift towards expected need and how the present need can promote health by building on effective health maintenance strategies and primary prevention. It is not simply a matter of pouring more and more money into the NHS, thereby perpetuating a growing demand as technology caters for what were once unrealised needs. A strong governmental stand is now required to redirect money from the high-tech, often tertiary, care sector to be invested in long-term health maintenance and health promotion. A sustainable health strategy cannot be realised if medium- and long-term strategies are not resourced. The old adage that prevention is better than cure holds true. Nevertheless, the Minister of State for Health, Alan Milburn, has argued that health care focuses on acute problems to the detriment of managing and indeed preventing chronic illness, which now affects around one in three people in the UK (Long-term Medical Conditions Alliance Conference, 2001). The new diabetes National Service Framework will be the first to focus on a chronic disease.

Economic efficiency is something that most national governments aspire to create for the benefit of society, but Kickbusch (1996) illustrates the point that economic efficiency is not the same as a caring society. Key players such as Rupert Murdoch and Bill Gates, for example, who respectively have a vast global telecommunications network and a software empire, are building a global marketplace. But building a caring society is much more than linking health gain with profit margins. Just think about the type of work undertaken by the Missionaries of Charity, founded by Mother Teresa of Calcutta. More recently, the world witnessed the terrorist destruction of the twin World Trade Centre towers in New York. Thousands of people were killed and many more lives were damaged, yet the resolve of the business community to carry on gave a sense of coherence to their grieving and purpose to their work while surrounded by destruction.

Socially determined deprivation damages health. The poor tend to be more socially isolated and lack the social support that tends to achieve health. Social cohesion and the sense of solidarity that this brings are perhaps the most important influences on health status. For example, the two World Wars of the twentieth century caused unprecedented distress and disruption, but the social solidarity, elimination of unemployment and diminishing differences of living standards rapidly increased life expectancy (Bradshaw, 1994). The notions of equal opportunity, social justice and **egalitarian principles** are required both across and throughout society to enable social health to be fully achieved.

> ## Activity 2
>
> The local community is often seen as a microcosm of the wider society. How does this constrain or enable the life chances of those in your social surroundings?

egalitarian principles
principles of equality of mankind

Environmental health

The environment in which we live, work and play has a direct impact upon the state of our health. Peterson and Lupton (1996) state that the shortage of rain, ozone depletion and the greenhouse effect place public health in a global dimension. International air travel has created what has been termed the 'global village', whereby a traveller can literally have breakfast in one continent, lunch in another and dinner in yet another. If the aircraft's cabin has not been spray-disinfested, so might some insects.

Public health experts and environmentalists have thus turned their attention to 'saving the sick planet'. Within this, the modern city has become the focal point for intervention because of its distortion of true nature. Its spaces and places have become sites for controlling pathology. There has been a rapid increase in the growth of modern mega-cities with high population densities and often inadequate safe water and sanitation. The link between urban conditions and health status has a nineteenth-century ring to it. In the UK, we take it for granted that our water supply is safe, yet a simple accidental mistake, as occurred for example in Camelford, Cornwall, when a very high level of aluminium entered the water supply, can cause long-term health problems for scores of people.

At the Earth Summit in Rio de Janeiro in June 1992, many world leaders signed a global environment and development action plan known as Agenda 21. The aim of this plan was to ensure that development to meet the needs of the present does not compromise the ability of future generations to meet their own needs. The WHO suggested that ecologically sustainable development should include the prevention and control of environmental health risks while ensuring equitable access to healthy environments. Five key areas of agreement covered a wide range of issues from climate change, biodiversity and sharing resources more equitably, to managing forests, economic growth and overseas aid.

More recently, at the New York Earth Summit, Irwin (1997) reported that these five main agreements had not been fulfilled. The freezing, at the 1990 level, of carbon dioxide emissions, mainly from exhaust fumes and industry, may be achieved by only Britain and Germany within the next few years, whereas most G7 countries will fail to met this objective. In the USA, emissions have actually increased by 13 per cent since 1995. The protection of endangered species to ensure biodiversity has had some modest success, but this is being achieved as deforestation destroys approximately three species every hour. Overseas aid for sustainable development has, instead of increasing, actually decreased. As national governments across the world change, a few powerful politicians seem to continue to delay environmental protection measures, perhaps heaping untold consequences on generations to come. So why is Agenda 21 important and relevant? Over two-thirds of the Agenda 21 plan cannot be delivered without the commitment and co-operation of local government, in which a lead role is played by local authorities. By 1996, each authority had been encouraged to have its own development strategy at the local level that should involve partnerships within the community.

Using food as an example, consider how the production and transportation of what we eat has changed over recent years. Many of our shops and supermarkets are located so far from our homes or workplaces that they require special trips to get there. The use of cars inevitably results in a lack of exercise, which contributes internally to the deposition of fatty tissue within our arteries, and externally to the burning of non-renewable fossil fuels, which contributes to air pollution (Lang, 1997). This last fact has, according to the UK government

Activity
3

What environmental issues sustain or prevent the achievement of good health in the city or town where you live or study? You may wish to draw up a list of the enabling and ruinous forces that interact on health.

How have these environmental issues affected people in your community, those whom you nurse?

(HM Government, 1993), been further compounded by the fact that the distance over which food is transported rose by over 50 per cent between 1979 and 1993. The growth in road freight transport conveying the commodities of food, drink and tobacco increased by more than one-third during this same period (MAFF, 1994).

Organisational health

Most employers stress that their workforce is their greatest asset. Employees spend as much as half of their adult lives at work, so the working environment and the nature of the work will clearly have a significant impact on health.

Figures produced by the Confederation of British Industry in 1999 on sickness absence during the previous year indicated that 200 million days were lost, an average of 8.5 days per employee. The cost of this loss of working time to British business was estimated to be around £10.2 billion for 1998. The Health and Safety Executive has estimated that at least half of all lost work days related to stress (Cooper et al., 1996). It seems that managers are not blind to stress in the workplace. In a survey by the Institute of Directors, 40 per cent of responding members stated that stress was a big problem, 90 per cent of them believing that working practices could be a factor affecting the level of reported stress. Further work reported by Cooper (1997) in a study examining working practices indicated that the most highly rated causes of workplace stress are:

- 60 per cent time pressures to meet deadlines
- 54 per cent work overload
- 52 per cent threat of job losses
- 51 per cent lack of consultation or poor communication
- 46 per cent understaffing.

Kasl and Cooper stated in 1987 that the chance of the word 'stress' fading from our vocabulary is as high as that of the communist state withering away from Russia! Stress has not only outlived communism, but has also found a firm place in our modern lexicon of work, even though it remains an emotionally charged term.

To be stressed, or to suffer stress, means different things to different people (Selye, 1983). 'Stress' has in recent years become casually tossed around to describe a wide range of 'discomforts' resulting from our hectic pace of work and domestic life. From an organisational perspective, Sheridan and Radmacher (1992) argue that 'we are in the midst of an epidemic of stress that is causing illness and even death, but few agree about how to define it'. You may already have found that dealing with people in the daily context of nursing can be stressful and that stress is a personal experience. The benefits of a healthier workforce should be viewed not purely in financial terms but as an integral part of good management. Health promotion at work is an investment in people.

Organisational health is complex and multifaceted. As an example involving a large organisation, health in the university will be examined as this is a place where students of nursing work, so it should provide readers with a familiar setting. A health-promoting university (HPU) is much more than a place where people go to be educated (although this is its main business): it is concerned with introducing a new culture, rather than just a few health-promotion projects, into our educational settings.

Its overall goal is a commitment to health promotion as a core value of its mission and the development of its organisation in total. Within this setting, health is viewed as being everyone's business. So why should a university be involved in a health-promotion concept?:

- Most universities are large employers, forming a significant part of the local community
- Both students and staff spend a large percentage of their time within the university environment
- Young adult students are at university at a time when they are forming attitudes, behaviours and beliefs that may stay with them throughout their adult life
- Students will themselves play a major part in influencing the health of others, as policy-makers, educators, parents, partners, employers and members of our future society
- There are potentially huge resource savings to be made by becoming more efficient and effective.

In 1995, the University of Portsmouth and the local health authority made a joint appointment of a health-promotion adviser to co-ordinate a university-wide health-promotion initiative. A health needs assessment was performed with both students and staff, which resulted in a report being published and a prioritised 3-year action plan developed. But although an assessment can identify problems, only doing something about them makes the exercise succeed. The health-promotion adviser is made available for students and staff by being situated in the students' advice centre. A short summary of the work already completed is set out below.

Work with a primary focus on student health
- Access to primary health care – ensuring that all new students register with a GP and dentist, student induction talks being supported by displays to

increase the uptake of registration. This information is also available on the World Wide Web under health on the university's home page, accessed from outside the university at http://www.port.ac.uk/departments/healthpro

- Peer education project on mental health
- World Aids Day education and clubbing events
- Development of a sexual health peer education project
- Women's health issues
- Men's health issues
- Guidelines for drugs, alcohol and tobacco
- Meningitis awareness campaigns – especially during the first weeks of each new academic year
- Sensible drinking promotion
- Physical activity, sport and exercise promotion
- Non-smoking as the norm in parts of the students' union
- Exam-time summer health fair.

Work with a primary focus on staff health
- Lunch-time sessions for stress management
- Stress management workshops for departments
- Drugs education and development of a framework for residential staff
- Sexual health
- Smoking cessation
- Increasing physical activity.

Activity 4

Being a full-time student impinges on family and social life. What organisational support do you get to enable you to achieve your potential as a nurse?

The aims of these initiatives are to enable students and staff to fulfil their potential through:

1. Reduced levels of absenteeism.
2. Achieving personal organisational goals.
3. Improving morale, especially the staff's – whereas stress is an individual experience, organisational stress affects groups of staff in similar ways.
4. Better social relationships throughout the university.
5. Increased networking across faculties and departments.
6. Reduced utilisation of clinical services (through awareness).

The HPU initiative works very closely with a variety of local and national organisations, creating new networks with key partners including the WHO. At a local level, the HPU is part of the district-wide health improvement programme taken up by the local primary care trust. There is much more still to be done to achieve a healthier potential for everyone who experiences university life, but at least a start has been made, as has an organisational commitment to accomplish this.

Political health

Since the creation of the NHS over 50 years ago, which was arguably the greatest politically egalitarian act in recent times, successive governments have sought to make it more effective and efficient. The past two decades have witnessed a drive to make it perform like a business.

The White Paper *Our Healthier Nation* (DoH, 1998b) set out the government's strategy for improving health for those in England, laying out a set of priority health targets. The notion of 'health gain' is built upon, first, the reduction of premature mortality, thus increasing life expectancy; and second, the addition of 'life to years', ameliorating morbidity. These ideas originated from the Health for All initiative (WHO, 1985), in which the following six principles were highlighted:

- Right to health
- Equity
- Empowerment
- Community participation
- Accountability
- Partnerships.

Modern health care is now becoming focused on a primary care-led NHS. The pattern of health promotion and health education is shifting away from an illness model to one that seeks to underpin health from a much wider perspective. The opportunities to help and advise individuals, families and communities are unparalleled and will undoubtedly become a focus and a challenge for the future. A brief description of the key areas will be given before illustrating how health authorities and primary care Trusts can build on these targets for specific local needs.

Our Healthier Nation covers four key areas (DoH, 1998b):

1. Coronary heart disease and stroke.
2. Cancers.
3. Mental illness.
4. Accidents.

Each local health authority area is also required to set local targets, including those related to health inequalities, specifically tailored to meet local needs, for example teenage pregnancy. Because HIV and AIDS were targets in the earlier White Paper *The Health of the Nation* (DoH, 1992) and present a significant threat, they will also be briefly discussed here.

Activity 5

Students' unions are dynamic and lively places, usually exhibiting a diversity of ages, cultures and ethnic groups. What health issues do you think need addressing? What is being done about these issues? How could you become involved?

CONNECTIONS

Chapter 14 discusses this process further.

Many of the priorities of the health improvement programme have targets that have been set at national level; other priorities are set at local level.

1. Coronary heart disease and strokes
2. Cancers
3. Asthma
4. Perinatal mortality
5. Mental health (suicides)
6. Accidents
7. Waiting lists/times
8. Developing primary care
9. Promoting independence
10. Reducing health inequalities

In addition to these priorities, the health improvement programme has key objectives related to smoking reduction, drug and alcohol use, teenage pregnancy and services for older people and children. For example, the delivery of services targeted at preschool children and their parents (Sure Start) is included under the reducing inequalities programme.

Figure 2.4 ● Health improvement programme priorities: an example of local health authority priorities guided by *Our Healthier Nation* (Portsmouth and Southeast Hampshire, Department of Public Health, 2000)

The government's role has been to facilitate action at a high level, providing networks for health across all ministerial departments (DoH, 1999). For example, the Department for Education and Employment and the DoH jointly fund the National Healthy School Standard (DfEE, 1999). This standard provides a process of quality, ensuring that local services provided to schools support whole-school practice and are therefore more likely to impact on pupils' health, learning opportunities and achievement (see the Healthy Schools website http://www.wiredforhealth.gov.uk). Translating this activity into practice to promote health at a local level will be the responsibility of health authorities working with local education authorities, local authorities and others. Figures 2.4 and 2.5 outline the response of one local authority to this strategy.

Coronary heart disease and stroke

Coronary heart disease and stroke account for a third of all deaths in men and one-fifth of all deaths in women. Major risk factors include cigarette smoking

(DoH, 1998a), a raised plasma cholesterol level, elevated blood pressure and a lack of physical activity. The potential for reducing both morbidity and mortality through modifying these risk factors seems obvious. The coronary heart disease National Service Framework (DoH, 2000b) sets out a number of standards to reduce heart disease (standards 1 and 2), to prevent heart disease in high-risk patients in primary care (standards 3 and 4), and finally to treat those with heart disease to minimise the impact and rehabilitate people as part of secondary prevention (standards 5–12).

Cancers

Although there are many types of cancer, each with a different aetiology, the potential to prevent, treat and cure them varies considerably. The *Our Healthier Nation* overall target is to reduce the death rate from cancer in people under 75 years by at least a fifth by 2010. A national Cancer Action Team will drive progress to achieve this reduction in mortality.

aetiology
the cause of a condition; also the study of all the factors involved in the development of a disease

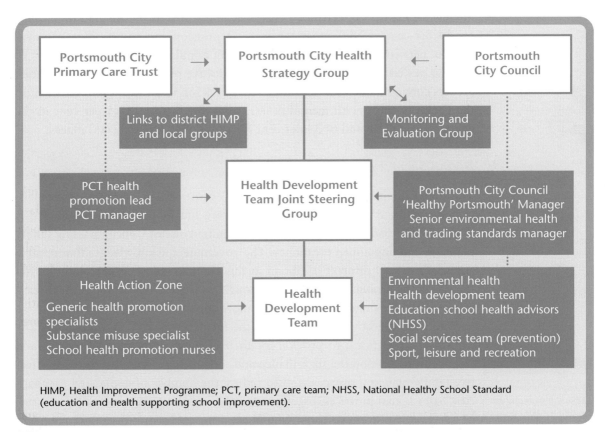

Figure 2.5 ● **Portsmouth City Health Development Team initiative** (adapted from Richens, 2001)

- *Breast cancer:* around 14,000 women die from breast cancer each year. Breast cancer screening is likely to be extended to include the routine screening of women up to 69 years of age to provide earlier diagnosis and treatment
- *Colorectal cancer:* this is the second most common cancer in England, about 30,000 new cases being recorded each year, with a lifetime risk of 1 in 25. Pilot screening studies have commenced using faecal occult blood as an indicator for further investigation
- About 1,000 women die from *cervical cancer* each year, a figure that seems to be falling by around 7 per cent per year. The NHS cervical screening programme set up in 1988 is based on a computer call and recall system for all women aged 20–64 years
- *Skin:* the aim is to halt the year-on-year increase by 2005
- *Lung:* the target of *Our Healthier Nation* is to reduce the mortality rate by 30 per cent in men and 15 per cent in women under 75 years of age by 2010.

Mental illness

Mental illness is a leading cause of disability and ill-health, resulting in approximately 14 per cent of certified cases of sickness. It is also estimated to account for 14 per cent of NHS inpatient costs. Depression and anxiety have a prevalence of between 2 and 7 per cent in the adult population, with a lifetime risk of over 20 per cent. Psychotic illnesses, like affective psychosis and schizophrenia, are less common albeit more severe. The aim is for a significant improvement in the health of those with mental illness, with a reduction of 15 per cent in the overall suicide rate and of 33 per cent for those with severe mental illness.

HIV/AIDS and sexual health

The human immunodeficiency virus (HIV) causes the acquired immune deficiency syndrome (AIDS). This key area, targeted in the earlier White Paper (DoH, 1992), deals also with sexually transmitted diseases, encompassing family planning and unplanned pregnancy. The government acknowledges that reliable statistics are very difficult to obtain in this complex area: no-one really knows the size of the problem in England, although, as we learn more about the disease process, the epidemiology is becoming more sophisticated.

The main objectives are: to reduce the incidence of HIV and other sexually transmitted infections; to provide for their effective prevention, diagnosis and treatment; to develop the surveillance and monitoring systems; to provide effective family planning services; and to reduce the number of unplanned pregnancies. Safer sexual practices, together with the use of condoms to reduce the risk of infection, are stressed. Those who inject drugs and share equipment are noted to be at significant risk of HIV as well as hepatitis B and C.

CONNECTIONS

Chapter 7 explores sexual health and its relationship to body image.

Accidents

Accidents cause death and a high incidence of morbidity, especially among people under 30 years of age. The number of deaths of children under 15 years, young adults aged between 15 and 24 years and people aged over 65 have been separately targeted, with reductions of 33 per cent, 25 per cent and 33 per cent respectively being proposed by 2005. The government has based its strategy on a better co-ordination of agencies to prevent accidents, for example local authority involvement in planning, building control, highways, housing, social services, education, environmental health and the emergency services. Also involved are public health promotion in terms of accident prevention, to enable people to be better informed, taking action on specific types of accident and considering vulnerable groups.

Health promotion receives a relatively small amount of the entirety of the health budget, and the prevailing political philosophy towards societal health needs will affect the relationship between national and local government. At her first major speech to the Royal College of Midwives on 15 May 1997, Tessa Jowell, then Minister for Public Health (a new post created by the incoming Labour government), set out to tackle the inequalities that give rise to ill-health alongside the service that provides treatment and care. By tackling the wider influences that detract from health, such as poverty, poor housing, unemployment and polluted environments, government can make an impact on health inequalities.

Smoking has been recognised as the greatest single cause of preventable illness and premature death in the UK, yet the powerful tobacco lobby has managed to convince politicians that banning tobacco advertising is not in their political interest. Many people still smoke, the largest increase in smoking rate being seen in teenagers, especially girls. Maternal smoking during pregnancy has consistently shown a significant statistical relationship to the risk of sudden infant death syndrome. The planned ban on tobacco advertising and the consequent removal of tobacco sports sponsorship is undoubtedly a courageous and long overdue political step.

> **Activity 6**
>
> Giving power back to clients or patients and working with them to meet their needs must lie at the very heart of nursing, suggest Brown and Piper (1997), as these approaches represent the aggrandisement of human care by enabling potential to be fulfilled.
> In which ways does the political agenda enable or hinder nurses in working in partnership with their clients?

Spiritual health

A person's spiritual dimension enables him or her to move from self-interest to care for another, as well as allowing a greater enjoyment in the fullness of life. Although the word 'spirituality' has an association with religious activity, it is 'to be that state in which a person finds his view of life (spiritual life) to be matched by his experience within it' (Langford, 1993). The spiritual dimension perhaps acts as a means of integrating the other dimensions of life. It is ultimately concerned with issues and life principles, and is often seen as a search for

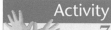

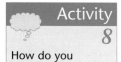

Activity 7

Find out what support is available to help meet clients' spiritual needs. Make a note of the services and any useful contact addresses.

How could you help someone who has a value base different from your own?

Activity 8

How do you recharge your spiritual batteries?

CONNECTIONS

Chapter 9 explores spiritual health in more detail.

meaning. Spirituality, it may be argued, therefore permeates every aspect and moment of living. It involves eating, drinking, working, creating, showing love, sharing laughter and tears, worshipping and dying. Langford (1993) goes on to suggest that all these activities are equally 'spiritual' occasions.

Nursing can be both physically and emotionally draining as dealing with life-and-death situations can be both rewarding and exhausting. Nurses perhaps need four things to assist them in assisting others:

1. A *confidant*, a friend, preferably someone outside the family, with whom they can share deeply issues concerning work and their emotional reactions to them. A confidant enables a person to be aware of him- or herself and keep a balance by being alert to possible problems.
2. *Peer support* offers mutual support and the chance to talk through issues that others can understand because they share the same experience. A student cohort provides a variety of characters, each person then being able to relate to someone who is right to help them.
3. Doing *something completely different* – taking time out, developing a hobby or going on holiday – can help to recharge nurses' spiritual batteries.
4. Developing their *spiritual base* to withstand a multitude of questions, pressures and changes as they progress through their nursing careers.

Individual health

An individual's life chances for health will be dependent on the five other aspects of health (social, environmental, organisational, political and spiritual) and how they interrelate. We have already considered the basic essentials for health maintenance: no wars, threat of terrorism or civil disturbance, assured personal safety, good housing, safe clean water and sewage disposal, and nutritious uncontaminated food.

Our current health status is not fixed but is instead highly dependent upon what has gone before and, to some extent, what the future holds. Although we cannot predict the future with absolute accuracy, a future without hope would be severely detrimental. Conversely, when individuals are given hope for their future, they can overcome enormous threats and challenges to their health: think back to Annie with the ovarian cancer or to young Samantha waiting for her heart transplant.

Individuals' past health history may show a balance in their personal life or there may be a negative health course, as in the case of Sam. The current health balance depends on the six aspects contributing to well-being and functioning as determined by the individuals concerned and those who share life with them.

Future health potential is dependent upon a strong integration of these six aspects of health, supporting and enabling a positive self-concept, having developed coping skills as part of the individual's health resource repertoire.

Let us take an everyday example of a life skill and relate this to individual health and the potential to maintain or improve it. In a study undertaken on behalf of the National Food Alliance by MORI (1993), fewer than half the national sample of children could boil an egg or bake a potato. We are all consumers of food, but individuals are being deskilled or underskilled when it comes to preparing and cooking. Conversely, however, there is an abundance of advice within the media, from television programmes to magazines, on how to cook. Convenience and fast foods have played a part in the deskilling process, but fast food can be nutritious. Fast Food Fit (http://www.port.ac.uk/departments/healthpro) is a campaign developed by Portsmouth City Council to help families on low budgets to cook nutritious food. It has a number of healthy recipes that can be prepared quickly and at a low cost. This scheme now covers university students, many of whom find cooking boring, cannot afford decent wholesome food or prefer a 'liquid diet', with all the threats to health that this may bring.

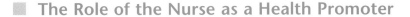 The Role of the Nurse as a Health Promoter

Investment in the health sector is rapidly becoming an amalgam of public and private partnerships, some key individuals being involved in joint societal efforts. Although it is evident that the responsibility for health promotion does not lie with the health sector alone, nurses nevertheless have an unequal contribution to make to alliances created in the pursuit of health. Within the UK, this is especially true as nurses form the largest body of health-care professionals orchestrated by the NHS, with an immeasurable number of client and patient interactions.

The Nursing and Midwifery Council *Code of Conduct* (NMC, 2002) has set standards within a professional framework to regulate the conduct of members. Eight core statements make up the code, which is founded upon the practitioner being personally accountable in safeguarding and promoting the interests of individual patients and clients within the context of society. These core values and characteristics of acceptable practice act in a way to protect the public. Specifically practitioners must:

Promote and protect the interests and dignity of patients and clients, irrespective of gender, age, race, ability, sexuality, economic status, lifestyle, culture and religious or political beliefs [point 2.2] ...Recognise and respect

Activity
9

Make a list of the aspects of your own life in which good health could be improved. Be realistic. From this list produce a plan that could be implemented over a 4 week period. Think about how the success of your plan could be evaluated.

Implement the plan and, after 4 weeks, evaluate it. Within health promotion, we need short-term gains to encourage and motivate us towards longer-term benefits.

the role of patients and clients as partners in their care and the contribution they can make to it. This involves identifying their preferences regarding care and respecting these within the limits of professional practice, existing legislation, resources and the goals of the therapeutic relationship [point 2.1].

Health promotion is not simply something that is done to the client or patient, as in changing a dressing, giving drugs to prevent auditory hallucinations or taking a blood pressure, but instead informs and pervades all aspects of nursing care in enhancing health through:

- Needs assessment
- Planning health gain
- Evaluating interventions and strategies for effectiveness and efficiency.

Knowing those whom we seek to support within our professional capacity as nurses will help us to understand their health needs. 'Knowing the client/patient' has become a buzz phrase within contemporary nursing, but understanding the individual's status in terms of health, beliefs, values and attitudes, along with the structural determinants of health and outside influences, will form a starting point for a needs assessment.

Within the acute illness setting, a nurse's professionalism may be the sustaining presence in the facilitation of the patient's own coping abilities. This contrasts with the episodic and often interventionist nature of the medical relationship. In planning health gain, the power that nursing possesses is often very subtle. As Campbell (1993) points out, the positive power of nursing:

> is one which knows when to hold and support without possessiveness, and when to motivate and let go, without bullying or rejection.

It is, or should be, the nature of nursing care that empowers the client or patient, and Campbell goes on to suggest that nursing is a form of health promotion. The notion of health gain lies at the centre of health promotion as a core value.

Giving power back to clients or patients and working with them to meet their needs must, suggest Brown and Piper (1997), lie at the very heart of nursing as it represents the aggrandisement of human care by enabling potential to be fulfilled.

Within nursing practice, an awareness of the nuances of the patient or client is essential, especially if the observant nurse is to pick up on these cues to potentiate health. Because awareness makes demands upon us, usually in the form of some action, but also equally by just providing a listening ear, it costs us in terms of our time. Continually responding to the demands of others requires effort, patience and a degree of self-denial. It can be painful, especially when you are busy and this is the umteenth time that Mrs Moon has had a commode, or in the community, when you are dressing Miss Patel's leg ulcer and her cat walks across your sterile field. Nurses may lapse into deaf or partially sighted mode as a coping mechanism. It is important that individual nurses are realistic in terms of what they can achieve within their professional role. One way is through the use of praxis (reflective practice and action) to prevent the adoption of second-rate or diminished care by lowering standards through a lack of awareness or inaction. Professional dialogue in terms of a discussion with qualified staff and peers often helps to clarify issues before they become problematic.

Under the framework of the English National Board's Higher Award (ENB, 1991), 10 key characteristics form the structure within which nurses can develop their practice. The sixth of these characteristics is health promotion (Chart 2.1). Although this award is designed for experienced postregistration nurses, it provides a useful structure within which the novice nurse can begin to build his or her practice. Four principles underpin this framework:

- *Reviewing* practice, knowledge, skills and expertise
- *Identifying* continuing education needs
- *Designing* modular programmes
- *Assessing* continuing education activities.

Reviewing practice is something that all nurses need to do. It is particularly valuable for students of nursing as it links very closely with the identification of their learning needs. Designing modular programmes does not, at first glance, seem to fall within the remit of student nurses, but within a supervised capacity, students should develop ways and means of involving patients and clients in strategies to make health gains. These strategies may be individualised (designed specifically for the client) and form part of the client's overall care.

Chart 2.1 ● English National Board key characteristic 6: health promotion

Promote understanding of health promotion, preventative care, health education and healthy living	Understand and apply the principles and practice of health promotion in the work setting and create, maintain and take responsibility for a healthy work environment	Facilitate responsibility and choice among clients for healthy living, and their ability to determine their own lifestyles	Develop and implement strategies for health care based on understanding of the impact of health trends on resources

Planning for health through raising awareness in an enabling way is crucial. There should be no place for 'victim-blaming', in which often rushed and ill-informed judgements are made based on stereotypical and partial information. Health-promotion strategies will need to be assessed for effectiveness and evaluated in terms of how well they meet the clients' needs and the normative needs of the health professionals involved. A schematic model of how this could be approached within nursing is outlined in Figure 2.6.

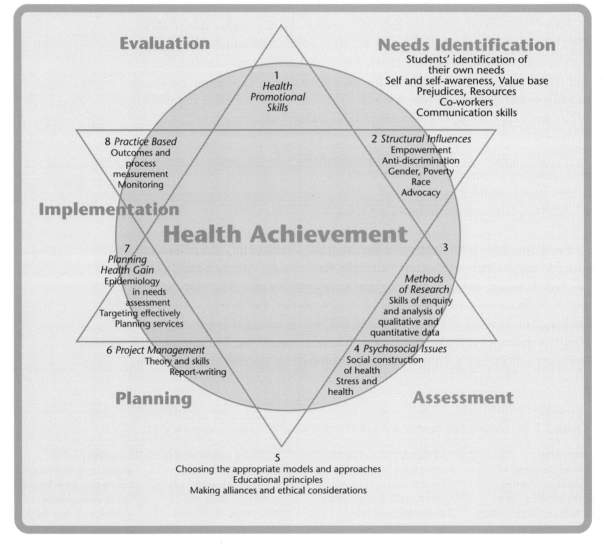

Figure 2.6 ● The role of the nurse in promoting health could include these key areas from planning to evaluation

Chapter Summary

This chapter has explored what health is as a dynamic concept within a situation of flux. It can be a slippery concept to grasp. Contemporary challenges to health have been discussed and some theoretical concepts explained. A model utilising six aspects of health – social, environmental, organisational, political, spiritual and individual – has provided the framework for expanding on these concepts. The activities in these sections will enable readers to relate them to their own setting. In doing so, it is hoped that a greater understanding can be achieved.

Real-life examples have been drawn on to illustrate key points. An overview of the *Our Healthier Nation* strategy for England has provided a baseline against which national progress towards a healthier nation can be measured. Finally, a discourse of the role of the nurse as a health promoter and evaluator of health has attempted to ensure that health is seen in the context of everyday nursing practice. Health promotion is not an add-on extra but should be integrated into care and internalised by practitioners as the foundation of good nursing practice.

● Test Yourself!

Choose someone you know (not a client but a family member or close friend) who is willing to answer some personal questions.

1. What are their health needs?

2. How do they perceive them?

3. Take one of these expressed needs and plan a strategy to meet it. See how many of the six aspects of health you can incorporate into this.

4. Implement the plan, working in partnership with your respondent.

5. On completion, how does your respondent feel?

6. Evaluate the process and outcomes. What went well? Did anything unexpected happen? If you were to do this again, what would you change?

Further Reading

Naidoo, J. and Wills, J. (2000) *Health Promotion – Foundations for Practice*, 2nd edn. Baillière Tindall, London.

Scriven, A. and Orme, J. (eds) (1996) *Health Promotion: Professional Perspectives*. Macmillan – now Palgrave Macmillan, Basingstoke.

Tones, K. and Tilford, S. (2001) *Health Promotion: Effectiveness, Efficiency and Equity*, 3rd edn. Nelson Thornes, Cheltenham.

References

Bradshaw, J. (1994) The conceptualisation and measurement of need. In Popay, J. and Williams, G. (eds) *Researching the People's Health*. Routledge, London.

Brown, P.A. and Piper, S.M. (1997) Nursing and the health of the nation: schism or symbiosis? *Journal of Advanced Nursing* **25**: 297–301.

Campbell, A.V. (1993) The ethics of health education. In Wilson-Barnett, J. and Macleod Clark, J. (eds) *Research in Health Promotion and Nursing*. Macmillan – now Palgrave Macmillan, Basingstoke.

Cooper, C.L. (1997) Crisis talks. In Arnold, H. *Personnel Today*, 2 October, pp. 29–32.

Cooper, C.L., Liukkonen, P. and Cartwright, S. (1996) *Stress Prevention in the Workplace: Assessing the Costs and Benefits to Organisations*. European Foundation for the Improvement of Living and Working Conditions, Dublin.

Department for Environment, Food and Rural Affairs (2001) *Bovine Spongiform Encephalopathy in Great Britain: A Progress Report*. http://www.defra.gov.uk/animalh/bse/bse-publications/progress/jun01/report.pdf [accessed 6 October 2001].

DfEE (Department for Education and Employment) (1999) *Healthy Schools: National Healthy School Standard*. DfEE, Nottingham.

DHSS (Department of Health and Social Security) (1980) *Inequalities in Health* (Black Report). DHSS, London.

DoH (Department of Health) (1992) *The Health of the Nation: A Strategy for England*. HMSO, London.

DoH (Department of Health) (1998a) *Smoking Kills*. HMSO, London.

DoH (Department of Health) (1998b) *Our Healthier Nation*. HMSO, London.

DoH (Department of Health) (1999) *Saving Lives: Our Healthier Nation*. HMSO, London.

DoH (Department of Health) (2000a) *The NHS Plan: A Plan for Investment. A Plan for Reform*. HMSO, London.

DoH (Department of Health) (2000b) *CHD National Service Framework*. HMSO, London.

DoH (Department of Health) (2002) http://www.doh.gov.uk/cjd/stats/apr02.htm [accessed on 19 April 2002].

Dubos, R. (1979) Mirage of health. In Black, N., Boswell, D., Gray, A., Murphy, S. and Popjay, J. *Health and Disease: A Reader*. Open University Press, Milton Keynes.

Emmerson, A., Enstone, J., Griffin, M., Kelsey, M. and Smyth, E. (1996) The second national prevalence survey of infection in hospitals: overview of the results. *Journal of Hospital Infection* **32**: 175–90.

ENB (English National Board for Nursing, Midwifery and Health Visiting) (1991) Professional Portfolio, Higher Award Learning Outcomes, Summary Card 2. ENB, London.

Graham, H. (1987) Women's smoking and family health. *Social Science and Medicine* **25**(1): 47–56.

HM Government (1993) MM20 Overseas Statistics. December. HMSO, London.

Irwin, A. (1997) The five failures. *Daily Telegraph*, 24 June, p. 13.

Kasl, S.V. and Cooper, C.L. (eds) (1987) *Research Methods in Stress and Health Psychology*. John Wiley & Sons, Chichester.

Kelly, M., Charlton, B. and Hanlon, P. (1993) The four levels of health promotion: an integrated approach. *Public Health* **107**(5): 320.

Kickbusch, I. (1996) New players for a new era: how up to date is health promotion? *Health Promotion International* **11**(4) (editorial).

Lang, T. (1997) *Food Policy for the 21st Century: Can it Be Both Radical and Reasonable?* Discussion Paper No. 4. Thames Valley University, London.

Langford, D. (1993) *Where is God in all this?*, 2nd edn. Countess Mountbatten House, Moorgreen Hospital, Southampton.

Long-term Medical Conditions Alliance Conference, Royal College of Physicians, 28 February 2001. http://www.doh.gov.uk/healthinequalities.

MAFF (Ministry of Agriculture, Fisheries and Food) (1994) *Agriculture in the UK 1993*. HMSO, London.

MAFF and FSA (Ministry of Agriculture, Fisheries and Food, and Food Standards Agency) (2001) *BSE Enforcement Bulletin 58*, May 2001.

MORI (1993) *Poll for Get Cooking Project*. National Food Alliance, London.

NMC (Nursing and Midwifery Council) (2002) *Code of Professional Conduct*. NMC, London.

Peterson, A. and Lupton, D. (1996) *The New Public Health*. Sage, London.

Pike, S. and Forster, D. (eds) (1995) *Health Promotion for All*. Churchill Livingstone, London.

Richens, I. (2001) *Portsmouth City Health Development Team*. Portsea Island Primary Care Trust. Unpublished report.

Seedhouse, D. (1986) *Health: The Foundations for Achievement*. John Wiley & Sons, Chichester.

Seedhouse, D. (1997) *Health Promotion: Philosophy, Prejudice and Practice*. John Wiley & Sons, Chichester.

Selye, H. (ed.) (1983) *Seyle's Guide to Stress Research*, Vol. 2. Van Nostrand Reinhold, New York.

Sheridan, C. and Radmacher, S. (1992) *Health Psychology: Challenging the Bio-medical Model*. John Wiley & Sons, Chichester.

WHO (World Health Organization) (1947) *Constitution*. WHO, Geneva.

WHO (World Health Organization) (1985) *Targets for Health for All by the Year 2000*. WHO, Copenhagen.

Web Pages

There is a huge amount of information about health and health promotion on the Internet. The quality of information varies so you will need to discern the good sites from the not so good.

The Department of Health (DoH) hosts an extremely useful website http://www.doh.gov.uk

It publishes, for example, monthly updates on the number of deaths and probable cases of CJD in the UK http://www.doh.gov.uk/cjd/stats

University of Portsmouth health-promoting university http://www.port.ac.uk/departments/healthpro

National Healthy School Wired for Health http://www.wiredforheath.gov.uk

Nursing and Midwifery Council http://www.nmc-uk.org/

SOMDUTH PARBOTEEAH

Chapter

Safety in Practice

3

Contents

Learning outcomes

This chapter will provide the reader with a broad introduction to moving and handling, infection control, basic food hygiene and the administration of medications. It is intended that this chapter will provide students with the essential knowledge to carry out nursing practice in a manner that will safeguard them and those patients/clients in their care. At the end of this chapter, you should be able to:

- Describe and explain the principles of moving and handling, infection control, food hygiene and drug administration

- Undertake a risk assessment

- Describe a range of strategies for the optimum safety for staff and clients when moving and handling

- Describe the role of the nurse in infection control

- Describe the importance of good food hygiene

- Extend your range of skills in drug administration.

> Throughout the chapter, you will be given an opportunity to undertake some exercises that will assist in further developing your competence, knowledge and skills. Some of these activities may require you to access and read additional policies and texts; suggested textbooks are listed at the end of this chapter.

Moving and Handling

This section describes the role of the nurse in the moving of patients and clients. By the end of this section, the nurse will:

- Have a full understanding of the policies and legislation affecting practice
- Be able to undertake moving and handling procedures
- Develop safe moving and handling techniques.

In professional work, there will be many times when there is a need to move clients/patients, equipment or other types of load, and these provide an additional risk to health-care workers.

The number of manual handling injuries sustained in the health service sector and reported to the Health and Safety Executive (HSE) under the Reporting of Injuries, Diseases and Dangerous Occurrences Regulations 1985 is shown in Table 3.1. The Disabled Living Foundation (1994) has indicated that one in four qualified nurses has taken time off with a back injury sustained at work, this for some meaning the end of their nursing career. Gladman (1993) reported that student nurses are at a high risk of injury and that the problem may be further compounded by the recent recruitment of older people, who may already suffer from back pain. It is therefore imperative to stop manual handling injuries taking their toll on nurses' health. The estimated annual cost to the NHS of back pain was approximately £480m in 1993, with lost production costs of £3.8bn and benefit payments of £1.4bn (Rosen, 1994).

The law as it relates to manual handling is regulated by statute principally in

Table 3.1 Manual handling injuries in the NHS, 1994–97

Manual handling inuries in the health services	Number of cases
Scotland	1,500
England	15,000

Source: HSE (1998).

the form of the Health and Safety at Work Act 1974 and the Manual Handling Operations Regulations 1992, the latter introduced under the provisions of the Health and Safety at Work Act to enable the UK to implement the requirements of European Directives on the manual handling of loads. Manual handling operations have been defined within the HSE directives (HSE, 1992) as:

> transporting or supporting a load, including lifting, putting down, pushing, pulling, carrying or moving by hand or bodily force. This also includes the intentional dropping or throwing of a load.

Under these regulations the employer has a general duty 'To ensure, so far as is reasonably practicable, the health, safety and welfare at work of all employees' (Health and Safety at Work Act 1974) and must avoid the need for hazardous manual handling operations. Employers' responsibilities are listed in Chart 3.1. Where this is not reasonably practicable, the HSE recommends that employers make a suitable and sufficient assessment and take appropriate steps to reduce the risk of injury to the lowest level reasonably possible.

Employees have a duty under the Act to take reasonable care of their own health and safety and that of other people who may be affected by their actions, and it is essential that all health-care workers adhere to these regulations. Failure on the part of any individuals to follow them may jeopardise patients' safety and cause serious injury to themselves, which may result in chronic ill-health.

As a student nurse preparing to take on a professional role and faced with moving and handling operations throughout your career, you will need to continue to review any relevant new legislation. All employers are required by law to update their employees annually on the principles and practice of moving and handling operations.

As the safety of the nurse and patient is paramount, nurse education will

> **Activity 1**
>
> Identify the training offered by the university. Find out who is moving and handling co-ordinator in your university and hospital.
>
> Identify clients who need to be moved and the resources available to do this.

Chart 3.1 ● Health and Safety at Work Act 1974 – general duties of employers

1. To ensure that employees are not exposed to foreseeable risks of injury

2. To develop a no manual handling policy in practice

3. The provision of information, instruction, training and supervision necessary to ensure health and safety

4. The provision and maintenance of a working environment that is safe and without risks to health and adequate as regards facilities and arrangements for welfare at work

include instruction on moving and handling operations, and guidance on local practice and the use of moving and handling equipment. Teaching staff have a responsibility to provide the correct information, as indicated by law, and students contracted within a school must, also by law, undergo regular updating. Failure to do so may affect their ability to practise.

Risk assessment

CONNECTIONS

Chapter 10 looks at assessing the risk of certain wounds developing.

In managing patient care, it is fundamental that a risk assessment is carried out as recommended by the HSE (1992) and the Royal College of Nursing (RCN, 1996). The four main factors to be considered in a risk assessment are:

- The task
- The load
- The work environment
- Individual capability.

The task

The nurse should consider whether the task involves:

- Holding the load at a distance from the trunk, for example moving a patient on a divan bed
- Unsatisfactory bodily movement or posture, as with a patient suffering from a stroke
- Excessive or sudden movement of the load, for example with an uncooperative patient
- Frequent or prolonged physical effort, as when moving a patient to give nursing care
- An insufficient rest or recovery period, for example when too many patients require toileting.

It is important to carry out a thorough assessment of the task in hand. Poor posture during moving and handling introduces the additional risk of a loss of control of the load and a sudden unpredictable increase in physical stress.

The load

Is the load:

- Heavy or difficult to grasp, for example an obese patient suffering from a stroke?
- Unstable or potentially damaging, for example a confused patient?

Within the health-care setting, the patient is referred to as the 'load'. Therefore, size, weight, shape, fragility, stability, the individual's ability to function both physically and mentally, and any attachments that may adversely affect movement, such as infusion pumps, should be considered. Human beings can display individual characteristics that may help or hinder moving and handling operations: elderly clients, for example, may suffer from arthritis.

The work environment

Aspects of the work environment to consider are:

- Space constraints preventing a good posture, for example working in a bathroom or toilet area
- Uneven, slippery or unstable floors, for example when wet
- Variations in the level of floors or work surfaces, for example a low divan bed
- Poor lighting conditions
- Inadequate or insufficient storage facilities.

A safe working environment may if necessary be created by removing obstacles from the vicinity of the patient and reporting aspects of the work environment that require structural modification. If the environment is not safe, the patient should be moved to a safer area.

Individual capability

Does the job:

- Require unusual strength or height, for example reaching out to a patient on a fixed height bed?
- Put at risk those who are pregnant or who have a health problem?
- Require special knowledge or training for its safe performance?
- Require protective clothing or personal protective equipment, for example nurses' belts, that can hinder posture or movement?

The Manual Handling Operations Regulations do not contain any weight limits below which moving and handling can be considered safe. The RCN (1996) recommends that all patient handling should be assessed by considering all risk factors rather than weight alone. The numerical guidelines (Figure 3.1) can be used to determine when an assessment is needed. It is assumed that the load can easily be grasped with both hands and that the procedure is being undertaken in a safe working environment.

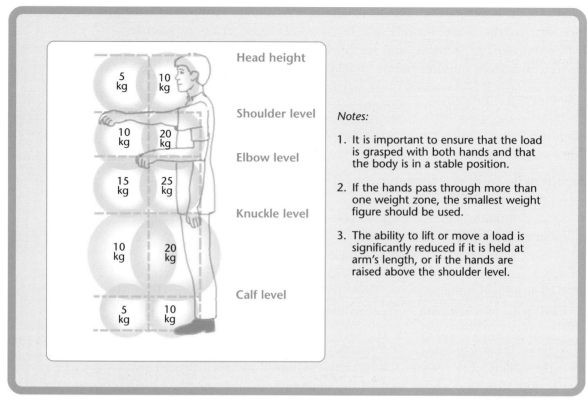

Figure 3.1 ● Guidelines for lifting and lowering for men

Casebox 3.1

Mr Jones, a 38-year-old man with learning difficulties has been admitted to your ward with right-sided paralysis and is unable to move his right arm and leg. He is conscious and aware of his admission but is unable to undertake any activities for himself. He weighs 80 kg and has also been suffering from urinary incontinence. He has been placed in a side room that has its own toilet facilities but reduced working space.

Undertake a risk assessment of the above scenario and discuss your findings with your manual handling co-ordinator.

What would you do if the nurse you were working with asked you to lift this patient manually rather than use the appropriate equipment?

■ Assessment should ascertain whether there is likely to be any risk of injury. A more detailed assessment will consider the task involved, the load, the environment and individual capability.

■ In this case, you should politely refuse to lift Mr Jones, referring to the Manual Handling Operations Regulations (HSE, 1992). An alternative method of moving the patient should be employed.

Ergonomics

Ergonomics can be defined as the study of the relationship between the working environment and the people within it; it is important in the prevention of injury resulting from manual handling activities, ensuring the optimum 'fit' between the people and the work.

Ergonomic processes include risk assessment and the identification and implementation of measures to reduce risk. Posture, the types of furnishing used, their height, position and manoeuvrability, the tasks undertaken and the environment are all assessed in order to ensure that the job is designed to fit the worker and thus reduce the incidence of manual handling injuries.

Assisting with patient movement

When moving and handling patients, for example postoperatively, the aim is actively to encourage independent movement, the health-care worker assisting as little as possible. Teaching the principles of normal movement can be undertaken collaboratively between the nurses and the physiotherapist so that continuity of care is maintained.

CONNECTIONS

Chapter 8 identifies the causes and consequences of impaired mobility and the nurse's role in mobilising patients.

Any normal movement that patients can undertake for themselves avoids the need for a full lift, and patients' preferences and ways of moving should be taken into account even if the process is more time-consuming. Elderly patients suffering from chronic arthritis may, for example, have developed strategies that help them to cope with daily activities and thus maintain their independence.

Principles of patient handling with equipment

The Manual Handling Operations Regulations (HSE, 1992) require that risks should be reduced by the introduction and use of appropriate equipment. As new pieces of equipment frequently become available, this section will not give any specific details of how to operate each one of them. Instead, principles relating to the use of equipment will be described:

- All equipment should be available with full instruction in its use
- All staff must be trained in the use of equipment they are expected to employ
- Equipment must be in good working order
- Equipment used in people's homes is often designed with regard to criteria different from those used in the hospital
- Equipment designed for shared use should have guidelines on disinfection.

Activity

2

Find out which manual handling equipment is used in your area and which types of equipment are most suited for certain tasks. Taking into account the four criteria for risk assessment, design a nursing action plan for moving a patient.

Equipment must be:

- Compatible with its surroundings
- Compatible with other equipment and mechanical aids
- Designed to avoid or reduce the need for manual handling
- Easy to use, move, adjust and maintain in the clinical area.

All staff require thorough training in the use of any equipment they will be using with the clients and patients in their care. They should have the opportunity to learn about and try out equipment before using it on a patient, and students should have the opportunity to practise and be supervised when using any equipment for the first time.

Team operations

Involving two or more staff may make it possible to carry out moving and handling operations that are beyond the capability of one person. Team operations can, however, introduce additional problems, and the following areas should be considered as part of the risk assessment:

- The percentage of load borne by each member of the team
- Whether members will impede each other's movement, for example during 'log rolling' a spinal injury patient
- A lack of good hand-holds, for example when dealing with a person who has collapsed in a toilet.

Introducing a safer handling policy

The RCN (1996) recommends that health-care workers in the hospital or the community should no longer have to lift manually; specialised equipment should be made available to minimise the risk of injury. While hospital Trusts are in the process of developing their policies, health-care workers should take all necessary precautions to ensure their safety.

■ Control of Infection

This section will describe the role of the nurse in the prevention of cross-infection. By the end of this section, the nurse will be able to:

- Describe hospital-acquired infection
- Understand the need for universal precautions

● Describe the role of the infection control team
● Discuss local infection control policies.

A **hospital-acquired infection** (HAI) is one that is neither present nor incubating at the time the patient is admitted to hospital. The National Audit Office (2000) has reported that there are at least 1,000,000 cases of HAI each year. At any given time, approximately 9 per cent of patients have an HAI (National Audit Office, 2000), patients who acquire an infection remaining in hospital for an average of 2.5 times longer than a non-infected patient, an equivalent of 11 extra days at a total estimated annual cost to the NHS of £1bn.

The most common hospital-acquired infections are of the:

1. Urinary tract (30 per cent), the majority being found in catheterised patients.
2. Lower respiratory tract.
3. Skin and wounds.

Resistant strains of *Staphylococcus*, difficult to treat and control, have recently become a major problem in hospitals. In addition to a greater morbidity and mortality, patients have a longer hospital stay and receive more expensive drugs, thus significantly increasing the cost.

The protection of patients

Modern-day care with increased surgical intervention and technological advances on an increasingly elderly population with a greater susceptibility to infection heighten the risk of acquiring infection while in hospital. Although it is unlikely that HAIs can be completely eradicated, Department of Health (DoH) guidance (DoH, 1995) suggests that 30 per cent of current HAIs are preventable.

The most likely means of transmission of infectious organisms from body fluids is by direct contact or the percutaneous inoculation of the infected fluid. Since it is impossible to identify which patients are infected, the DoH (1990a) recommends the adoption of 'Universal Precautions' (Chart 3.2) embodying the principles of good practice in the control of bloodborne infections and the spread of infection. In addition, the following basic measures should be taken in order to minimise the risk of patients acquiring an infection while in hospitals:

● Employ good hand hygiene
● Do not touch patients' wounds or dressings unless it is essential; if you have to do so, always wear gloves
● Ensure that all equipment for use on patients is sterile or disinfected

hospital-acquired infection

an infection neither present nor incubating at the time the patient is admitted to hospital, being instead acquired as a result of hospitalisation itself. It may not become evident until after discharge

Chart 3.2 ● Universal precautions

1. **Skin** – Cuts or abrasions of exposed areas should be covered with a waterproof dressing, which is also an effective viral and bacterial barrier
2. **Gloves** – Wear gloves
3. **Handwashing** – Thorough handwashing is necessary between procedures
4. **Aprons** – Wear disposable aprons if there is a possibility of splashing
5. **Eyes** – Eye protection should be worn if there is a danger of flying contaminated debris
6. **Sharps** – Extreme care should be taken during the use and disposal of sharps
7. **Needlestick injuries** – Follow guidelines to avoid injury; in the event of a needlestick injury, follow local policy
8. **Conjunctivae/mucous membranes** – If splashed, irrigate with copious amounts of water
9. **Spillages** – Follow local guidelines to deal with spillages. Gloves and aprons should be worn
10. **Waste** – All contaminated waste should be placed in yellow sacks and disposed of according to local Trust policy

Source: Adapted from DoH (1990a).

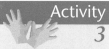

Activity 3

Identify local and national guidelines concerning the control of infection in hospitals and the community.

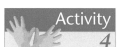

Activity 4

Identify the different methods of hand decontamination used in different areas of practice, such as hospitals, health centres and patients' homes.

● Ensure general standards of cleanliness
● Follow specific guidance for patients as required.

Hand hygiene

Many infections are spread by contact, the hands being a major vehicle in the transmission of infection (RCN, 1992). Normal skin has a resident population of micro-organisms, other transient organisms being picked up and shed during contact in the delivery of nursing care. The aim of handwashing is to remove these transient organisms or reduce their number below that of an infective dose before they are transmitted to a patient. It is the most important method of preventing spread by contact.

The RCN (1995) recommends thorough handwashing and careful drying on soft, high-quality disposable tissues to remove the majority of resident and transient micro-organisms. All jewellery should be removed before handwashing, and the nails should be kept short and clean. Antiseptic detergent solution used in handwashing will help to reduce the number of micro-organisms on the hands. As an alternative, a 70 per cent alcohol rub can be used in between proce-

Chart 3.3 ● Indications for handwashing

● Before and after aseptic techniques or invasive procedures
● Before contact with susceptible patients
● After handling body fluids
● After handling contaminated items
● Prior to the administration of drugs
● Before serving meals (see text)
● After removing aprons and gloves
● At the beginning and end of duty
● If in any doubt

dures, and staff must follow the recommended guidelines for its use. Hands should be washed following the procedures shown in Chart 3.3.

It is vital, too, that the patient's hands are kept clean. The nurse should, therefore, offer handwashing facilities after the patient has used the toilet, before meals and any other time they are requested.

Laundry

Soiled and contaminated linen can be a source of infection. Linen should be bagged at source when removed from the bed, and the hospital's policy for its disposal followed.

Waste disposal

Domestic and clinical waste is likely to contain and support the growth of Gram-negative bacilli, so all waste should be regarded as heavily contaminated and handled with care. The Department of Health and Social Security gives guidance on the safe disposal of clinical waste and on the colour-coding of waste containers.

The NHS has a legal responsibility for the safe disposal of hazardous waste. All waste is classified according to the following categories:

● *Domestic waste:* includes all materials not mentioned below. Domestic waste should be discarded into a black plastic bag that is securely closed
● *Clinical waste:* includes all materials contaminated with micro-organisms, for example dressings. Clinical waste should be sealed in yellow plastic bags and disposed of by incineration

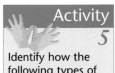

Activity
5

Identify how the following types of linen are dealt with in your hospital/community: used linen, soiled linen, infected linen, patients' personal clothing and duvets.

- *Sharps:* includes all needles and sharp instruments. Sharps should be discarded into a sharps box and disposed of by incineration. It may be necessary for a community Trust to organise the safe disposal of waste from the community
- *Human tissue:* immediately enclose in a yellow bin and transport to the hospital incinerator.

As it is impossible to cover here all the situations that will be encountered, readers are strongly urged to consult their infection control team and check their local policies for guidance.

Basic Food Hygiene

This section will describe the role of the nurse in food-handling in clinical areas. By the end of this section, you should be able to:

- List the key legislation regarding food safety
- Define food poisoning
- Identify the 10-point code for nurses
- Identify the action to take in the event of food poisoning.

In Great Britain, the Food Safety Act 1990 constitutes the main framework for food legislation and provides a wide range of regulations in respect of many activities relating to food itself and also to food sources and contact materials. In this way consumers' interests are protected. To further strengthen food safety procedures and policies, the Food Standards Agency (1998) was set up with the central aim of protecting the public amidst concerns over food safety. Secondary legislation is further imposed by the European Union.

In 2000, there were 65,209 laboratory-confirmed cases of food poisoning, attributed to the five most common bacterial pathogens: *Salmonella, Campylobacter, Listeria, Escherichia coli* 0157 and *Clostridium perfringens.* Food poisoning outbreaks are not uncommon in hospitals. Dryden et al. (1994) described a hospital-acquired outbreak of salmonellosis in two hospitals affecting 22 patients and 7 staff in 14 wards, the estimated cost of which was in the region of £33,000.

Food poisoning patterns have also become more complicated. The incidence of food poisoning caused by *Salmonella* and *Listeria* (Dryden et al., 1994) has decreased in the community, whereas the number of cases of *Campylobacter* infection has risen, this now being the most commonly reported type of food poisoning. Concern about food safety has now culminated in a recognition of the need for stricter controls and new legislation, as shown in Chart 3.4.

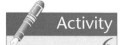

Activity 6

Have you been ill from eating contaminated food? What symptoms did you have?

Undertake a brief survey in your class to find out how many of your colleagues have been affected by food poisoning and what the source of infection was.

Chart 3.4 ● UK and EEC food safety legislation

● Food and Drugs Act 1955 (superseded by the 1984 Act)
● Food Act 1984
● Food Safety Act 1990
● EC Food Safety Legislation: Directive 89/397/EEC
● Food Standards Agency (1998)

Environmental health officers have the power to inspect all premises where food is prepared and consumed, and a failure to maintain safe practices may result in prosecution. Accordingly, all food handlers, including nurses, should receive training in food hygiene, the majority of cases of food poisoning being caused by ignorance, bad practice or poor management. The multiplicity of roles for nurses may include food preparation, food-handling and assisting clients with their meals; breaches of hygiene at any time can cause food poisoning.

A variety of diseases can be caused by eating food contaminated with pathogenic micro-organisms or their products, but not all of these diseases can be classified as food poisoning. **Food poisoning** has been described as an acute illness, normally with a short incubation period, caused by the recent consumption of food contaminated by pathogenic micro-organisms or their toxins. There is a disturbance of the gastrointestinal system within a few hours or days of consumption. Although diarrhoea, vomiting and abdominal pain are the most common symptoms of food poisoning, other clinical features such as pyrexia may be present. The clinical features may not all be present at the same time. The cause can be either microbial or non-microbial (Chart 3.5), although bacterial contamination is the most likely source.

food poisoning

an acute illness, normally with a short incubation period, caused by the recent consumption of food contaminated by pathogenic micro-organisms or their toxins

Chart 3.5 ● Sources of food contamination

● Foreign bodies: for example glass, hair and insects
● Chemicals: for example cleaning products
● Toxins: may be natural, for example red kidney beans
● Micro-organisms   – Bacteria, for example *Salmonella*
                      – Viruses
                      – Fungi
                      – Prions (identified as the agent causing the human
                        form of bovine spongiform encephalitis)

A review of over 500 outbreaks of salmonellosis in England during the 1970s and 80s (Sharp, 1992) showed the main contributory factors, several of which co-existed, to be:

- Food prepared too far in advance: 42 per cent
- Food stored at room temperature: 30 per cent
- Food cooled too slowly before refrigeration/freezing: 22 per cent
- Reheating food at the wrong temperature: 13 per cent
- Using contaminated food, and undercooking poultry or meat: 25 per cent
- Inadequate thawing of frozen food: 11 per cent
- Cross-contamination between cooked and uncooked food: 15 per cent
- Keeping hot food below 63°C
- Food handlers with symptomatic/asymptomatic infections.

Similar factors contribute in other forms of food poisoning, poor temperature regulation compounding all other contributory factors. Micro-organisms require suitable combinations of food, water, time and warmth to multiply (Figure 3.2); given a suitable environment, they can multiply every 20 minutes to a level potentially capable of causing food poisoning.

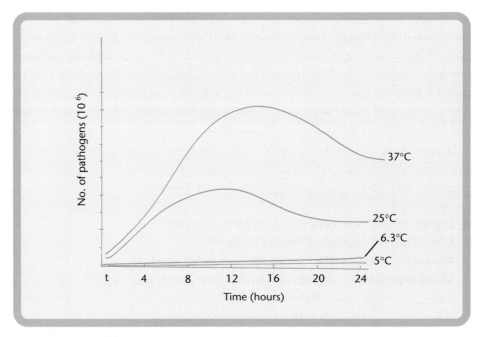

Figure 3.2 ● Diagrammatic representation of a growth curve of a food pathogen. Body and room temperature provide an ideal growth environment

Our knowledge of the sources of food poisoning bacteria and of routes of contamination can allow adequate precautions to be taken to prevent illness, especially in the vulnerable group of ill patients in the hospital and the community.

Ten-point code for nurses

1. WASH your HANDS
   – before touching food
   – after using the toilet or combing your hair
   – after administering to a patient's needs
   – after handling waste, bedpans or body fluids.
2. TELL your MANAGER immediately if you have any skin, nose, throat or stomach problems.
3. Cover cuts and sores with a brightly coloured waterproof dressing when handling food. (If the plaster is lost in the food, it can easily be identified.)
4. WEAR CLEAN clothing (plastic aprons for serving meals) according to hospital policy.
5. NEVER COUGH or SNEEZE over food. Do not pick your nose or touch your lips or mouth when serving food.
6. Keep equipment and utensils CLEAN. (Clean up as you go.)
7. KEEP food CLEAN and COVERED.
8. Touch food (both prepared and uncooked) as little as possible.
9. KEEP the lid on all waste sack holders and dustbins.
10. TELL your manager if you cannot follow the rules. Do not break the law.

(Adapted from DoH, 1990b)

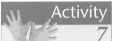
Activity 7

Describe the food service to patients in isolation and what extra precautions should be taken.

Identify whether any of your clients require any special eating or drinking utensils. Explore the range of utensils available for babies, children and those with a learning disability.

Food service on the wards

Lukewarm food is potentially dangerous. A moderate temperature allows food poisoning bacteria to grow rapidly, temperatures of between 5°C and 63°C being referred to as the 'danger zone'. While food is being held for service:

- Hot food should be kept hot at above 63°C
- Cold food should be kept cold at below 5°C
- Avoid the danger zone between 5°C and 63°C
- Meals should be served immediately upon arrival on the ward
- Should there be any delay (if the patient is out of the ward, for example), refer to hospital policy for requesting a fresh meal
- Microwaves should not be used to reheat or cook food in clinical areas.

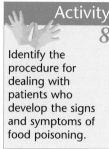

Activity

8

Identify the procedure for dealing with patients who develop the signs and symptoms of food poisoning.

The United Kingdom Central Council for Nursing, Midwifery and Health Visiting (UKCC, 1997) has declared that 'Nurses have an implicit responsibility for ensuring that patients are appropriately fed', and, under the Nursing and Midwifery Council (NMC) *Code of Professional Conduct* (NMC, 2002), nurses also have the responsibility to report to a senior person any circumstances in which the safe and appropriate care of patients and clients cannot be provided. Although the task of feeding may be delegated to junior members of staff, the overall responsibility remains with the registered nurse.

Ward fridges should be of the larder type, the temperature being checked daily and recorded on the relevant forms. Ice cream should not be stored in ward refrigerators, and overcrowding should be avoided. Cross-contamination between raw and 'high-risk foods' (for example trifle) must not be allowed.

Microwave ovens and ice-making machines in clinical areas should be of catering grade, and staff using these should follow the guidelines for their use, cleaning and maintenance. Some microwave ovens produce 'cold spots' in food, so a more even distribution of heat is required, which can be achieved by thorough stirring both during and after cooking. Staff must make every effort to use the hospital catering department to supply meals for patients.

Failure to follow the guidelines may result in prosecution under the Food Safety Act 1990 and may also be in breach of the NMC Code of Conduct (2002). The practical appication of food hygiene principles ensues that food given to patients and clients is safe and will cause them no harm.

■ Administration of Medications

This section will describe the role of the nurse in the practice of drug administration. By the end of this section, the nurse should be able to:

- Understand the legislation and local Trust policies governing the administration of drugs by health-care professionals
- Safely administer drugs to patients via a variety of routes
- Be involved in the storage and preparation of drugs
- Understand how drugs work.

The administration of medicines is considered to be one of the most important responsibilities of the nurse, nurses' professional responsibilities in terms of drug administration being set out in the UKCC document *Guidelines for Administration of Medicines* (UKCC, 2000). The nurse is responsible for assessing, planning, implementing and evaluating drug therapies as well as educating patients about their drug regimens. To be effective, the nurse must have an understanding of the fundamental principles of drug action, the purposes of drug use and the nursing actions necessary to bring about a beneficial outcome. The student is advised to consult other textbooks for more comprehensive information on drug actions and pharmacokinetics. Routes such as the intravenous and the epidural, using electronic devices such as pumps, are not described as they require further training at postregistration level.

The UKCC recommends that the administration of medicines should be undertaken by a First Level Registered Nurse/Midwife who has demonstrated the knowledge and competencies and who can speedily respond to contraindications and side-effects (UKCC, 2000). All practitioners, including student nurses, who are administering drugs must be responsible and accountable for their practice as outlined in the Code of Conduct (NMC, 2002).

In the UK, the range of substances intended for medicinal use must conform to standards specified in the *British Pharmacopoeia* or the *British Pharmaceutical Codex* and must satisfy the relevant government legislation, listed in Chart 3.6. The implications of these acts will be discussed below, and the reader with a keen interest for more details is recommend to consult a current copy of the *British National Formulary*. Failure to comply with the legal requirements, and any ensuing errors, may result in criminal prosecution.

Before any medication is administered, it is important that the nurse carries out a detailed assessment of the patient, including:

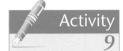

Activity 9

Take the medication history of a client you have cared for and discuss any relevant issues with your mentor.

- Medications that the patient is currently taking
- Their frequency and dosage
- Any home remedies being taken
- Other complementary therapies being used
- Allergies to any drugs
- Height, weight, blood pressure, temperature and respiration, as some drug dosages, for example dopamine infusion, are calculated on body mass, and side-effects can affect blood pressure
- General fitness and health as such information can influence decisions about the routes and methods of drug administration; an emaciated patient may not, for example, be able to tolerate deep intramuscular injections

Chart 3.6 ● Statutes controlling substances intended for medicinal use

- Misuse of Drugs Act 1971
- Poisons Act 1972
- Medicines Act 1968, 1983
- Prescription by Nurses Act 1992
- Misuse of Drug Regulations 1985

- Diet; if, for example, foods such as cheese, yoghurt, broad beans, Marmite, red wine and beer are administered to a patient who is receiving monoamine oxidase inhibitors, dangerous side-effects may ensue.

In the UK, certain drugs can be bought over the counter and others must be prescribed by a doctor. In hospitals, medicines should not be administered without a written prescription. Prescriptions should include information necessary for the safe administration of the drug. The prescription chart should detail:

- The name of the patient
- The date that the prescription was written and the signature of the prescriber
- The medication and dosage
- The route for administering the drug
- The time of administration
- Any specific information, for example that it is to be taken with meals.

Prescriptions are normally written on a standard prescription sheet (usually produced locally and differing between hospitals and in the community). Winslow (1997), in a study of medication prescription orders, found that 78 per cent of signatures were illegible or legible only with effort, thus increasing the risk of medication errors and patient harm. **The nurse should not administer any drug if the prescription is illegible.** It is important that all records of prescribed medicines should be kept together to prevent drug interactions and overdosage, and for monitoring purposes. The following criteria should be adhered to in order to prevent drug errors:

1. The prescription must be **legible**, and the approved or generic name should be used.
2. Details of the client's name and address, the dose required and the frequency and route of administration must be clearly stated. For certain drugs (for example antibiotics), the proposed duration of therapy should be stated.

controlled drugs

those drugs, such as morphine, subject to the prescription requirements of the Misuse of Drugs Regulations 1985

3. **Controlled drugs**, that is, drugs that are subject to the prescription requirements of the Misuse of the Drug Regulations 1985, should be clearly monitored.
4. A prescription should not be altered once it has been written and should be written out in full again if a change in dose or frequency is indicated.
5. When a prescription is to be cancelled, it should be crossed out and signed and dated by the doctor.
6. In emergencies, telephone orders for the administration of medicines can be accepted by a first-level registered nurse (providing there is local agreement) if the doctor is unable to attend the ward. The prescription must then be

written and signed by the nurse, stating that it is a verbal prescription. The doctor's name should be recorded on the prescription sheet, and the doctor should sign the prescription as soon as possible. No telephone orders should be repeated.

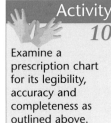

Activity 10

Examine a prescription chart for its legibility, accuracy and completeness as outlined above.

The nurse's first task is to check the prescription for completeness; he or she can then prepare to administer the drug. When preparing medications, it is important to ensure cleanliness of the hands, a clean surface and sterility of all the materials used. All the components must be assembled in a well-lit room and medicines prepared in a safe area away from distraction. A general guide to ensure patients' safety in the administration of medications is to check the 'five rights':

1. The right medication.
2. The right amount.
3. The right time.
4. The right patient.
5. The right route.

Right medication

After checking the prescription, the nurse selects the right medication, carefully checking the labels on the containers. Medications from a container that is unlabelled, defaced or illegible must never be used. The nurse should read any instructions pertaining to the medication and check the expiry date. Nurses must never administer a drug prepared by someone else because the nurse administering the drug will still be held accountable for any errors made by others during preparation. Medications must never be decanted from one container into another. The nurse should be familiar with basic information about the drug, including its action, contraindications and side-effects, and current reference books, such as the *British National Formulary*, should be available at all times.

Right amount

To prepare the right amount of medication, the nurse must be familiar with the different measurement systems and common abbreviations used (Chart 3.7).

When preparing liquid medications for oral administration, it is important to shake all suspensions and emulsions in order to ensure a proper distribution of the drug. A calibrated medicine pot or syringe may be used to draw up the right amount of medication. If the medication is poured from the container, the

Chart 3.7 ● Common abbreviations used in prescriptions

p.o. – by mouth	p.r.n. – given as necessary	caps – capsules
s.c. – subcutaneous	q.d. – daily	elix. – elixir
s.l. – sublingual	q.h. – every hour	I.U. – International Units
i.m. – intramuscular	q.d.s. – four times a day	kg – kilogram
i.v. – intravenous	t.d.s. – three times a day	g – gram
e.c. – enteric coated	b.i.d. – twice a day	mcg – microgram
s.c. – sugar coated	a.c. – before meals	mg – milligram
m.r. – modified release	p.c. – after meals	l – litre
stat – given immediately	tr. – tincture	ml – millilitre
	neb. – nebuliser	guttae – drops

medicine pot should be placed on a flat surface. To check for accuracy, the pot should be raised to eye level and the measurement read at the lowest point of the meniscus.

Some medications, for example eye drops, are measured with a dropper. The dropper must be held vertically, and the bulb should be slowly squeezed and released until the required dosage has been reached.

The administration of injections depends on the drugs prescribed. Some injectables, for example pethidine, are available in liquid form, and the required amount can easily be drawn up. Administering the correct amount also depends on the strength of the drug. Heparin, for example, is available in 5,000, 10,000 or 25,000 units/ml, so the amount injected will vary. Other injectables, such as penicillin, are produced in 'powder form' and require dilution before they can be administered. If fluid is to be added, the solution displacement value must be taken into account. This can be found in the literature accompanying the vial and is usually 0.02 ml. If this value is not checked, it can result in erroneous doses being administered. When drugs are supplied at strengths different from the dosages that have been prescribed, the nurse must determine the quantity of drug that is to be administered. Special formulae are available, but it is also essential for the nurse to have a basic knowledge of arithmetic. The student who is experiencing difficulty should consult one of the many drug calculation textbooks now available or seek help from lecturers or mentors.

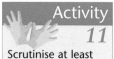

Activity 11

Scrutinise at least six prescription charts. Were you able to recognise the abbreviations used? Discuss your findings with your mentor.

Right time

In order to achieve maximum therapeutic effectiveness, the doctor will specify the number of times a day the drug is to be given. It is important to adhere to

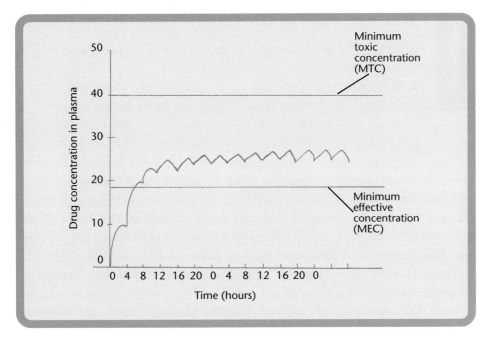

Figure 3.3 ● Plasma level versus time plot of a drug administered at 4-hourly intervals in order to keep the plasma concentration of the drug in an effective but not toxic range

this regimen as closely as possible in order to maintain a relatively constant blood plasma level of the drug (Figure 3.3). Drugs often have to be given with or after meals, and it is important to ensure that the patient understands the reason for this.

Right patient

It is important to identify the right patient or client, and in a busy hospital or community setting, this is even more important. The following should be employed as a matter of routine regardless of the number of patients involved:

● In acute care settings, check the wrist identity bracelet and the name band on the bed
● If patients are not confused, ask them to tell you their name but never prompt or say, 'Are you Mr/Mrs...?
● If the patient questions the dosage, appearance or method of administration, always double-check the prescription and medication
● Never leave drugs for a patient who is not there.

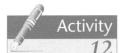

Activity

12

Undertake a survey of your patients to find out whether they receive their medications on time. Discuss your findings with your mentor.

What effects will a delay have on the treatment programme?

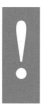

SPECIFIC POINTS ON CHILDREN'S MEDICATIONS

- If the child is too young, ask the parents to tell you the child's name.
- Children and/or parents have a right to know about the treatments, and they should always be addressed by name.

Right route

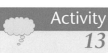

Activity

13

Discuss with your mentor the importance of administering medicines via the prescribed route.

What information is given to the patients in anticipation of the procedure?

The doctor will usually specify the route by which the medication is to be administered, and the nurse administering the drug has the responsibility of ensuring that this is followed. If there are any discrepancies, the doctor should be consulted. If the nurse is concerned about the safety of administering a particular drug, the doctor should be asked to prepare and administer the drug.

Drugs may be administered in a number of ways (Chart 3.8), but not all drugs may be administered by all the possible routes. When a drug is available in more than one form, the choice of route depends on factors such as the rate of absorption required, the speed of onset, the patient's general condition and any side-effects.

Nurses are not responsible for the administration of drugs by all of these routes but may have to assist doctors, for example with intrathecal administration.

Chart 3.8 ● Routes of drug administration

- **Oral** – by mouth
- **Sublingual** – under the tongue
- **Injection** – intramuscular, subcutaneous, intradermal (into soft tissues)
- **Rectal** – into the rectum
- **Vaginal** – into the vagina
- **Topical** – onto the skin or mucous membranes
- **Inhalation** – via the respiratory tract
- **Optic** – into the eye
- **Aural** – into the ear
- **Nasal** – into the nose
- **Intra-articular** – into the cavity of a joint
- **Intrathecal** – into the spinal fluid
- **Intravenous** – into a vein
- **Epidural** – into the epidural space
- **Intracardiac** – into the heart

Oral medications

The **oral route** is the most frequently used route for drug administration. Oral medications are either in liquid (for example elixir) or solid (for example tablet) form. Some tablets (enteric coated) are covered with a substance that does not dissolve until the medication reaches the small intestine. These tablets should never be crushed or chewed because the medication will irritate the gastric mucosa. The administration of oral medication may be carried out by one or two registered nurses, depending on local policy.

oral route
via the mouth

Guidelines for oral drug administration

1. Wash your hands.
2. Check the prescription for completeness of date, time, drug to be given, dosage, route, frequency and duration of therapy. Check that the drug has not already been given and is due.
3. The nurse must have a basic understanding of the effects of the drug to be administered.
4. Select and check the required medication for discolouration, precipitation, contamination and expiry date.
5. Prepare the dosage as prescribed. Do not crush enteric-coated, sublingual or sustained-action tablets. Empty the required dose into a medicine pot. To prevent contamination, avoid touching the preparation. If dispensing liquid, the bottle should be held with the label towards the palm of the hand to prevent spillage obscuring the name of the drug.
6. Check the labels on the containers again.
7. Take the medication and the prescription chart to the patient. Check the patient's identity (as described earlier) and the drug to be given.
8. Position the patient as upright as possible to aid swallowing, and instruct the patient accordingly. A glass of water or juice (50 ml or more) should be given to facilitate swallowing. The nurse must ensure that the patient has swallowed the medication. Infants and young children should be supported firmly to avoid spilling the medication.
9. Make the patient comfortable and ask him or her to stay upright for a few minutes.
10. Immediately complete all the necessary records.
11. Clear all the equipment away.

> **CONNECTIONS**
> *Chapter 4 outlines the principles of managing a nasogastric tube.*

Some patients with a nasogastric tube may have their oral medications administered through it. The procedure for administering the drug via a nasogastric tube is described in Chart 3.9. Liquid medications will flow easily

Chart 3.9 ● Administering drugs via a nasogastric tube
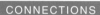

1. If possible, elevate the patient's head 30–45 degrees to avoid aspiration during and following administration

2. Check the placement of the nasogastric tube either by aspirating a small quantity of the gastric contents and testing for acidity or by inserting a small amount of air into the tube while listening with a stethoscope for the entry of air into the stomach

3. Flush the tube with 30 ml of water for adults and 20 ml for children

4. Administer the medication* through a syringe barrel connected to the tubing, as shown in Figure 3.4. Hold the barrel of the syringe about 15 cm (6 inches) higher than the patient's nose and allow the fluid to flow into the stomach by gravity

5. Between medications flush the tube with 5 ml of water

6. If the patient is receiving continuous feeding, feeding is recommenced; otherwise the tube is clamped

CONNECTIONS

Chapter 4 contains a section on enteral feeding via a nasogastric tube.

* Follow the guidelines for preparing drugs as outlined above.

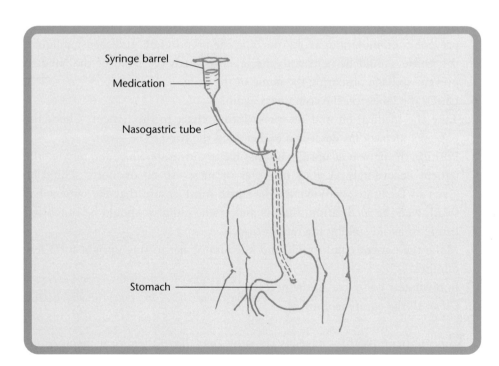

Figure 3.4 ● Administration of medication via a nasogastric tube. The fluid is allowed to flow into the stomach by gravity

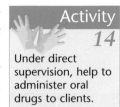

down the tube; tablets and other solid medications should if possible be avoided but can otherwise be crushed and combined with a liquid in order not to obstruct the lumen. The medication should not be added to the 'feed'; instead, the continuous feeding should be interrupted and resumed after administration of the drug. The tube should be flushed with water prior to and after administering the drug. Enteric-coated tablets and similar drugs should not be crushed.

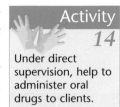

Activity 14

Under direct supervision, help to administer oral drugs to clients.

 ## SPECIFIC POINTS ON CHILDREN'S MEDICATIONS

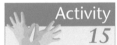

■ Flush the nasogastric tube with 20 ml of water.

Parenteral medications

The term 'parenteral' refers to the act of administering drugs by a route other than the alimentary canal. The term is most commonly used to indicate injection routes such as intramuscular, subcutaneous and intravenous. Less common ways by which drugs are administered include intrathecally, intra-articularly, intracardiac and intra-arterially, these more specialised procedures being performed by doctors. Drugs given parenterally have a more rapid effect than those given orally. It is also easy to achieve high plasma levels for effective treatment. Some drugs (for example insulin) may, if given orally, be destroyed.

parenteral route
a route other than via the alimentary canal

When administering drugs by injection, it is important first to select and assemble the correct equipment:

- The patient's prescription
- The medication
- A clean tray
- A sterile syringe and needle
- Alcohol swabs
- **Gloves if necessary.**

Activity 15

Identify the different gauge needles that are used for intradermal, subcutaneous, intravenous and intramuscular injections, and for drawing up medications.

There are many different syringes and needles, suiting many different procedures (Table 3.2). It is important to choose carefully according to the procedure; the length and gauge of the needle must, for example, be suitable for the injection site, the type of injection, the volume of medication, the viscosity of the drug and the patient's condition. Syringes for injections range from 0.1 to 5 ml, depending on the volume of drug to be administered.

Gloves should be worn to prevent cross-infection or if the drug is likely to cause skin sensitisation with frequent use: dermatitis can, for example, be caused by frequent contact with drugs such as penicillin, streptomycin and

Table 3.2 Selection of needles for different types of injection

| Type of injection | Suggested needle gauge | | Size of syringe |
	Adult	Child	
Intradermal	26 G x ⅜" (0.45 x 10 mm)	26 G x ⅜" (0.45 x 10 mm)	1 ml calibrated in 0.1 ml divisions
Subcutaneous	25/26 G x ⅝" (0.45 x 16 mm)	26 G x ⅝" (0.45 x 16 mm)	1 ml calibrated in 0.1 ml divisions
Intramuscular	21 G x 1½ " (0.8 x 40 mm)	23 G x 1¼" (0.6 x 30 mm)	5 ml calibrated in 0.2 ml divisions

Activity 16

Describe the policy for the safe disposal of used needles, syringes, vials and glass ampoules. Describe the actions to be taken in the event of an accidental needle injury.

chlorpromazine. When cytotoxic drugs are given, vinyl gloves should be worn; goggles and a mask may also be necessary.

Intramuscular injection

intramuscular route

into a muscle

The **intramuscular route** is used to administer medications that are irritating or painful. Skeletal muscles are well perfused with blood and have fewer pain receptors, so pain is minimal, and up to 5 ml of injectate may be given into the large muscles (1–2 ml into the deltoid muscle for example). To give an intramuscular injection:

1. Collect and check all the equipment to ensure sterility. If the outer packaging is damaged, replace the pack.
2. Wash your hands.
3. Prepare the needle(s) and syringe(s) on a tray. Check for any defects.
4. Check the patient's prescription(s) for completeness.
5. Select the drug and verify it against the prescription.
6. Prepare the drug, using gloves if necessary.
7. Administer the intramuscular injection.

Drawing medication from a single-dose ampoule

● Check the ampoule for cracks, cloudiness and precipitation
● Gently tap the upper area of the ampoule to release any medication trapped at the top of the ampoule
● Cover the neck of the ampoule or use an 'ampoule breaker' when snapping it open

- Insert the needle into the ampoule and withdraw the required amount. Avoid contaminating the medication
- Change the needle and dispose of it as per hospital policy
- Tap the barrel to dislodge any air bubbles towards the needle and expel the air.

Drawing medication from a multidose vial solution

- Remove the metal cover from the vial and inspect the medication as above
- Clean the rubber cap with antiseptic solution and let it dry
- Withdraw the prescribed amount of solution. Two methods can be used to draw up the solution:
  - *Method 1:* insert a 19 G needle into the cap to vent the vial. Insert the assembled needle and syringe, and draw up the required amount
  - *Method 2:* assemble the needle and syringe. Fill the syringe with the same volume of air as the medication that will be withdrawn. Insert the needle through the rubber stopper, holding the vial at an oblique angle, and inject the air into the vial. Keep the needle in the solution, invert the vial and allow the medication to enter the syringe. The volume can be adjusted by using the plunger, and the needle is removed when the required amount has been drawn up
- Change the needle as it may have become blunted/damaged
- Tap the barrel to dislodge any air bubbles towards the needle and expel the air.

Reconstituting a powdered medication

- Clean the rubber cap with an antiseptic and allow it to dry
- Add the required amount of diluent, that is, sterile water, carefully down the wall of the vial, and allow an equal amount of air to escape into the syringe
- Check for the displacement value of the drug
- Remove the needle and syringe
- Shake the vial to dissolve the powder
- The reconstituted solution can now be withdrawn as described for removing solutions from a multidose vial.

> **Activity 17**
>
> Under direct supervision in the skills laboratory or clinical area, prepare a powdered medication for injection.

Guidelines for intramuscular injection

1. Identify the patient and explain the procedure. It is important to gain the patient's co-operation.
2. Position the patient for easy access to the injection site, comfort and privacy. Infants and children should be firmly held so that they do not move and thus receive an injury during the procedure.

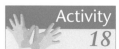

On a model, identify the sites for intramuscular injections. Did your patients have a preference for which sites were used?

Observe patients during an intramuscular injection and discuss your findings with your supervisor.

3. Clean the site with antiseptic and let it dry.
4. Holding the needle at 90 degrees (Figure 3.5), quickly thrust the needle into the muscle. Leave a third of the needle shaft exposed. If the needle breaks from the hub, it can thus be removed safely.
5. Pull back the plunger. If blood appears, withdraw the needle and repeat the procedure with a sterile needle. Explain to the patient what is happening.
6. If no blood appears, depress the plunger and inject the drug slowly.
7. Quickly withdraw the needle and apply gentle pressure over the puncture site.
8. Position the patient comfortably.
9. Dispose of the needle and syringe as per hospital policy.
10. Complete all the necessary records.

Sites for intramuscular injection

Various sites on the human body may be used for giving an injection. When choosing a site, it is important to identify the relevant anatomical landmarks in order to avoid injuring nerves, striking bones or puncturing blood vessels. The site must also be inspected for its suitability, for example:

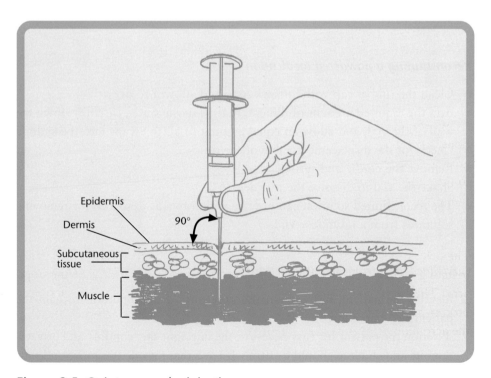

Figure 3.5 ● Intramuscular injection

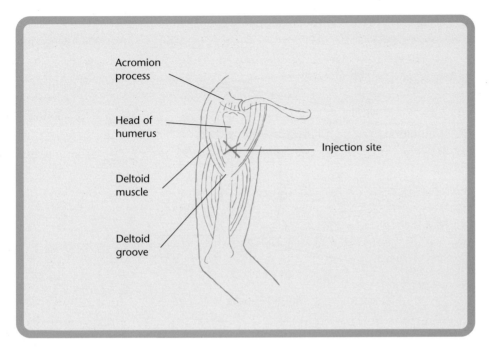

Labels in figure:
- Acromion process
- Head of humerus
- Deltoid muscle
- Deltoid groove
- Injection site

Figure 3.6 ● Deltoid injection site

- Is there sufficient muscle mass?
- Does the area to be injected have a good blood supply?
- Is there any skin damage?
- Is there evidence of fibrosis or infection?

When patients are receiving frequent intramuscular or subcutaneous injections, for example of insulin, it is important to rotate the injection site to obtain greater drug absorption, decrease tissue fibrosis and cause minimal discomfort to the patient. A rotation chart may be useful in implementing an effective rotation programme. The most frequently used sites are outlined below.

The deltoid muscle in the upper arm

The deltoid is used for small quantities of injectate, 1 ml or less, of clear non-irritating medication. The muscle is located in the lateral aspect of the upper arm. The injection site (Figure 3.6) is located 4–5 cm below the acromion process and above the deltoid groove in adults, and approximately 2 cm below the acromion process in older children.

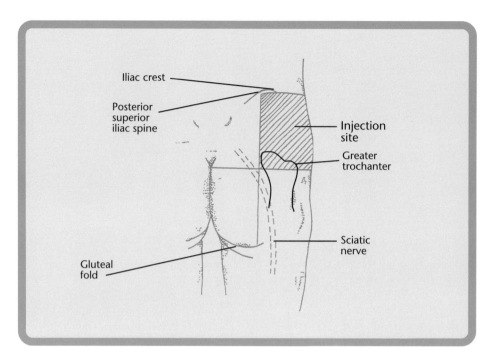

Figure 3.7 ● Dorsogluteal injection site

The dorsogluteal site in the buttocks

This site (Figure 3.7) is frequently used for injections into the gluteus maximus muscle, this larger muscle mass being the preferred site for larger volumes. The patient should be asked to lie prone with the toes pointing inwards to relax the buttocks. The injection site is identified by palpating the anatomical landmarks of the posterior superior iliac spine and the greater trochanter (at the head of the femur). A line is drawn between these two points, a safe injection site being in the area above and lateral to this line. The area below this line should be avoided to prevent damage to the sciatic nerve. This site should not be used in infants or children who have not been walking for at least 1 year since this muscle is not developed.

The ventrogluteal site in the hip area

The injection is given in the gluteus medius and gluteus maximus muscles. The patient is placed on his side or can be allowed to stay in the supine or prone position. To find the injection site on the right hip (the most convenient site for right-handed practitioners), palpate the greater trochanter, the iliac crest and the anterior superior iliac spine. Place the palm of the left hand on the greater trochanter and the left index finger towards the anterior superior iliac spine

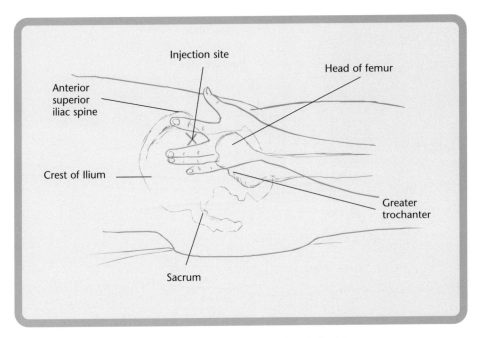

Figure 3.8 ● Ventrogluteal injection site on the right hip

(Figure 3.8). Move the middle finger away from the index finger to form a V between the fingers. The injection is given into the centre of the V. This is the preferred site for infants and children who have not been walking for a year (Beecroft, 1990; Whalley and Wong, 1995) because the pelvis is concave below the iliac crest and contains a relatively large muscle mass.

The vastus lateralis in the thigh

The vastus lateralis muscle is situated in the lateral thigh and can be used for both adults and children. This site (Figure 3.9) is preferable because there are no major blood vessels or nerves in the area. The patient is asked to lie in the supine position with the thigh well exposed, pointing the toe inwards to give a better exposure of the lateral aspects of the thigh. The injection site can be located by dividing the thigh horizontally and vertically into thirds by imagining lines drawn one hand's breadth below the greater trochanter at the top of the thigh and one hand's breadth from the knee. The thigh is then measured vertically, this time by marking out one hand's breadth along the middle of the inner side of the thigh and one hand's breadth on the outer side of the thigh, thus creating a rectangle in the middle where it is safe to inject. This strip is between 2 and 4 cm long in children and about 7 cm long in adults. The needle is directed into the tissues at a right angle.

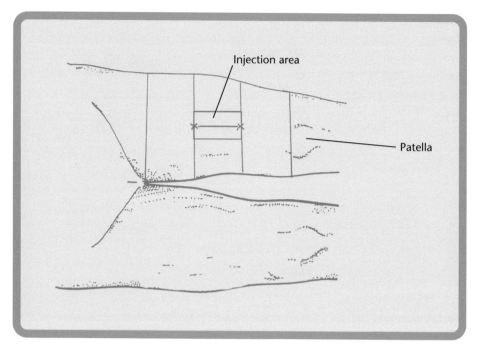

Figure 3.9 ● Vastus lateralis injection site

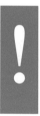

SPECIFIC POINTS ON CHILDREN'S INJECTIONS

■ *Sites for intramuscular injection in infants and children who have not been walking for 1 year*
1. Vastus lateralis in the middle third of femur (Figure 3.9)
2. Ventrogluteal (Figure 3.8)
3. Mid-anterior thigh: injection given into the rectus femoris muscle. This muscle is located on the anterior aspect of the thigh and is quite visible in infants.

■ *Sites for intramuscular injection in older children who have been walking for more than 1 year*
1. Vastus lateralis (Figure 3.9)
2. Dorsogluteal site in the gluteus medius muscle (Figure 3.7)
3. Deltoid muscle for older children (Figure 3.6).

Z-track intramuscular injection

This technique for intramuscular injection has been primarily reserved for use with medications such as iron preparations that are known to be particularly irritating and can permanently stain the subcutaneous tissue. During this procedure, there is lateral displacement of the cutaneous tissue prior to injection, and the tension is released immediately after injection. When utilising the Z-track technique, the nurse grasps the muscle and pulls it laterally about 2.5 cm until it is taut, holding the tissue in this position. The needle is inserted at a 90 degree angle. After ensuring the position of the needle, the medication is injected. Following withdrawal of the needle, the skin is immediately released.

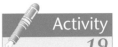

Activity 19

Undertake an Internet search to find out more about the complications of intramuscular injections and discuss your findings with your mentor.

Complications of intramuscular injections

The nurse should be aware of the possible complications of injections and make every effort to prevent them.

Infection

The introduction of infection via a needle may lead to local (abscesses) or systemic (septicaemia) complications. It is important to maintain strict asepsis during all invasive procedures. All equipment should be sterile, and good handwashing is essential.

Muscle myopathy

Intramuscular injections, by their very nature, cause injury to tissues. Needle myopathy damage can be prevented by a good injection technique using the optimum-sized needle. Focal myopathy can be caused by the injectate and by using an injectate of neutral pH.

Wrong route

Injectates may accidentally be given into a vein or an artery, resulting in a rapid physiological response. Depending on the drug used, severe complications and even death may occur. The syringe should therefore always be aspirated before the drug is injected: if blood appears in the barrel of the syringe, the needle should be withdrawn and an alternative site used. The patient should be informed of the reason for this. Drugs injected into an artery may cause thrombosis, with disruption of the blood supply.

Nerve damage

Damage to the sciatic nerve in the dorsogluteal region should be avoided. The nurse should identify the landmarks, as shown in Figure 3.7, and select a safe area for injection. Alternatively, the nurse can select another site, such as the vastus lateralis, which carries the least risk.

Skin preparation for intramuscular injections

The cleaning of injection sites with alcohol swabs and by other means has been debated for a number of years (Dann, 1969; McConnell, 1993; Campbell, 1995). In a classic study of over 5,000 patients, Dann (1969) reported that cleansing with an alcohol swab is not always necessary and does not result in infection at the injection site. The risk of infection may, however, be increased in immuno-compromised patients, and Mallett and Dougherty (2000) advise nurses to cleanse the skin prior to injection. As the procedural guidelines recommended by Mallett and Dougherty have been adopted by many hospitals in UK, the cleansing of the intramuscular injection site should continue in line with these recommendations.

Subcutaneous injections

subcutaneous route

under the skin

The sites for administering subcutaneous injections include the lateral aspects of the upper arm, the abdomen on either side of the umbilicus, the middle and outer area of the thigh and the back (Figure 3.10). It is important to allow diabetic patients to maintain their own subcutaneous injections while in hospital.

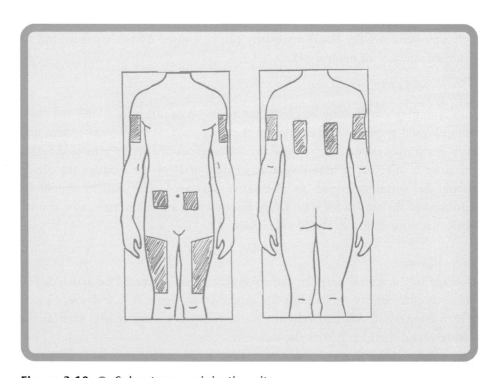

Figure 3.10 ● Subcutaneous injection sites

Guidelines for administering a subcutaneous injection

1. Explain the procedure to the patient and gain his co-operation.
2. Select the site and assist the patient into position to maintain his comfort and dignity. Expose the injection site; at a viable injection site, the nurse should be able to pinch at least 2.5 cm of subcutaneous tissue. Check the rotation chart if one is in use.
3. Wash your hands thoroughly to prevent infection.
4. Prepare the medication, selecting the correctly sized needle (Table 3.2).
5. Clean the injection site with isopropyl alcohol 70 per cent and allow it to dry. For subcutaneous insulin and heparin injections, alcohol swabs are contraindicated as they interfere with drug action and toughen the skin, making subsequent injections difficult.
6. Grasp the skin firmly between the thumb and forefinger, as shown in Figure 3.11.
7. Maintain the fold and insert the needle almost to its full length at an angle of 45 or 90 degrees depending on the drug being administered, the latter position being used for subcutaneous insulin and heparin. Pull back on the plunger to check whether any blood appears (check the manufacturer's instructions on this point first). If no blood appears, slowly push the plunger. When the syringe is empty, quickly and smoothly withdraw the needle and apply gentle pressure to prevent the formation of a haematoma. Studies of subcutaneous injection techniques by McGowan and Wood (1990) have shown no difference with respect to bruising outcome when heparin was administered without aspirating the syringe or using pressure at the site.

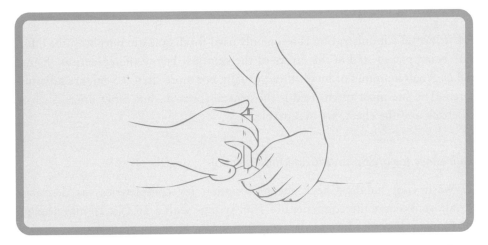

Figure 3.11 ● Current recommended method for injecting insulin at right angles with the skin pinched

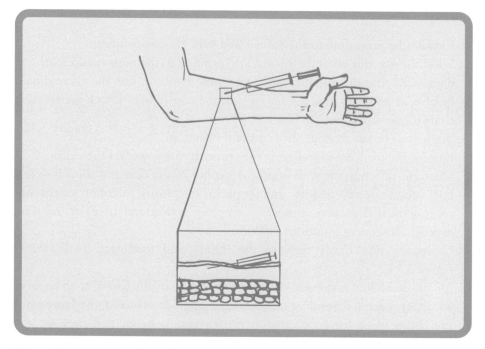

Figure 3.12 ● Intradermal injection

8. Safely discard the syringe and needle.
9. Wash your hands.
10. Complete all the relevant records.

Intradermal injections

intradermal route
___
within the layers of the skin

CONNECTIONS

A more detailed diagram of the skin can be found in Figures 8.3 and 10.1.

Intradermal administration is frequently used for diagnostic purposes, the injectate being placed within the layers of the skin just below the epidermis (Figure 3.12). Small amounts of medication, usually not more than 0.5 ml, are administered. The site most often used is the central forearm, but other areas, such as the back and the chest, are acceptable.

Guidelines for giving an intradermal injection

1. Wash your hands. Check the prescription for completeness as described above. Prepare the equipment (a 1 ml syringe with a 26 G × 16 mm needle).
2. Explain the procedure to the patient and gain his co-operation.
3. Select the site and assist the patient into position to maintain his comfort and dignity. Select a site with minimal, or preferably no, hair and skin blemishes.

4. Clean the area with antiseptic solution. Avoid using iodine solutions as the residual stain may interfere with interpreting the results of the skin test. If the skin is oily, cleanse the area with acetone to remove any fat deposits. Allow the skin to dry.

5. Support the patient's arm and stretch the skin taut.

6. Place the bevel of the needle almost flat against the patient's skin and insert the needle with the bevel side up at an angle of 10–15 degrees (Figure 3.12). The needle should be about 3 mm below the skin surface. The medication is slowly injected while watching for a wheal to develop.

7. Once the wheal appears, withdraw the needle.

8. The area should never be massaged as this may interfere with the test results.

9. If the test is carried out to determine sensitivity, follow the test instructions to determine, for example, signs of local reaction.

10. Discard the equipment.

11. Wash your hands.

12. Complete all the relevant records.

Topical medications

Topical administration refers to the application of medications to the skin or mucous membranes to achieve local or systemic effects. The medication may be incorporated into a base such as an oil, lotion or cream, which is rubbed into the skin (inunction), the area being cleaned with soap and water before application. The inunction can be applied with the fingers and hands, or using cotton wool balls or gauze swabs. If there is a risk of infection or application is to the mucous membranes, gloves should be worn.

topical
applied to the skin or mucous membranes

inunction
rubbing a drug mixed with a fatty base into the skin; also the name given to the mixture

CONNECTIONS

Chapter 6 discusses methods of delivering drugs by inhalation.

Guidelines for the topical administration of drugs

1. Wash your hands. Check the prescription as discussed above before administering the drug.

2. Explain the procedure to the patient, who is positioned to expose the area and carry out any assessments. Observe for any changes. The patient's privacy and dignity should be maintained.

3. Prepare the equipment, and follow aseptic guidelines if there is risk of infection. Remove solid or semisolid medications with a sterile spatula.

4. Apply the medication to the site.

5. Inform the patient if the preparation is likely to stain the skin or soil the clothing.

6. Complete the appropriate records.

Guidelines for application of transdermal medications

transderaml route

application directly on to the skin, the substance applied then being absorbed via the skin

More drugs are now becoming available for administration via the **transdermal route**, for example glyceryl trinitrate derivatives (Transiderm-Nitro), opiates and some analgesics (Durogesic, Emla). Following the application of the patch, the drug is absorbed through the hair follicles and sweat glands, entering the bloodstream.

Before any patch can be applied, the previous application must be removed from the patient's skin, and the prescription is then checked to ensure the patient's safety. The new patch is applied to a clean non-hairy skin surface, the most frequently used sites being the chest wall, the upper arms, the backs of the hands and the antecubital fossae, depending on the intended use of the medication. The patches should have labels indicating the date and time of application and the signature of the practitioner.

To prevent inflammation and irritation, the site should be rotated and recorded on a rotation chart. If the patch has been properly applied, the patient is able to shower or bath.

Eye medication

Eye medications are available in two forms: eye ointments and eye drops. The administration of eye drops and eye ointment will initially be the responsibility of the nurse, but he or she may also be involved in instructing the patient as well as other family members in the administration of the medication.

It is important that the correct eye is treated. The prescription must be carefully checked and any abbreviations verified. The patient should be informed if her vision is going to be affected after the procedure. Although the eye is not sterile, it is important to use an aseptic technique when performing eye treatment. If infection is present in both eyes, the least affected eye should be treated first to prevent cross-contamination. The following general guidelines should be used when administering eye drops and eye ointments.

1. Explain the procedure to the patient, emphasising that her nose may feel as if it is 'running' because the punctum of the eye drains into the nasal space. The patient may also get a taste of the drug at the back of her throat.
2. The patient should ideally lie flat with her head tilted backwards to allow easy access to the eyes. The nurse should stand behind the patient's head as it is easier to administer the drug from that position.
3. Prepare all the necessary equipment. Warm the eye drops and/or ointment to room temperature.
4. Wash your hands and put on gloves if necessary.
5. Check the eye and perform eye toilet as necessary.

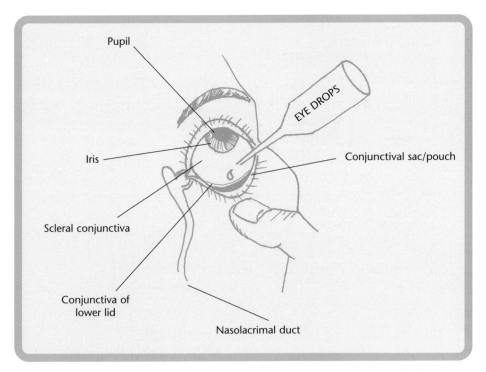

Figure 3.13 ● Instilling eye drops or ointment into the conjunctival sac/pouch

6. Gently pull down the lower lid to form a pouch, as shown in Figure 3.13. Drop the required number of drops gently into the pouch. Ask the patient to close the eye gently and blink several times. The nurse must wait for 2 minutes before instilling another drug. For eye ointment, start from the angle near the nose (the inner canthus) and work towards the ear, gently squeezing the tube along the inner edge of the lower lid. Avoid touching the eye with the sharp nozzle. An eye pad may be applied if requested. Separate tubes or bottles should always be used for the two eyes.

7. The patient should be advised not to rub or squeeze the eye. Leave the patient comfortable.

8. Remove any gloves and wash your hands.

9. Complete all the necessary documentation.

SPECIFIC POINTS ON CHILDREN'S MEDICATIONS

■ The nurse should get extra help so that the head can be held still during eye and ear treatments, to prevent the child rubbing his eyes or ears, and to provide comfort and reassurance.

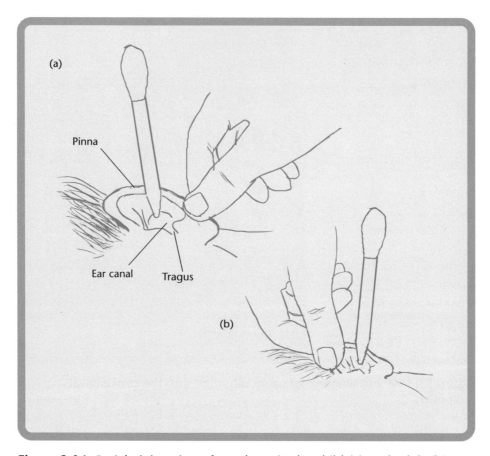

Figure 3.14 ● Administration of ear drops in the child (a) and adult (b)

Ear medications

1. Wash your hands and put on gloves if necessary.
2. Prepare all the necessary equipment and check the prescription for completeness.
3. Warm the medication to room temperature.
4. Clean the outer canal if necessary. Normal saline may be used.
5. Ask the patient to lie on the side with the ear to be treated facing upwards.
6. In adults and children over 3 years old, gently pull the pinna upwards and backwards and instil the prescribed number of drops into the ear canal (Figure 3.14b). In children below 3 years of age, gently pull the pinna downwards and backwards and instil the prescribed number of drops (Figure 3.14a).
7. Advise the patient to remain in that position for 5 minutes.

8. When patient is allowed to sit up, cleanse the external ear of any spillages or leakages, and make the patient comfortable.
9. Remove gloves and wash your hands.
10. Complete all the relevant records.

If both ears are to be treated, wait for 15 minutes between instillations.

Nasal medications

A number of drugs, for example nitroglycerine and ephedrine, are available for use as nasal sprays or nasal drops. These should be used appropriately or the drug's effectiveness will be diminished.

Nasal drops may flood the sinuses or dribble down the throat and be ingested. The patient should be advised to expectorate any drug going down the throat rather than swallow it. The timing of these drugs is important: they should be administered 20 minutes before meals so that the nasal passages will be clear during feeding.

1. Wash your hands and put on gloves if necessary.
2. Prepare all the necessary equipment and check the prescription for completeness.
3. Get the patient to clear his nasal passages; provide some tissues.
4. For a nasal spray, keep the head and spray container upright. Squeeze the container as instructed and, following each spray, ask the patient to take a deep sniff. Repeat with the other nostril. For nasal drops, it is better if the patient is lying down. Instil the required amount of medication, inserting the dropper approximately 0.5 cm into the nostril. The tip of the dropper should not become contaminated. Young children may be held on the lap with the neck extended.
5. Provide the patient with tissues and make him comfortable.
6. Complete all the relevant documentation.

Rectal medications

The **rectal route** is frequently used for the administration of drugs in adults and children. The action of the drug can be local (for example lubricant suppositories) or systemic (as with aminophylline). These medications are in the form of a suppository, cream or solution. It is vital that children receiving such medication have been prepared for the procedure, using phrases that they can understand.

rectal route
via the rectum

1. Wash your hands.
2. Prepare all the equipment and check the prescription for completeness.
3. Explain the procedure to the patient and provide privacy.
4. Position the patient on his left side and only expose the buttocks.
5. Put gloves on.
6. The suppository is lubricated with a water-soluble lubricant (KY-Jelly).
7. The buttocks are separated to expose the anus.
8. Ask the patient to take a deep breath and insert the suppository past the anal sphincter. Clean away any excess lubricant.

If a suppository is being used to obtain a systemic action (for example aminophylline), it should be inserted blunt end first to minimise rectal discomfort or irritation and maximise the retention period. For local action, for example to promote defaecation, suppositories should be inserted in the conventional manner with the pointed end first.

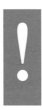

SPECIFIC POINTS ON CHILDREN'S MEDICATIONS

- When giving a suppository to an infant or toddler, he can lie on his back with his legs flexed. For children over 3 years, the suppository is inserted using the index finger. With children of 3 years or less, the little finger may be used.

9. Ask the patient to refrain from pushing the suppository out and make him comfortable. Children and infants may be held or cuddled to distract them. (A commode should be available to avoid any embarrassment.)
10. Dispose of all equipment, and wash your hands.
11. Complete all the relevant records.

Vaginal medications

vaginal route

into the vagina

Medications intended for administration via the **vaginal route** are available in many forms – pessaries, creams and medicated douches – most of which can only be administered using special applicators.

The patient should be encouraged to empty her bladder as she is expected to remain lying down for 20 minutes after insertion of the medication.

1. Wash your hands.
2. Prepare all the equipment, and check the prescription for completeness.
3. Explain the procedure to the patient and provide privacy. Select the appropriate position, either supine with the knees drawn up and legs parted, or left lateral with the knees drawn up.

4. Wash your hands and put on gloves.

5. Lubricate the pessary or applicator.

6. Insert the pessary along the posterior vaginal wall and into the top of the vagina. If using an applicator, insert the barrel of the applicator into the vagina as far as it will go. Squeeze the tube to insert the drug while holding the applicator steady. Withdraw the applicator and make the patient comfortable.

7. Provide the patient with sanitary towels and advise her to remain in position for 20 minutes.

8. Discard the equipment or clean it for reuse.

9. Remove gloves and wash your hands.

10. Complete all the relevant documentation.

Activity

20

Discuss with your mentor the benefits of administering drugs rectally. What are the ethical issues when administering drugs via the rectal and vaginal routes?

Identify which drugs are routinely given via these routes.

Patient education and compliance in drug administration

Drug therapy can be effective only when the patient co-operates with the drug regimen and takes all the prescribed drugs correctly. In hospitalised patients, drug treatment is closely supervised, but there is a wealth of evidence indicating that, once discharged from hospital care, many patients fail to continue with their treatment because of:

- Forgetfulness
- A lack of understanding of the illness and/or drugs
- Unclear instructions
- The cost of the medication
- Non-acceptance of the diagnosis
- Inconvenience, such as when at school
- A confusing cocktail of medications
- Side-effects of the drugs, including a fear of addiction.

Failure to complete a course of treatment may result in a poor outcome with a detrimental effect on the patient. The doctor will be concerned at the lack of progress with the drug treatment and may opt to increase the dosage, change to a different drug or question the original diagnosis. The nurse can take positive steps to ensure that the patient co-operates with the drug programme by:

- Effective patient education
- Using 24 hour containers to ensure that required drugs are taken at the appropriate times
- Starting self-administration while the patient is still in hospital
- A written record of the regimen.

Patients should be individually assessed for their willingness to learn about their medications, this information being used by the primary nurse to produce an effective teaching programme ensuring that the patient continues with the treatment following discharge.

General principles when administering medications to children

It is essential to provide safe and effective drug therapy to children. Because of anatomical and physiological differences, the drug's pharmacokinetic properties – absorption, distribution, metabolism and excretion – may be affected. For more details of drug pharmacokinetics in children and infants, the reader is advised to consult textbooks on paediatric pharmacology.

General guidelines for giving medications to children

1. It is important to establish a trusting relationship with the child and to identify any preferences. Always be honest regarding painful injections or distasteful medications. Remain calm.
2. Adequate time should be allowed before and after drug administration to comfort the child. Explaining the procedure to children and giving any instructions that they must follow to enhance the effectiveness of therapy may take longer than expected.
3. The nurse should be kind but firm when approaching the child.
4. Organise help to control and support children. Do not interrupt what the child is doing; make medicine-taking a part of it.
5. Identify the child correctly, checking with the parents. If possible, organise drug administration when the parents are present.
6. Explain the procedure to the child and parents. Parents may provide information on how the child likes to take her medication. Offer a choice, for example taking it from the parent or the nurse.
7. Avoid mixing medications in milk or essential foods as the child may then avoid those foods and develop malnutrition or dehydration.
8. If possible, allow children to participate, for example choosing the juice to be drunk with the medicine.
9. Reward children for taking their medications but avoid punishing children who are uncooperative.
10. Do not anticipate difficulty: the child quickly picks up your anxiety.
11. Never make a promise you cannot keep.

Specific guidelines when giving injections to children

1. The aseptic and safe-checking procedures should be followed as discussed.
2. Prepare the equipment and check the prescription for completeness.
3. Explain the procedure to the child in a manner consistent with the child's age and understanding. Audiovisual aids such as booklets or dolls may be used to get the message across. Parents should be informed and involved in supporting the child.
4. Appropriate restraint, for example a blanket, may be required.
5. Select the injection site (see above).
6. The procedure should be undertaken quickly and gently.
7. Support should be provided as necessary by the nurse and/or parents.

Giving medications to clients with learning disabilities

Clients with learning disabilities may have varying degrees of mental and physical disability, and it may be as difficult for the nurse to explain as it is for the patient to understand. Following the five 'R's of drug administration (see above) should secure the client's safety. The client may also suffer from physical deformities that may require adapting the methods and in some cases changing the form of the drug and the route of administration. The pharmacist may be able to help with special preparations. Liquid preparations are safer than tablets or capsules. If no alternative forms of medication are available, the tablets should be crushed and mixed with soft foods for easy swallowing. Swallowing may also be stimulated by gentle downward stroking motions over the larynx.

Medication errors

Finally, although medication errors should be avoided at all costs, they may occur. Incidents should immediately be reported to the nurse in charge and the doctor. The patient should be monitored for any side-effects and be informed of what has happened. Preventative measures may be taken to control the effects of the drugs. The incident is usually investigated, and if the nurse has been found to be negligent, disciplinary action may be taken by the employing authority and the NMC. The patient can also take legal action against the nurse or the employer. The advice is thus to be a safe practitioner.

Administering medication without the patient's consent

Although the UKCC recommends seeking the patient's consent for the administration of medicines, it has also recommended (UKCC, 2001) that in situations in
which patients or clients lack the mental capacity to consent or refuse treatment,
for example when they cannot take in or retain information about treatment,
cannot believe that information or cannot weigh up the information as part of a
decision-making process, medicines may be administered in a covert way such as
by mixing them with food, without the patient being aware of this. The UKCC
policy also urges practitioners to seek legal advice and to debate the ethics of the
situation before deciding that the covert administration of medicines is in the
patient's interest.

Avoiding the risks of sharps injury

Sharps injuries are the major cause of the transmission of blood-borne organisms from patients to health-care staff, so all personnel involved with sharps
should follow the national and local policies to prevent injury. Evidence indicates that injuries occur during use, after use, during disposal and while
resheathing needles. Sharps injuries can be avoided by developing safe working
practices, the key principles of which include:

- Eliminating the unnecessary use of sharps
- Using automatically retracting needles or lancets in place of non-retracting ones
- Not resheathing needles manually
- Having a range of sharps boxes available
- Avoiding overfilling sharps boxes
- Taking sharps boxes to the point of use and having them available at all
  locations
- Assembling devices with care and not taking them apart unless this is
  unavoidable
- Using a tray to carry devices such as syringes and needles
- Disposing of sharps directly into a sharps box.

◼ Chapter Summary

This chapter has revealed some of the key aspects of safe practice when moving
patients, preventing cross-infection and food poisoning, and administering medicines. Every activity that the nurse undertakes carries considerable risk to the
patient as well as to the nurse. By applying the principles described in this chapter,
the nurse can ensure that nursing procedures are carried out safely for all.

● Test Yourself!

1. Find out the rate of HAI in your hospital.

2. Who are the members of the infection control team?

3. Undertake a survey of hand hygiene in your area of practice.

4. Describe the precautions that nurses should take to reduce the incidence of food poisoning.

5. Describe the signs and symptoms of food poisoning.

6. What precautions should be taken in the event of an outbreak of food poisoning on the wards?

7. Describe the responsibilities of the nurse in drug administration.

8. Identify at least three intramuscular/subcutaneous injection sites.

9. What special precautions should you take when administering injections to infants and children?

Further Reading

Ayliffe, G.A.J., Collins, B.J. and Taylor, L.J. (eds) (1993) *Hospital Acquired Infections*, 2nd edn. Cambridge University Press, Cambridge.

Burden, M. (1994) A practical guide to insulin injection. *Nursing Standard* **81**(29): 25–9.

Campbell, J. (1995) Injections. *Professional Nurse* **10**(7): 455–8.

Corlett, E.N., Lloyd, P.V., Tarling, C. et al. (1997) *The Guide to Handling of Patients*. National Back Pain Association and Royal College of Nursing, London.

Humphries, J.L. and Green, J. (1999) *Nurse Prescribing*. Macmillan – now Palgrave Macmillan, Basingstoke.

Palmer, S.R. and Rowe, B. (1983) Investigation of salmonella in hospitals. *British Medical Journal* **287**: 891–3.

Russell, P. (1997) Reducing the incidence of needlestick injury. *Professional Nurse* **12**(4): 275–88.

▓ References

Beecroft, P.C. (1990) Intramuscular injection practices of paediatric nurses: site selection. *Nurse Educator* **5**(4): 23–8.

Campbell, J. (1995) Injections. *Professional Nurse* **10**(7): 455–8.

Dann, T. C. (1969) Routine skin preparation before injection: an unnecessary procedure. *Lancet* **ii**: 96–8.

Disabled Living Foundation (1994) *Handling People: Equipment, Advice and Information.* DLF, London.

DoH (Department of Health) (1990a) *Guidance for Clinical Health Workers; Protection against Infection with HIV and Hepatic Viruses. Recommendations of the Expert Advisory Group on Aids.* HMSO, London.

DoH (Department of Health) (1990b) *Food Handler's Guide.* HMSO, London.

DoH (Department of Health) (1995) *Hospital Infection Control: Guidance on the Control of Infection in Hospitals.* DoH, London.

Dryden, M.S., Keyworth, N., Gabb, R. et al. (1994) Asymptomatic foodhandlers as the source of nosocomial salmonellosis. *Journal of Hospital Infection* **28**: 195–208.

Food Standards Agency (1998) *A Force for Change.* Stationery Office, London.

Gladman, G. (1993) Back pain in student nurses – the mature factor. *Occupational Health*, February, pp. 47–51.

HSE (Health and Safety Executive) (1992) *Manual Handling Operations Regulations – Guidance on Regulations.* HMSO, London.

HSE (Health and Safety Executive) (1998) *Manual Handling in the Health Services: HSC Guidance.* HSE Statistics. HMSO, London.

McConnell, E.A. (1993) Clinical do's and don'ts: how to administer a z-track injection. *Nursing* **23**: 18.

McGowan, S. and Wood, A. (1990) Administering heparin subcutaneously: an evaluation of techniques used and bruising at the site. *Australian Journal of Advanced Nursing* **7**(2): 31–9.

Mallett, J. and Dougherty, L. (eds) (2000) *The Royal Marsden Hospital of Clinical Procedures.* Blackwell, Oxford.

National Audit Office (2000) *The Management and Control of Hospital Acquired Infections in Acute NHS Trusts in England.* NAO, London.

NMC (Nursing and Midwifery Council) (2002) *Code of Professional Conduct.* NMC, London.

RCN (Royal College of Nursing) (1992) *Safety Representatives Conference Committee. Introduction to Methicillin Resistant* Staphylococcus aureus. RCN, London.

RCN (Royal College of Nursing) (1995) *Guidance on Infection Control in Hospitals.* RCN, London.

RCN (Royal College of Nursing) (1996) *Manual Handling Assessments in Hospitals and the Community – an RCN Guide.* RCN, London.

Rosen, M. (1994) *Back Pain: Report of a Clinical Standards Advisory Group.* HMSO, London.

Sharp, J.C.M. (1992) Epidemiology. In Eley, A.R. (ed.) *Microbial Food Poisoning.* Chapman & Hall, London.

UKCC (United Kingdom Central Council for Nursing, Midwifery and Health Visiting) (1997) *Responsibility for Feeding of Patients.* UKCC, London.

UKCC (United Kingdom Central Council for Nursing, Midwifery and Health Visiting) (2000) *Guidelines for the Administration of Medicines.* UKCC, London.

UKCC (United Kingdom Central Council for Nursing, Midwifery and Health Visiting) (2001) *New Guidance on Covert Administration of Medicines.* UKCC, London.

Whalley, L.F. and Wong, D.L. (1995) *Nursing Care of Infants and Children*, 4th edn. C.V. Mosby, London.

Winslow, E.H. (1997) Just how illegible are physicians' medical orders? *American Journal of Nursing* **97**(9): 66.

4

Eating and Drinking

Contents

Learning outcomes

The purpose of this chapter is to encourage you to apply the essentials of nutrition and hydration to your everyday life and that of your clients. At the end of the chapter, you should be able to:

- Describe and explain the principles of a healthy diet and fluid intake

- Enable others to make healthy changes to their food and fluid intake

- Assess clients' nutritional and hydration status

- Assist clients in achieving optimum nutrition and hydration

- Suggest a range of helpful strategies for use when feeding and hydrating clients

- Extend your range of skills in promoting effective nutrition and hydration

- Promote the dignity of the client needing nutritional support.

There will be reflective activities, activities for you to undertake, reading activities, case histories and review questions to ensure that you interact with the material in a useful and practical way.

Supporting texts you will find particularly helpful are:

Bender, D.A. (1997) *Introduction to Nutrition and Metabolism*, 2nd edn. UCL
    Press, London, or another introductory nutrition text.
Department of Health (1991) *Dietary Reference Values for Food Energy and
    Nutrients for the United Kingdom. Report of the Panel on Dietary Reference
    Values of the Committee on Medical Aspects of Food Policy*. HMSO, London.
Rutishauser, S. (1994) *Physiology and Anatomy*. Churchill Livingstone, Edin-
    burgh, or your own preferred anatomy and physiology text.

What Is a Healthy Diet?

Food is fundamental to physical survival. It is needed for growth, repair and the
manufacture of the elements that protect us from disease. Humans will literally
eat almost anything to satisfy extreme hunger. Once survival has been ensured,
other factors, for example age, culture, history, religion, access, taste and preferences, come into play. Most of us believe that we are eating a balanced diet.

At the rock-bottom physiological level, there are certain fundamentals that
the body needs in order to function effectively, not just today but next week and
next year, in order to stay healthy into later life. Exclusive breastfeeding is, for
example, recommended for at least the first 4 months of life to enable the best
possible start as it protects against respiratory diseases and gastroenteritis.
Clients' ability, motivation or knowledge may, however, be impaired, in which
case it is the nurse's responsibility to assist, empower and educate. The United
Kingdom Central Council for Nursing, Midwifery and Health Visiting (UKCC)
reminded us in the 1997 'Feeding of Patients' letter that even if this task is delegated to others, the responsibility remains with the nurse, who is accountable for
all aspects of nursing care.

Concepts of a balanced diet have steadily altered across time in response to
beliefs and research, and at no other time in history have we had access to so
much hard evidence of the impact of food on the human body, from starvation
to the so-called diseases of affluence, such as obesity. For some considerable
time, **nutritional** advice was aimed solely at preventing deficiency diseases. The
war-time diet, for example, kept people remarkably healthy on surprisingly low
levels of protein, fat and sugar.

nutrition

the study of the effects
of food and drink on the
body

Despite considerable 'hype' from those with vested interests and frivolous
speculation from irresponsible journalism, there is a clear consensus about a
balanced diet, which has remained relatively consistent over the past few years.
The Committee on Medical Aspects of Food Policy (COMA) published comprehensive recommendations for nutrient consumption in its 1991 report *Dietary
Reference Values for Food Energy and Nutrients for the United Kingdom* (DoH,

1991). This replaced the single-figure ('one size fits all') recommended daily allowances (RDA) by a range of tables for different populations. In 1992, the government published *The Health of the Nation* (DoH, 1992), a national strategy that set health targets, including those for eating behaviour, nutritional status and diet-related diseases. A better diet has also been mentioned in *Saving Lives: Our Healthier Nation* (DoH, 1998). The message here is that, whatever you read in the lighter end of the press, experts agree on the information given in the most recent nutrition textbooks. But, unfortunately, consensus does not sell newspapers.

Food substances can be divided into macronutrients, which make up the bulk of our energy and nutrient intake, including carbohydrates, proteins and fats (lipids), and essential micronutrients, which are the vitamins and minerals. These will be dealt with in turn below.

■ Macronutrients

Carbohydrates

carbohydrates

a group of organic (carbon-containing) compounds, comprising starches and sugars, that make up the body's main source of energy

Carbohydrates are needed for fuel and can be divided into two main groups: starches and sugars. Starches are made up of long chains of sugar units called polysaccharides.

The most useful starchy foods include bread, rice, cereals, pasta, potatoes, flour, pizza base, cornflour, crispbread, chapattis, poppadums and porridge. These tend to be filling, which is not so good for toddlers, rather than nutrient dense, so it is what you add to them that makes the difference. Other sources of starch include cakes, biscuits and pastry. These tend to have more energy per portion because they contain high levels of hidden fat as well as sugar. Sugars may be monosaccharides (for example glucose, fructose and galactose) or disaccharides (sucrose, lactose and maltose) and can be divided into:

- *Intrinsic sugars*, which are contained within plant cell walls
- *Non-milk extrinsic sugars*, which have been extracted from the natural cellular matrix, as in fruit juice, table sugar and honey in food.

Processed foods, chocolates, sweets and snacks are dense sources of sugar. There is evidence that a high sugar intake is a factor in maturity-onset diabetes, atherosclerosis, obesity and dental caries (COMA, 1989).

A healthy adult diet is a varied one that contains enough starch to provide 50 per cent of the total energy while reducing the contribution of extrinsic sugars. Infants should gain 40–50 per cent of their total energy from carbohydrates, 40 per cent of this being lactose (milk sugar). Children need about 50–100 g of non-milk sugars per day, 1 g of carbohydrate providing 16 kilojoules (kJ), or 3.75

kilocalories (kcal), of energy. The 1991 COMA recommendation was to reduce the contribution of non-milk extrinsic sugars, especially sucrose, to 11 per cent of food energy. For the average adult, this is 60 g per day. Identifying how much sugar in its various forms can be found in processed foods can help you to determine your sugar intake.

Proteins

Proteins are found in meat, fish, eggs, pulses (peas, beans and lentils), nuts, tofu, soya and textured vegetable protein. They are also found in smaller amounts in bread (11 per cent protein in wholemeal, 9 per cent in white), other cereals and potatoes.

> **proteins**
> organic nitrogenous compounds essential as a building material for growth and repair

Protein is needed to supply nitrogen for growth (in children), defence and repair, such as wound healing and replacing blood loss. A small amount of protein is continually lost from the body throughout life in hair (adults losing more than 100 hairs a day), shed skin scales (a large proportion of dust), shed gut lining (a major constituent of faeces) and enzymes and other proteins secreted into the gut and incompletely digested. There is also a turnover of body proteins as tissue proteins are continuously broken down and replaced. Although there is no change in the total amount of protein in the body, an adult with an inadequate intake of protein will be unable to replace any loss and will thus use up tissue protein. This is broken down into urea and excreted as nitrogenous waste in the urine, faeces and sweat. For healthy adults, an intake of 0.75 g protein per kg body weight (0.75 g/kg) per 24 hours is generally considered to be acceptable, requirements increasing during pregnancy and breastfeeding. Protein intake is crucial to the growth of children, so they may need early referral to a specialist dietitian in illness.

> **CONNECTIONS**
> *Chapter 10 describes the factors needed for wound healing.*

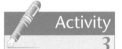

> **Activity**
> **3**
> List the sources of protein in your diet. If you weighed your daily intake, how would it compare with your carbohydrate intake?
>
> Check your finding against the 'tilted plate' (Figure 4.2). Do you need to make any adjustments?

Protein is made from 20 or so different **amino acids**, which are classified into:

- *Essential*, which cannot be synthesised in the body
- *Semi-essential*, which can be supplied by the metabolism of certain amino acids providing these are consumed in adequate amounts
- *Non-essential*, which can be synthesised from carbon and other precursors in the body.

> **amino acids**
> the building blocks from which proteins are constructed; the end-products of protein digestion

For further details, consult Bender (1997).

There is some evidence that a diet with a high proportion of protein from animal sources (high biological value or 'first-class' protein) is associated with kidney stones and osteoporosis. If the protein intake is over twice the reference nutrient intake (that sufficient for 97 per cent of population), it has been noted that calcium appears in the urine. Thus, if you find that you are eating a lot of animal protein compared with carbohydrate, it is expensive financially, physiologically and ecologically.

It is perfectly possible to get all the protein you need from vegetable sources, providing that the right amount, combination and range of protein-containing foods are consumed, that is, proteins from different plant sources are eaten together. These include:

- Nuts and cereal: a peanut butter sandwich, or muesli with nuts
- Beans and rice: a casserole or salad
- Beans and cereal: for example, hummus (chickpea spread) and bread
- Lentils and rice: as in soup.

These are known as complementary combinations. The major principle of a vegetarian diet, therefore, is that pulse dishes must be eaten with bread, rice or other cereal foods.

One gram of protein provides 16 kJ (4 kcal) of energy.

Fats

fats

a group of energy-rich organic substances comprising triglycerides, cholesterol and fatty acids, which are needed for cell structure and function

The major dietary **fats** are triglycerides, cholesterol and fatty acids. Fat is found in solid fats and liquid oils, in dairy products and as hidden fat in food, for example between the muscle fibres in meat, as oils in nuts, cereals, vegetables and fruit (especially avocados), or as fat used in the processing and cooking of foods.

There is a requirement for essential fatty acids, which play an important role in cell structure and function. These cannot be formed in the body so must be gained from the diet. The two essential fatty acids are linoleic acid (an omega-6 fat; see below) and alpha-linolenic acid (an omega-3 fat; see below).

Vitamins A, D, E and K are fat soluble so are found in fatty or oily foods (see below). Their absorption from the gut requires an adequate amount of fat in the diet since they are absorbed dissolved in this fat.

For adults and older children, it is recommended that no more than 33 per cent of the total energy should come from fat. This can be subdivided into:

- 10 per cent from saturated fatty acids, for example butter
- 6 per cent (10 per cent maximum) from polyunsaturated fatty acids, for example sunflower oil or sardines
- 12 per cent from mono-unsaturated fatty acids, for example olive oil
- 2 per cent from *trans*-fatty acids, in for example biscuits and pastry (as hydrogenated vegetable oil or fat).

A restricted dietary fat intake is not recommended for those below the age of 5 years.

The fatty acids that make up the fats in our diet can be, in chemical terms, saturated or unsaturated. Saturated fatty acids have only single bonds between the carbon atoms that make up the molecule, whereas in unsaturated fatty acids there may be one (mono-unsaturated) or more (polyunsaturated) double bonds between carbon atoms. In general, fats that contain mainly saturated fatty acids are solid at room temperature, whereas those which contain mainly unsaturated fatty acids, especially mono-unsaturates, are liquid at room temperature even though they solidify when chilled.

Saturated fats are mainly of animal origin and encourage the body to produce more low-density lipoprotein (LDL; see below) cholesterol, increasing the risk of heart disease. They may also make the blood more prone to clotting. Certain cancers, such as those of the bowel and breast, have been linked to a high intake of saturated fats (Sanders, 1994; Field et al., 2001).

Polyunsaturated fatty acids lower the total blood cholesterol level by decreasing the concentration of LDL cholesterol and high-density lipoprotein (HDL) cholesterol (see below). The two main types of polyunsaturated fatty acid are omega-3 and omega-6. Omega-3 fatty acids have either a short or a long chain structure, the latter tending to reduce the inflammatory response, which can help those with rheumatoid arthritis. They also make the blood less likely to clot, thus reducing the risk of a heart attack (Sanders, 1994). One or two servings of oily fish or 14 g of walnuts a week are recommended. Omega-6 sources include polyunsaturated margarine and corn, sunflower, rapeseed and soya bean oils, and it is recommended that linoleic acid should provide 12 per cent of dietary fat intake. The proportion of polyunsaturated fat must not be increased above 10 per cent of food energy as it is the ratio of saturated to unsaturated fat that is important. The current advice is to replace saturated fats with a mixture of poly- and mono-unsaturates.

inflammatory response
the body's non-specific immune response to injury, characterised by redness, heat, swelling and pain

Mono-unsaturated fat reduces LDL ('lethal') cholesterol but maintains or slightly increases HDL ('healthy') cholesterol. HDL cholesterol actually removes fats from the walls of arteries and from other body tissues, ferrying it to the liver where it is broken down into bile. HDL cholesterol also protects against oxygen-related tissue damage (oxidation), thought to contribute to heart disease, cancer and rheumatoid arthritis (Sanders, 1994; Field et al., 2001).

Trans-fats are polyunsaturates that have been artificially hardened by adding extra hydrogen; this can occur in food processing and in frying. They are thought to be at least as unhealthy as saturated fat and have been linked to an increased risk of heart disease and rheumatoid arthritis. Trans-fats increase LDL cholesterol and may reduce the level of HDL cholesterol (Sanders, 1994). Hydrogenated fats/oils can be noted on processed food labels. Chart 4.1 gives

Chart 4.1 ● Examples of types of fat and their sources

- Saturated: red meat, dairy products, lard, suet, palm and coconut oils
- Polyunsaturated:
  - Omega-3: oily fish: mackerel, halibut, pilchards, sardines, herrings, trout, salmon; walnuts, soya oil
  - Omega-6: polyunsaturated margarine, corn oil, sunflower oil
- Mono-unsaturated: olive oil, rapeseed oil, peanut oil, avocados, nuts
- *Trans*-fatty acids: hard margarine, biscuits, cakes

Activity 4

Look at the food labels on your groceries. How many foodstuffs contain *trans*-fats? Do the food labels identify how much saturated fat is present? Does the fat contribute more than 33 per cent of the total number of calories?

This can help you to identify whether more than 33 per cent of your food energy comes from fat.

examples of types of fat and their sources, and Table 4.1 identifies the percentages of these in common sources of fat in the diet.

Cholesterol is essential for life, being present in the membranes of animal and plant cells, and is also important in the formation of oestrogen and other sex hormones. Most cholesterol in the body is manufactured in the liver from saturated fatty acids contained in digested meat and dairy products. Once the fatty acids have been produced, globules of fat cling to proteins in the blood to form lipoproteins. These ferry the cholesterol around the bloodstream. It is only when the level of these is too high or too low that health is at risk; this is especially so for LDL cholesterol, which is related to the development of atherosclerosis and ischaemic heart disease.

The main dietary factor that affects the concentration of cholesterol in the plasma is fat intake. Sources of cholesterol in the diet include eggs, offal and shellfish. The current advice is to take no more than the equivalent of one egg per day. Both the total amount of fat and the relative amounts of saturated and

Table 4.1 Percentages of fats in common sources

	Mono-unsaturated	Polyunsaturated	Saturated
Butter	33	3	64
Hard margarine	49	13	38
Soft margarine	44	23	33
PUFA margarine	17	63	20
Coconut oil	7	2	91
Corn oil	31	52	17
Olive oil	74	11	15
Sunflower oil	34	52	14

Source: Adapted from Bender (1933).
PUFA, polyunsaturated fatty acid.

unsaturated fat affect the concentration of cholesterol in LDL cholesterol. A high intake of total fat, especially saturated fat, is associated with an undesirably high concentration of LDL cholesterol. A relatively low intake of fat, with a high proportion in the form of unsaturated fat, is associated with a desirable lower LDL concentration. Regular aerobic exercise appears to increase the HDL cholesterol level. The balance in the bloodstream should be, for example, less than 4.0 mmol/l of LDL and more than 1.0 mmol/l of HDL (Higgins, 1997).

It is difficult to eat enough of a very low-fat diet to meet energy requirements, so it is inappropriate for growing children. Infants need to gain 40–50 per cent of their total energy from fat in the first year of life. Most people in the UK have too much fat in their diet, averaging 40 per cent of total energy, which may contribute to obesity and other diseases of affluence. The flavour and lubrication of many foods come from the fat component, enhancing the pleasure of eating, the 'mouthfeel' of chocolate being an example.

One gram of fat provides 38 kJ (9 kcal) of energy. It is therefore the most energy-dense form of food.

Energy

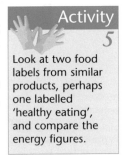

Activity

5

Look at two food labels from similar products, perhaps one labelled 'healthy eating', and compare the energy figures.

Energy output is measured in Joules, but this is not practical when studying human nutrition so kilojoules (kJ; 1000 joules) and megajoules (MJ; 1,000,000 joules or 1000 kJ) are used instead.

In human nutrition kilocalories (kcal) are also encountered. One calorie is the amount of heat needed to raise the temperature of 1 g of water by 1°C, and one kilocalorie – 1000 calories – the amount needed to raise 1 kg of water by 1°C.

Conversion: 1 kcal = 4.184 kJ; 1 kJ = 0.239 kcal

The metabolic fuels are fats, carbohydrates, protein and alcohol. For people whose body weight lies within the healthy range, energy intake should be enough to maintain a reasonably constant body weight when an adequate amount of exercise is taken. Requirements are also related to age, sex, race and level of physical activity. Women, for example, have a slower metabolism than men, black women have a slower metabolism than white women, people with well-developed muscles have a faster metabolism than sedentary people, old people have a slower metabolism than young people, and people of the same height and weight can vary in their daily requirement by as much as 4.184 MJ (1000 kcal) per day (Johnson, 2001).

A physically active body with lots of metabolically active muscle requires more energy than a relatively sedentary one with a higher percentage of body fat. A baby boy of 4–6 months of age needs about 2.89 MJ (690 kcal) per day, and a girl of the same age 2.69 MJ (645 kcal). By the time the boy is 11–14 years old, he will need about 9.27 MJ (2220 kcal), whereas the girl will need 7.92 MJ (1845 kcal). The average daily energy requirement for adults aged 19–50 years is 10.60 MJ (2550 kcal) per day for men and 8.10 MJ (1940 kcal) per day for women, male physiology being metabolically more active as it is geared to laying down muscle. Breastfeeding may increase a woman's energy requirements by as much as 2.30 MJ (550 kcal) per day. As we get older, our metabolism slows down; women, for example, need 209 kJ (50 kcal) per day fewer for every 5 years after the age of 27.

If a person does not consume enough energy, tissue breakdown will take place to make up the deficit. If too much energy is consumed, it is stored as glycogen or fat. If you look at how active you were 10 or more years ago, before the advent of mobile phones and remote controls, you probably expended more energy than now, getting up to answer the telephone or change the television channel. You may also have used the bus and walked or cycled more than at present.

Although we have a requirement for energy in our diet, it does not in theory matter how the requirement is met. There is no necessity as such for a dietary source of carbohydrate, for example: the body can make as much as it requires from proteins, albeit expensively. Similarly, there is no need for a dietary source of fat apart from the essential fatty acids. And a dietary source of alcohol is non-essential (see below). Some dietary elements are, however, needed for specific purposes, for example fibre, which used to be called roughage.

non-starch polysaccharides

indigestible substances in plant cells that aid the transit of food through the gastrointestinal tract; also commonly known as fibre or roughage

The terms 'roughage' and 'fibre' should be replaced by 'non-starch polysaccharides' (NSPs). NSPs are a collection of indigestible substances found in plant cells, the main action of which is to aid the passage of food through the bowel and ease elimination. Sources include fruit and vegetables, whole grains, wholemeal bread, cereals, beans and pulses. There is no fibre in animal food sources such as milk, meat, cheese and eggs. The COMA report of 1991 (DoH, 1991) recommended an increase in the average consumption of NSP from 12 to 18 g per day in adults in order to reduce constipation, diverticular disease and the risk of colorectal cancer. The minimum intake should be 12 g per day.

There are two sorts of NSP: soluble and insoluble.

- *Soluble NSP* dissolves in the gut and helps to maintain a healthy blood glucose level by a sort of slow-release effect. The richest sources are pulses, oats (for example porridge), barley (for example pearl barley in soups), rye (for example in bread), beans and lentils, but it is also found in fruits and vegetables. Soluble NSP may help to decrease a high blood cholesterol level, probably by combining with bile acids and cholesterol in the intestine and preventing their being absorbed.

● *Insoluble NSP* soaks up moisture as it travels through the digestive system, forming bulk that aids the easy passage of waste products. It is found in wheat-based breakfast cereals, bread, rice, maize, pasta, fruits and vegetables. Bran hurries the food through, reducing the absorption of micronutrients (vitamins and minerals) and producing a sort of scouring pad effect; it should thus be used with great caution.

Taking enough NSP in the diet means eating a *varied* selection of fruits and vegetables as whole and unpeeled as possible. Take account of current recommendations about pesticide residues on skins, cutting the tops and tails off and peeling them as appropriate. A **minimum** of five different fruits and/or vegetables a day is recommended for most people (Figure 4.1).

The diet should contain plenty of whole grains (rather than completely white, refined versions), wholemeal bread (as brown and granary bread is coloured

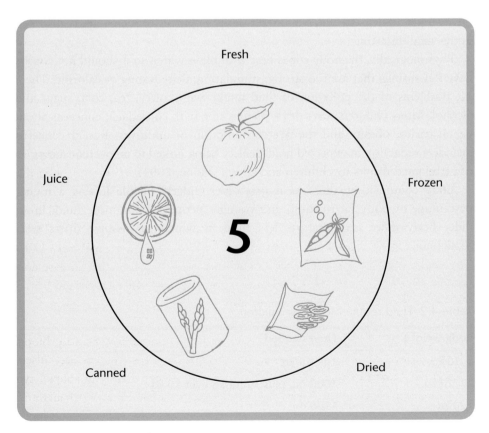

Figure 4.1 ● Five a day

with caramel or burnt sugar), cereals, rice and pasta. Enough NSP will cause easy bowel actions; too much will lead to diarrhoea and wind, the action of colonic bacteria upon NSP producing methane. Any increase in NSP should be gradual, and fluid intake may have to be increased.

Activity

6

Look up water and electrolyte balance in your preferred anatomy and physiology text (for example Rutishauser, 1994, pp. 237–52).

Why is a detailed knowledge of normal fluid and electrolyte balance necessary for nurses?

CONNECTIONS

Chapter 5 outlines the functions of the gastrointestinal and renal systems in relation to elimination.

Fluid

Water is the main constituent of the body, comprising about 60 per cent of adult body weight. The body gains some water from foods, but adults need to drink another 1.5–2.0 litres of fluid daily to replenish the water in every cell of the body and ensure efficient functioning at all levels. The healthy adult's fluid requirement can be estimated as 30–35 ml/kg per day. Children (Table 4.2) and people with cardiac or renal problems may need less. Much of this water can be gained from foods with a high water content.

One way to tell whether the fluid intake is correct is to check that the urine is pale and plentiful: dark and scanty urine is a sign of dehydration. The body needs more fluid if it is sweating, as a result of hot conditions or pyrexia, or if it is losing fluid through diarrhoea and vomiting. Nine litres of fluid pass through the average adult gastrointestinal tract daily, 7.7 litres of which are reabsorbed in the small intestine.

Physiologically, the body copes best with plain water, so it should not always have flavourings that are too strong, stimulating, dehydrating or calorific. There are problems of the pollution of fluid intake with coffee, tea, cola, sugar and alcohol. Many children never drink plain water, with consequent concerns about dental caries, obesity and the overconsumption of additives. Recent concerns include a reduction in expected bone density being linked to an overconsumption of carbonated drinks by children and adults (Milne, 2001).

Body composition alters as it gets older, elderly people having a higher percentage of body fat to fluid, and younger people having more fluid. In an older body there is, therefore, less fluid in which to dissolve drugs such as alcohol.

Activity

7

Work out the fluid requirement of one of your clients from the information given above. How do you know that he or she is drinking enough fluid?

Remember not to include alcohol in your calculations as it is dehydrating.

Table 4.2 Fluid requirements for children

Body weight	Fluid needed
1–10 kg	100 ml/kg
11–20 kg	1000 ml, plus 50 ml/kg over 10 kg
<20 kg	1500 ml
>20 kg	1500 ml, plus 20 ml/kg over 20 kg

Casebox 4.1

Tania is 9 years old and lives with her parents and younger brother in a terraced house with a small garden in a large town. The children are driven to school, to church and to various activities with their friends. They are allowed to take any food or drink from the kitchen whenever they want. Tania's parents are concerned that she is getting very overweight for her height but are frightened of the possibility of **anorexia nervosa**. Tania's ankle and knee joints are beginning to be painful, and her skin shows stretch marks. Her parents have taken her to see their GP, who has referred them to the practice nurse for some advice.

What would be the main principles of this advice?

- As Tania is still growing, she must not lose weight but slow the rate of gain.

- Activity levels must be considerably increased, building up steadily over time, to the benefit of the whole family.

- Food freely available to the children will have to be 'healthy', high fibre, low sugar and low fat.

- Tania can be encouraged to drink water, rather than cola, juice or carbonated drinks, when she is thirsty and with her meals.

- Energy-dense foods will have to be reserved for treats, and any changes made must not compromise the growth and development needs of Tania's younger brother.

- The practice nurse may be involved in supporting this process.

anorexia nervosa

A psychiatric disorder characterised by an intense fear of becoming overweight, even when emaciated

Micronutrients

Leaving the macronutrients, we will now turn our attention to the micronutrients: vitamins and minerals.

Vitamins

Vitamins are relatively complex organic compounds that have essential functions in metabolic processes and are needed in very small amounts. Some cannot be synthesised in the body so must be provided by the diet. There is a constant turnover of vitamins so they must be replaced. Vitamin C, for example, is water soluble, needing constant replenishment as there is no storage facility in the body. Water-soluble vitamins are absorbed from the upper intestine, and fat-soluble vitamins are absorbed with fat in food.

vitamins

complex organic compounds vital to metabolic processes

For estimated average requirements, see *Dietary Reference Values for Food Energy and Nutrients for the United Kingdom* (DoH, 1991). The supplements that many people take are controlled by food legislation, which is less restrictive than drug legislation. As a result, vitamin labels may still refer to a single-figure

RDA even though these were replaced in 1991 by precisely targeted dietary reference values tables (DoH, 1991).

The main vitamins are discussed below.

Vitamin A (retinol, carotene)

Vitamin A (retinol) is needed for promoting vision and cell differentiation, for maintaining the health of epithelial tissues and skin and for a healthy immune system. In children, it helps to ensure correct bone development and growth. It is one of the antioxidants, which may help to protect against bowel cancer and heart disease. Vitamin A is fat soluble and is found in liver, milk, fortified margarine, butter, eggs, fish liver oils, carrots and leafy green vegetables. It is stored in the liver and released when needed.

Vitamin A can be obtained in two forms: retinol in animal foods, and carotenoid pigments from red and yellow fruits and vegetables, especially carrots, the carotene being more accessible in cooked than raw carrots. Beta-carotene is found in green and orange vegetables; vegetarians can convert this to vitamin A.

A high vitamin A intake has been associated with birth defects in infants, so women in the UK who are, or might become, pregnant, are advised not to take vitamin A supplements without medical advice, or to eat liver or liver products.

Vitamin B group

These are water-soluble vitamins.

B1 (thiamin)

Vitamin B1 (thiamin) is needed for the metabolism and release of energy from carbohydrate, fat and alcohol. It is found in pork, ham and other meats, fortified breakfast cereals, broccoli, green peas and tomato juice.

B2 (riboflavin)

B2 (riboflavin) is necessary for energy metabolism. Sources include liver, milk, fortified breakfast cereals, eggs, plain chocolate, some fish and yoghurt.

B3 (niacin, nicotinic acid, nicotinamide)

Vitamin B3 (niacin, nicotinic acid, nicotinamide) is required for tissue oxidation. It is found in meat products, tuna, chicken breast, liver, potatoes, bread and fortified breakfast cereals.

B5 (pantothenic acid)

B5 (pantothenic acid) is needed for energy metabolism. Although it is found in all living matter, good sources include liver, kidney, yeast, egg yolk, peanuts and some vegetables. It is not found in sugar, confectionery, cola, margarine, lard, corn starch or alcoholic spirits.

B6 (pyridoxal, pyridoxamine)

B6 (pyridoxal, pyridoxamine) is needed for protein metabolism, the nervous system and the regulation of action of some hormones. It can be found in liver, whole-grain cereals, bananas, beans, legumes, nuts, seeds (especially sunflower seeds), chicken, beef and fish, including tuna. Small amounts are found in fruits, such as watermelon, and vegetables, especially green leafy vegetables. Intestinal flora synthesise a large amount of the vitamin, some of which is available for absorption.

B12

Vitamin B12 is essential for red blood cell production and a healthy nervous system. It is also needed for the synthesis of deoxyribonucleic acid (**DNA**) and ribonucleic acid (**RNA**). Sources include offal, other meat and meat products, fish and eggs, only small amounts being found in dairy products and fortified soya milk.

DNA and RNA
molecules that carry and transmit genetic instructions

Vitamin B12 is absorbed in the terminal ileum, deficiency most often being caused by a lack of absorption. Intrinsic factor, produced by the parietal cells of the stomach, is needed for the absorption of vitamin B12. As there are no plant sources except algae, strict vegetarians and vegans may be short of this vitamin without suitable supplementation. Yeast extract may be helpful.

Post-gastrectomy patients will require injections of B12. Tapeworm infestation or bacterial overgrowth may make the vitamin unavailable as the bacteria assimilate it for their own use. High doses of vitamin C can also interfere with vitamin B12 availability, converting it to an inactive form (Barasi, 1997).

Folate/folic acid

Folate/folic acid is necessary for red and white blood cell production, the health of the cells lining the gastrointestinal tract and the synthesis of DNA. It can be gained from offal (which must not be consumed during pregnancy; see vitamin A above), raw green leafy vegetables and whole-grain cereals.

A lack of folate/folic acid during the first few weeks of pregnancy can lead to neural tube defects such as spina bifida (a failure of the spinal column to close), so all women of childbearing age need to ensure a good folic acid intake. Those planning to become pregnant should take folic acid supplements for 3 months before abandoning contraception.

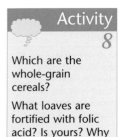

Activity
8

Which are the whole-grain cereals?

What loaves are fortified with folic acid? Is yours? Why is this relevant?

Vitamin C (ascorbic acid)

Vitamin C (ascorbic acid) is required for the integrity of the connective tissues, hormone synthesis and wound healing. It is an **antioxidant**, is water soluble and can be found in potatoes (especially their skins), fruit juice, citrus and other fruits, and green vegetables. It helps to increase iron absorption from vegetable sources. Smokers and those taking the contraceptive pill have an increased requirement as a result of increased excretion and decreased storage.

A deficiency of vitamin C causes scurvy, resulting in bleeding gums, loosening and loss of the teeth, delayed wound healing, lowered resistance to infection and damage to bone and connective tissue. Untreated scurvy is fatal. British sailors used to ransack the colonies looking for fruits high in ascorbic acid, hence the nicknames Pom (short for pomegranate) in Australia and Limey (for limes) in America. Those at risk of deficiency include the elderly and children from low-income and larger families who are unlikely to eat many fruits and vegetables or drink natural fruit juice. Faddy eaters of any age are at risk if they eat few fruits or vegetables.

Over 1000–2000 mg per day of vitamin C can cause diarrhoea and gastric upset. High doses may trigger oxalate kidney stones in those who are susceptible. Suddenly stopping a high intake may cause rebound scurvy because of an enhanced turnover of the vitamin.

> **CONNECTIONS**
>
> *Chapter 10 identifies the other factors necessary for wound healing.*

> **Activity 9**
>
> Why might a client confined to bed become deficient in vitamin D? What could be the long-term effects? (See also Chapter 8.)

Vitamin D (cholecalciferol, ergocalciferol)

Vitamin D (calciferol, ergocalciferol) regulates calcium absorption and utilisation for healthy bones and teeth. Fat soluble, it is synthesised mostly from the action of sunlight on skin. Vitamin D food sources include fortified margarine, oily fish, eggs, fortified breakfast cereals, fortified milks and butter.

A prolonged deficiency of vitamin D results in rickets in young children and **osteomalacia** in adults. A low vitamin D status can be common among children of Asian origin as a result of a vegetarian diet, a low calcium intake and limited exposure to the sun. Islamic girls are particularly at risk. A diet high in phytate (insoluble fibre from plant cell walls) may reduce the absorption of calcium, which may be a factor in **rickets**. Chronically ill children and elderly, housebound people may also be at risk of deficiency. Women who have had multiple pregnancies may have a higher risk of osteomalacia, in which their bones become demineralised. In addition, clinical conditions that impair fat absorption will reduce vitamin D absorption.

Overdosage over time can cause vitamin D to accumulate in the body, causing a high blood calcium level and symptoms such as headache and appetite loss.

Vitamin E

Vitamin E is needed for the protection of cell membranes and lipids against oxidative damage and can help to guard against heart attacks. Vitamin E is fat soluble, being found in polyunsaturated plant oils, avocados, whole-grain cereals, eggs, nuts, seeds and dark green leafy vegetables. The amount needed by the body depends upon the intake of polyunsaturated fatty acids.

Vitamin K

Vitamin K is essential for blood clotting and energy metabolism. A fat-soluble vitamin, it is found in vegetables, especially cabbage, sprouts, cauliflower and spinach, margarines and vegetable oils and animal liver.

A lack of vitamin K may cause the blood to take longer to clot. This can be noted in clients who have been on a very low-fat diet because of stones in the gallbladder, giving rise to pain when they eat fatty foods, or in those taking warfarin. A small number of newborn babies may have a low vitamin K level and are at risk of haemorrhagic disease of the newborn. To reduce this risk, it is usual to supplement the mother or administer a single oral prophylactic dose of vitamin K to the neonate.

prophylactic
preventing infection or disease

Vitamins are more effectively acquired from food than from supplements as there are all sorts of subtle elements and interactions in whole foods not necessarily present or active in supplements. If a supplement is really necessary, check that the dose is appropriate, make sure that it is taken with food and spread it out across the day rather than taking it all at once. Fat-soluble vitamins must be taken with fatty foods for maximum absorption, but avoid megadoses as they are stored in the body, which could lead to toxic effects.

Minerals

In addition to metabolic fuels, protein and vitamins, the body has a requirement for a variety of mineral salts (**minerals**) in very small (trace) amounts. The requirements of a growing child will be greater than those of a healthy adult who simply has to replace body losses from mineral turnover. A sick person or pregnant or lactating mother will have an increased requirement of these micronutrients.

minerals
naturally occurring inorganic substances needed in trace amounts in the diet

Calcium

Calcium (Ca) is needed for the growth and development of bones and teeth, the correct functioning of nerves and muscles, and blood clotting. It is found in

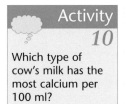

Activity 10

Which type of cow's milk has the most calcium per 100 ml?

CONNECTIONS

Chapter 8 mentions the effects of osteoporosis in limiting mobility.

milk, cheese, yoghurt, nuts, pulses, green leafy vegetables and canned fish. The body requires an adequate level of vitamin D to absorb and regulate calcium. Absorption may be reduced by excess NSP intake and phytate.

In deficiency states, bone calcium is mobilised to maintain essential functions, leading to rickets and osteoporosis. If a child has a low calcium intake, he may fail to achieve peak bone mass by the age of 30, which will increase the likelihood of osteoporosis in later life. Those at risk include children who dislike or do not take milk and dairy products, and fail to replace them with a calcium-fortified milk substitute (for example soya). Acute deficiency may cause tetany (muscle spasms) due to a loss of neuromuscular regulation.

Phosphorus

Phosphorus (P) is a component of all cells, necessary for energy storage, membrane function, growth and reproduction. Eighty-five per cent of the body's stores are found in bone. Sources include milk, milk products, bread, cereal products, all animal tissues, peanut butter and almonds.

Sodium

Sodium (Na) is needed for the maintenance of a constant body water content and plays an important role in the conduction of nervous impulses. It is found in many foods.

Chloride

Chloride (Cl) is required for the maintenance of a constant body water content. It is found in many foods.

Sodium chloride

The current recommendation for sodium chloride (NaCl, salt) is a maximum of 6 g of salt per day for an adult (10 g being equivalent to 2 teaspoonfuls of salt). Too much salt is thought to cause hypertension (raised blood pressure) in those susceptible to it. Processed foods and snacks tend to contain a high level of NaCl.

Potassium

Potassium (K) is necessary for the maintenance of a constant body water content, for acid–base balance and for nervous conduction. It is abundant in vegetables and fruit, including juice. Potassium is also found in meat, milk and almonds.

Iodine

Iodine (I) is needed for the functioning of the thyroid gland, which controls the metabolic rate of the body. It is found in seafish, bread and dairy products, and table salt in the UK is fortified with iodine. A deficiency is possible in those living far from the sea with no access to seafish.

Iron

Iron (Fe) is essential for red blood cell formation, oxygen transport and transfer, enzyme activation and drug metabolism. There are two sorts: organic/haem iron, found in meat, and inorganic/non-haem iron gained from bread, flour and cereal products, potatoes, green leafy vegetables, red wine, dried apricots and chocolate. Balti cooking is a good source because the food absorbs iron from the cooking pot. Haem iron is more accessible and more easily absorbed than non-haem iron. Vegetarians may, therefore, be at risk of deficiency. Iron is best absorbed with vitamin C, so the 2 mg of iron found in your fortified breakfast cereal is better absorbed with a glass of orange juice than a cup of tea. Keep that for later in the day (see below).

A lack of iron causes **iron deficiency anaemia**. Those at risk include vegetarians, faddy toddlers on self-restricted diets, especially those drinking a large amount of cow's milk and squash, with little solid food, and schoolchildren eating mostly chips, crisps and cola.

Iron supplements can cause gastric irritation, tarry stools and constipation. Overdosage of iron in those genetically susceptible to iron overload can increase the risk of heart disease.

iron deficiency anaemia

a reduced amount of haemoglobin in red blood cells, causing fatigue, glossitis and paraesthesia (sensations of numbness, prickling or tingling)

Zinc

Zinc (Zn) is needed for bone metabolism, enzyme activation, the release of vitamin A, growth, healing, healthy immune and reproductive systems, taste and insulin release. Sources include shellfish, fish, meat and meat products, milk and milk products, whole-grain bread and cereal products, vegetables and peanut butter.

Features of zinc deficiency include **anorexia**, failure to thrive in infants and children, weight loss, tremor, **dermatitis**, fine brittle hair, alopecia (hair loss), hypospermia (a reduced sperm count), **pica** and impaired taste and smell as well as delayed wound healing. At risk of zinc deficiency are faddy toddlers, children on a vegan diet and older children eating predominantly chips, crisps and cola. One solution is to snack on fortified breakfast cereals, cheese and yoghurt, and to eat two portions of protein daily (animal or green leafy vegetables and pulses).

CONNECTIONS

Chapter 10 identifies other factors necessary for wound healing.

anorexia

loss of appetite

dermatitis

inflammation of the skin, shown by itching, redness and skin lesions

pica

eating materials unsuitable as food, for example soil

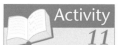

Activity

11

Look up the structure and function of the gastrointestinal tract, particularly digestion and absorption, in your preferred anatomy and physiology text (for example Rutishauser, 1994, pp. 107–35, 253–74).

Too much zinc can cause gastrointestinal irritation, including diarrhoea and nausea, and may disturb the balance of other important minerals, such as iron and copper, in the body.

Selenium

Selenium (Se) is necessary for part of an enzyme involved in the protection of membranes and lipids against oxidative damage. It is one of the antioxidants found in cereals, fish, offal, meat, cheese, eggs and milk. High-protein sources contain the most selenium. Selenium deficiency is closely related to lack of vitamin E, and supplementing with one can, in part, compensate for a lack of the other (Barasi, 1997).

Casebox 4.2

Ms Cohen, a retired civil servant of 60, underwent major hip surgery 2 weeks ago. She has little interest in food and was identified on admission as being underweight and malnourished.

How may this affect her progress after surgery?

What advice would be needed for her convalescence to be an opportunity to improve her nutritional status?

- Malnutrition will delay her recovery and increase the likelihood of complications. It interferes with respiratory function, partly by a loss of diaphragm muscle mass and strength, making Ms Cohen more likely to develop a chest infection.

Cardiac and immune function are depressed, so she will be at high risk of a wound infection or even a heart attack (myocardial infarction). Ms Cohen's grip strength will be diminished, making it harder for her to mobilise on crutches. Her bone density may also be very much diminished. Malnutrition has psychological effects such as apathy, depression and loss of the will to recover (Rollins, 1997), making Ms Cohen less likely to co-operate with her rehabilitation regimen.

- Ms Cohen needs to be fed as a matter of urgency or she is unlikely to get better. Nutritional support may need to be directed

along the lines of food as medicine, and considerable effort should be employed to coax her to eat and drink, little and often, high-calorie and nutrient-dense foodstuffs. Vitamin supplements may be an option. Her belief systems need to be identified: as she is an Orthodox Jew, is kosher food available? An education programme needs to be implemented to gain her interest in 'eating for convalescence'. Family, friends or neighbours could be encouraged to bring in her favourite foods – Jewish chicken soup is said to boost the immune system. Her community nurse may be recruited to monitor her nutritionally.

Mineral tailpieces

- *Phytates*, found in high levels in unprocessed wheat bran and soya, can lead to the malabsorption of minerals, especially calcium and zinc
- *Tannins* (polyphenols), found in tea, can reduce mineral availability
- *Oxalates*, found in high levels in spinach and rhubarb, can reduce mineral availability.

It is easy to assume that you or your clients are eating a 'balanced' diet, with very little evidence to support this. It is also possible to be confused by technicalities and unnecessary details when looking at nutrition. This chapter is about eating, so we will now look at the *foods* that make up a balanced intake. In the first student activity, you were asked to 'guestimate' the relative amounts, by weight, of food groups that your body needs. This can be summarised either by a diagram of a 'tilted plate' (Figure 4.2) or by percentages:

- Fruit and vegetables: 33 per cent
- Starchy foods, such as breads, cereals and potatoes, containing complex carbohydrates: 33 per cent

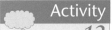

Activity 12

Did you know that there are over 500 different species of fungi and bacteria that live in your gut? They weigh 2 kg in an adult. What are they for? (See, for example, Rutishauser, 1994, pp. 123–4.)

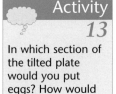

Activity 13

In which section of the tilted plate would you put eggs? How would you classify potatoes?

Figure 4.2 ● The tilted plate

- Milk and dairy products: 14 per cent
- Meat and alternatives: 12 per cent
- Oils, fats, foods with a high proportion of fats, sugars, foods with a high proportion of sugar (and alcohol, if taken): 8 per cent.

▣ Alcohol

Alcohol has a long history of bad and good press (Simpson, 1992). It is high in energy and carbohydrate, and, when taken in excess, can be a factor in obesity and vitamin deficiency, especially that of vitamin B1. It is dehydrating so is unhelpful in maintaining the body's fluid balance: hangovers are largely the result of dehydration.

A moderate alcohol intake is associated with a raised level of HDL cholesterol, a protective factor against heart disease (see above). The antioxidant components of alcohol are found, for example, in grape skins, so red wine is a good source of these. Red wine is thought to protect against heart attacks by preventing arteries furring up with deposits of LDL cholesterol. Polyphenols, abundant in red wine, are believed to block the oxidation of LDLs and thus stop them accumulating on the arterial walls (Coghlan, 1997). The best pattern for health is alcohol absorbed slowly with meals, which is one basis of the Mediterranean diet.

An excessive alcohol intake leads to long-term problems affecting every body system, for example brain atrophy, stroke, liver damage, cancer of the oesophagus, heart disease, premature ageing of the skin, a loss of secondary sexual characteristics, muscle wasting and bone demineralisation (Bonner and Waterhouse, 1996). Damage is exacerbated by binge drinking.

One unit of alcohol is equal to 8 g of pure alcohol. For example, 500 ml of 5 per cent alcohol lager will contain 25 ml of pure alcohol, that is, about 3 units. The unit system for a healthy intake needs to be applied with flexibility. According to government guidelines issued in December 1995, women can take up to 2–3 units per day (unless they are pregnant) and men up to 3–4 units per day (DoH, 1995). Marmot (1995), however, disagrees with this from the health point of view, suggesting that these values are too high and proposing a return to something like the former maximum of 14 units in a week for women and 21 units a week for men. Two alcohol-free days are encouraged to allow the body to recover. One gram of alcohol provides 29 kJ (7 kcal) of energy.

▣ Getting Enough Nutrients

COMA, in its 1991 report (DoH, 1991), produced ranges for different dietary components, using the following guidelines:

- *Dietary reference values* (DRVs) is a general term that must be used as it comprises a more precisely focused and evidence-based system than RDAs, which produce a single figure for each nutrient, covering every age group
- *Reference nutrient intake* (RNI) is the amount of a nutrient that is sufficient for up to 97 per cent of the population
- *Estimated average requirements* (EARs) are the estimated average requirements of each nutrient sufficient to meet the needs of half the population
- *Lower reference nutrient intake* (LRNI) is the amount of nutrient needed for people with a low need. If people consistently consume less than their LRNI, they may be at risk of deficiency.

Changing requirements across the life span

'Nutrient requirements and eating behaviours vary according to health status, activity patterns and growth' (DoH, 1991); it is, therefore, impossible to be totally precise when identifying specific needs for each age group. A baby, for example, has half the energy requirement of an elderly person but is much less than a third of his or her body weight: growth has great energy demands, as has sucking and crying. The peak of energy need is between 15 and 18 years of age for both sexes, and there is also the growth spurt at puberty to contend with. Energy demand depends on activity level too.

The EAR is calculated using a physical activity level (PAL) of 1.4 (Table 4.3), which equates to most of the UK population, and basal metabolic rate (BMR) in the formula:

$$BMR \times PAL = EAR$$

basal metabolic rate
the metabolic rate measured at rest, after sleeping and 12 hours after eating, with no exercise or excitement preceding the test

Assessing nutritional status

One way of checking whether someone is well nourished is to get him or her to keep a food diary (see Figure 4.4 below) and then rate it against the 'tilted plate'

Table 4.3 Physical activity level (PAL) for those over 18 years of age

PAL		
1.4		Very little activity at work and in leisure time
1.6	Female	Moderate activity at work/leisure
1.7	Male	Moderate activity at work/leisure
1.8	Female	High levels of activity at work/leisure
1.9	Male	High levels of activity at work/leisure

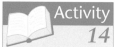

Activity 14

Look up metabolism in your preferred anatomy and physiology or nutrition text (for example Rutishauser, 1994, pp. 266–72).

What is the difference between **anabolism** and **catabolism**? Why is this relevant to eating and drinking?

anabolism

the building up of body substance; the constructive phase of metabolism

catabolism

the breakdown of body substance; the destructive phase of metabolism

(Figure 4.2). One day's intake is not enough information on which to make a judgement, unless it is typical of a very consistent intake, so the more information that can be gained, the more accurate the resulting baseline. In order to monitor a client's food and fluid intake, most units have food and fluid charts of varying degrees of formality. It is important that they are completed with the highest degree of accuracy possible and that the intake is added up and related to the client's needs by someone with the knowledge and interest to ensure that findings are acted upon.

There are also local and national nutritional awareness and assessment tools, some research based and validated, many not. Most have a series of questions to be answered, these being scored to identify the client's level of risk of malnutrition. The questions need to cover the clients' abilities to eat and drink, from mental status, appetite and food preferences, through to the state of dentition and the chewing and swallowing ability. Problems such as food intolerance, allergy, fatigue, pain, nausea, constipation, breathlessness, anorexia or the requirement to fast for tests or surgery will diminish a person's ability to take adequate food and fluids. Malabsorption, pyrexia, surgery, burns, diarrhoea, vomiting and excessive losses will increase requirements. The disease process and any medication taken may also have metabolic implications. The client's ability to access food and drink normally, in terms of shopping, storing, cooking or cutting up food, must also be assessed.

Observation of clients will include a subjective global assessment to see whether they appear well nourished, and will include looking at the fit of their clothes, the condition of their skin, eyes, hair and nails, how they move and how alert or apathetic they appear. Hand grip strength may be a useful indicator.

General lifestyle questions will include an assessment of their activity and exercise levels, how much time they spend out of doors, whether they smoke and what their alcohol consumption is. At the very least, every client should, on admission or assessment, be asked the following questions:

1. Have you unintentionally lost weight recently?
2. Have you been eating less than usual?
3. What is your normal weight?
4. How tall are you?

body mass index

a figure derived from a person's height and weight, which indicates whether his or her weight is acceptable

Body mass index

Questions 3 and 4 above enable the nurse to calculate **body mass index** (BMI; Chart 4.2), which is a better indicator of health than is weight alone. BMI relates height to weight to indicate a healthy range of weight.

Chart 4.2 ● Body mass index (BMI)

BMI calculation = weight (kg)/height^2(m)
Reference ranges for desirable BMI =
    18.5–24.9 normal range
    25–29.9 overweight
    30+ obese

A BMI below the acceptable range indicates undernutrition (or dehydration), one above the range indicating overweight/obesity (or oedema). This measure is not suitable for infants, children, pregnant women and amputees, and can be difficult to apply in the shrunken older person. If a person has a great deal of muscle, he may appear 'obese'. Another way of determining whether body build is healthy is to use the waist:hip ratio (Sakurai et al., 1995) or waist circumference (Lean et al., 1995, 1998).

Questions 1 and 2 above are essential as unintentional weight loss is significant even if the client has a 'normal' or 'high' BMI. A greater than 10 per cent loss in body weight in less than 3 months signifies that the client is malnourished and should be referred for specialist nutrition advice as there is a risk of increased **morbidity** and mortality; that is, he or she is more likely to suffer disease, complications and death.

morbidity
the state of being diseased

■ Assisting with Nutrition and Hydration

The aim of any help is to ensure, in a reasonable manner, that clients have an optimum food and fluid intake, maintaining their dignity in the process. The only food that is of any use to clients is that which they actually eat and retain, remembering that 'You are what you eat.' Assisting someone with their nutrition and **hydration** can be placed into four broad areas – social, ergonomic, economic and nutritional (SEEN):

hydration
the state of fluid balance of the body

- *Social:* the sociable side of eating
- *Ergonomic:* the study of work and its environment and conditions to achieve maximum efficiency, as applied to nutrition
- *Economic/educational:* the best use of time and resources; involves health promotion and education
- *Nutrition function:* especially important for the vulnerable client.

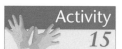

Activity 15

Most big chemists hold a range of feeding aids and catalogues of equipment. Get hold of some catalogues to see what can be provided for clients.

Look at the four 'SEEN' headings in the text and list as many helpful ideas/equipment as you can in 10 minutes.

Identify at least one negative event you have encountered in practice.

Social

Food can and should be an enjoyable break, a pause or punctuation, in the day rather than just fuel. Arrange a change of scene and company if possible by taking clients to a dining room or day room. Gather people around tables with upright chairs, away from beds, clatter, telephones, staff and clinical equipment. Identify for each individual the best setting to encourage them to eat, digest and absorb the most nourishment: watching someone else's food going round like socks in a washing machine may not enhance appetite. A person who needs help with feeding may be best served in privacy to reduce embarrassment and distractions. Involve clients in decisions about their food and drink – its timing, amount and so on (Shepheard, 1998).

Remember that presentation counts. Consider the cleanliness of the surroundings, ensuring that smells are neutral, fresh air is available and the food looks appealing. For blind clients use the 'clockface' to describe what is where on the plate. Braille or large-print menus may also be available.

Sherry can be particularly useful as an appetite stimulant for elderly clients (Simpson, 1992).

Staff can eat their meals with clients to enhance the social function. This can be a useful reminder to those with limited memory who just forget to eat without the external prompt of seeing others doing so.

Activity 16

Look up swallowing in your preferred anatomy and physiology text (for example Rutishauser, 1994, pp. 506–8; see also the structure and function of the gastrointestinal tract, especially digestion and absorption, pp. 107–35, 253–74).

Ergonomic/physiological

Ergonomics is the study of people, work and its environment, and the conditions to achieve maximum efficiency. It is necessary to know how swallowing works and the physiology of the gastrointestinal tract in order to help the client most effectively in this area.

Gravity feed is the most useful idea on which to base good practice. Sitting the client as upright as possible allows the first third of the oesophagus to generate the wave of peristalsis that takes food and fluid (and drugs) into the stomach. If possible, an upright chair drawn up to a table of comfortable height should be used. The client in an armchair may find even an adjustable bed-table too high. In such a case, consider putting a firm pillow under the client to raise him to a more comfortable height. Other strategies include putting the tray on to the edge of the bed if the client can turn to one side in the armchair, or sitting the client on the edge of the bed with her feet on the floor if she can support herself, and bringing the bed-table over her knees. Lap-trays with 'beanbag' backs can be used on any height of chair or in bed. For some clients, adjustable chairs should be placed in a more upright position for meals and drinks, and not put back to recline for at least 15 minutes afterwards; this will reduce the chance of **reflux**.

reflux

a backward flow of food and fluid up the gastrointestinal tract

Clients in bed need to be sitting upright with their pillows arranged so that they can lean forward. Clinical equipment may need to be moved out of the way or covered up. Consider the physiological implications of the client being frightened, nauseated or in pain. The effects of stimulation of the gastrointestinal tract by the **sympathetic nervous system** include a decrease in motility and a drying up of secretions, including a dry mouth, leaving clients unable to utilise what is taken in.

sympathetic nervous system

part of the autonomic (automatic) nervous system activated in response to fright and other unpleasant stimuli

If clients need help with feeding, sit at the same level so that you can reach comfortably. Try not to rush them or give them too much at a time. Between one half and a full teaspoonful per mouthful is plenty and is best placed in the stronger side of the mouth. Ensure that the client can close his lips as the lipseal needs to be maintained to trigger swallowing. Allow two swallows per mouthful to ensure that the mouth is empty. Ask the client to clear his throat to clear the airway; then wait a few seconds before offering the next mouthful. After every few mouthfuls, ask the client to cough, and to do so again at the end of the meal. Listen to his voice, asking him to say 'Ah' after every few mouthfuls. A 'wet' or gurgly-sounding voice is an indication to **stop** feeding, as this is a sign of aspiration into the respiratory tract; in such a situation, call for qualified assistance.

When the meal has been safely completed, check the mouth for retained food, which might give trouble later, and remove it with a swab or toothbrush. If the client can cope, a drink or mouthwash will help. After eating or drinking, the client should stay sitting upright for at least half an hour. Blood is diverted to the gut to digest food, so the client may feel chilly after eating. If indigestion is a problem, consider the use of ginger ale (also good for nausea) or peppermint.

Economic/educational

- It helps to know when mealtimes are in order to plan a break in the workload
- Try to ensure that those needing help with elimination have been encouraged to perform well before mealtimes in order to reduce unpleasant noises and smells, which act as an appetite suppressant
- If someone needs a commode at a mealtime, wheel them out to a bathroom for privacy
- Remove bedpans, urinals, commodes and toilet rolls from bed-tables and bedsides
- It is very important for staff and patients to wash their hands
- If the family want to visit and help, they can bring in favourite treats if policy allows

CONNECTIONS

Chapter 3 discusses the issue of food hygiene.

- It might be necessary to discourage other visitors at mealtimes as this will distract the client and divert the energy needed for eating
- Is the mouth clean and are the dentures in place?
- Do the dentures fit?
- Ensure that pain relief or antiemetic medication is given in time for it to be working well
- Does the patient need insulin or another medication before meals?
- Employ strategies to reduce breathlessness
- Time any nausea-inducing therapy so that it occurs after meals
- Ensure that ventilation is adequate to waft away body smells during meals and the smell of food afterwards
- Exploit educational opportunities when setting up menu choices
- Cut up food for those who need it
- Rearrange the contents of the tray so the client can reach everything. Lift heavy lids and peel off fiddly tops. Are salt and pepper available? Can the client hold the cutlery provided (indeed, is it all there?) or does she need built-up handles or other special cutlery?
- Is fresh water available?
- If a hot drink is delivered too early, put a lid on it and check it again later
- Supplement the paper napkin with additional protection if needed
- Would a straw help? This is of no use for stroke patients as their orbicularis oris muscle (the muscle around the mouth) is weak, making their suction power low; straws with valves or a feeder cup may help
- Does the client need an occasional prompt or gentle reminder, constant attention or feeding?
- Use your awareness of the gastrocolic reflex (the fact that putting food in at the top causes the system to shunt into activity) to anticipate patients' needs. Some clients who cannot tell you what they need may go red in the face after tea, coffee or meals, which can mean that they need to defaecate
- Keeping hot foods hot and cold foods cold enhances their palatability; cold food most improves swallowing
- If a client has problems with swallowing, has she been referred to a speech and language therapist?
- The easiest consistency to eat is a smooth texture. Soft solids such as ice cream, yoghurt, custard, purée, baked beans (without toast) and mashed potato are acceptable. Normal solids and thickened liquids are more difficult; these include thick milkshakes, yoghurt drinks and thickened soups. Jelly and bananas may help to supplement the fluid intake
- Food types to be avoided by the client with eating or swallowing difficulties are those which are stringy, crumbly, tough or of mixed texture, as well as such items as peas, nuts, sweetcorn and chips.

Nutrition function

- What are we trying to do for this patient? Are we using nutrition as therapy for:
  - weight gain
  - weight maintenance
  - weight loss
  - wound healing
  - enhancing fibre intake
  - ensuring a balanced intake
  - correcting malnutrition?

CONNECTIONS

Chapter 10 identifies other factors necessary for wound healing.

- Do we need to keep a food chart so that it can be checked against the 'tilted plate' for:
  - fruit and vegetables: 33 per cent
  - complex carbohydrates/starchy foods: 33 per cent
  - milk and dairy products: 14 per cent
  - proteins: 12 per cent
  - fats, fatty foods, sugars, sugary foods and alcohol: 8 per cent?

If there are any doubts about intake, keep a food and fluid intake chart of what has actually been consumed and retained by the patient.

Activity
17

Rate a client's 24 hour food intake against the 'tilted plate' (see Figure 4.2 above).

Are any deficits apparent? What suggestions can you make to remedy these?

- Is the nutrition therapy featured in the care plan? If not, why not?
- Ensure the adequate completion of menu cards, checking for portion size and balance
- Are we going for the easy option of soup and ice cream? This can be a nutritional disaster if allowed to go on for more than a couple of days, as it is low in nutrients
- Think about supplements and snacks
- Avoid tea or coffee just before or with meals as they can fill patients up too much
- Lots of fluid with food can overfill clients. This can be helpful if one is trying to reduce weight but is unhelpful if trying to enhance the intake of nutrients
- 1001 ways with mince is very boring, so build in some variety
- Little and often may help some, so order a sandwich or fruit to be eaten later
- How flexible are your catering arrangements? Can you get an omelette, sandwich and so on at any time?
- What are the limits? Can a meal be saved and heated in a microwave later on when it suits the patient? Food hygiene regulations must, of course, be taken into account.

CONNECTIONS

Chapter 3 reviews the relevant legislation and its application to food hygiene.

- Use dietitians appropriately. If there is a problem, they can be more helpful than the catering department
- Does the person need a soft or puréed diet? Keep component foods separate so that an unappetising greyish sludge is avoided

anosmia

loss of sense of smell

- Those with anosmia and diminished or altered taste sensation (which may be the result of drug therapy) may need to add extra pepper, salt (but not if they have high blood pressure), spices, herbs, vinegar, sauces or garlic. Relatives could provide these or they could be bought from ward/unit funds

hemianopia

blindness in half the field of vision of one or both eyes

- Have an awareness of particular client problems. Hemianopia after a stroke, for example, means that the client will ignore one side of the plate, so the plate should be rotated. Paralysis of one side of the face means that food is left in one cheek like a hamster. The client may need help to work the jaw at intervals
- Medication may be administered disguised in food or drink, but this must only take place in exceptional circumstances, and local policy must incorporate the UKCC guidelines. A pharmacist must be involved as adding medication to food or drink can alter its chemical properties and therefore affect its performance (Nicholls, 2001).

CONNECTIONS

Chapter 3 covers this issue and outlines general guidelines for giving medication to children.

Appetite and Choices

Activity
18

What emotions may be evoked by the smell of frying onions, brewing coffee or baking bread?

What does your favourite person smell of? When you smell this, how do you feel?

The psychology of eating is highly complex, so the reader is advised to consult a psychology text (for example Lyman, 1989) in addition to reading this section. This is also an extremely important area because food and eating are essential parts of the social and moral aspects of society.

There are four principal taste sensations, sweet, sour, bitter and salty being all that the tongue can detect. Monosodium glutamate (umami), which enhances flavours, may be considered. What adds subtlety to taste is the sense of smell. Taste and smell together make up the flavour system, which can evoke strong emotional responses, the association of odours with emotion being to a certain extent learned.

Flavour also includes other characteristics of food, such as temperature and texture. Variety in food seems to stimulate the appetite, and flavour motivates eating by the pleasure derived from its taste, smell and 'mouthfeel'. For this reason, children often come to prefer foods with a high fat content. Social situations and other people also provide cues that stimulate the appetite for certain foods, the presence of other people also generally tending to induce one to eat more. In addition, changes in people's nutritional state can affect their motivation to consume certain foods.

The selection and preparation of food requires a number of psychological processes, including choice, cognition, knowledge and attitudes. Two theories

(Lyman, 1989) help to explain how we might select food to produce nutritional balance. One idea postulates an innate recognition of foods containing deficient nutrients, the other that learning occurs to recognise food that makes one feel good and avoid food that makes one feel bad. The other important mechanism in food choice is the tendency to be suspicious of but interested in new foods. We classify food as edible or inedible, having developed attitudes about what makes an object appropriate and desirable as food.

Three factors account for food rejection and acceptance:

1. *Sensory-affective factors:* like and dislike are based on sensory attributes such as taste, smell and sometimes appearance. Good tastes are accepted; those which are unappealing are rejected as distasteful.
2. *Anticipated consequences:* acceptance or rejection is based on beliefs about the consequences of ingestion. An elderly person may, for example, believe that 'eggs are binding' or that 'bread is fattening'. The rejection of an item because of perceived negative consequences is based on its 'dangerous' nature. Conversely, the acceptance of an item is based on its anticipated beneficial effects.
3. *Ideational factors:* items are accepted or rejected because of our knowledge of what they are, their origins and their symbolic meanings. Ideational factors are mostly concerned with food rejection. There are two categories of

Activity 19

What food and drink selections have you made in the past 24 hours? Can you identify some of the factors influencing those selections?

Casebox 4.3

Miss Quinn, aged 82, has progressive dementia and has lived in a residential care home for 2 years. She wanders restlessly all round the clock and rarely spends more than a few minutes at anything. The staff are concerned that she appears to be losing weight.

What steps could be taken to ensure that this does not become a problem?

■ Make every mouthful count, so avoid wasting eating and drinking time on low-calorie fillers.

■ Use the fact that she has limited memory to encourage nutritious snacks around the clock instead of expecting her to concentrate for a full meal.

■ Instead of a cup of coffee made with water, she could be offered a cup of coffee made entirely with full-cream milk, a little more sugar being added over time.

■ Always present a cup of tea with a biscuit, small cake or sandwich.

■ Fluid supplements may be prescribed for her and served chilled or heated.

■ Has she chocolates, fruit and crisps in her room for constant access?

■ Meals can be enriched to enhance the calorie count by adding butter, cream or sugar as appropriate.

rejected food: inappropriate and disgusting. An example of the latter is many children's attitudes to vegetables.

Thus, in summary:

- Psychological categories of rejection (strongly linked to the biological) include distaste, danger, inappropriateness and disgust
- Psychological categories of acceptance include good taste, benefits and appropriateness
- We consume food because of the perceived benefits or for its own sake, because it tastes good or for comfort
- We avoid foods because of their dangerous properties, because of our intolerance or allergy to them, or because of dislike or unfamiliarity.

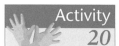

Activity 20

Give an example of your own food choices for each category. Try to identify why your choice has developed this way.

Then do this activity with a client.

Social factors are important in determining how we come to like or dislike certain foods. Parental choice can, for example, influence children one way or the other. People develop long-term food preferences that are stable over long periods of time and unaffected by changes in their mood or environment; these can be highly resistant to change if a more healthy diet is advised. Some food preferences change from day to day and are more likely to be affected by mood. Lyman (1989), for example, identified how people tended to prefer healthy foods when experiencing positive emotions and junk food when feeling negative. It was also noted that crunchy foods were most likely to be associated with anger, boredom and frustration. We might, for instance, treat ourselves to a favourite food after a hard day at work.

◼ Political, Social and Economic Influences

Many people are, for social, economic, geographical and other reasons, unable to access the basics of a healthy diet without considerable difficulty. Many groups, such as elderly people, the homeless, refugees, the unemployed or those with children, may be living below the poverty line. They may, for example, live on large housing estates, planned without amenities such as shops, clubs, churches or pubs, and shopping for food may involve a bus journey to add to the cost in time and money. Local shops will be more expensive and have a more limited choice than supermarkets. Low-income families are less likely than higher-income families to eat fresh fruit and vegetables, fish or fresh meat, and more likely to eat fatty foods and starchy 'filler' foods such as white bread, jam, cakes, biscuits and sweets. Vitamin and mineral status is often compromised. Shopping basket surveys have shown that a healthy diet may cost up to 35 per cent more than an unhealthy one. The loss of free school milk and free

Casebox 4.4

Raul is 15 years old and has learning disabilities and many physical problems. He is moving to a new care home, and the opportunity is being taken to reassess his needs.

How can the team assess his nutritional status and identify what assistance Raul requires?

■ Measure his height and weight, and calculate his BMI.

■ Keep a food record over a week to check for likes, dislikes and overall balance.

■ Is Raul getting enough fluid? What are his preferences?

■ What capacities has he for chewing and swallowing? Should he be assessed by a speech and language therapist? What state are his teeth and gums in?

■ Could the drugs that he is taking (for example phenytoin) interact with his food?

■ How is Raul best positioned for meals, and how much can he do for himself? Does he need a special tilted chair? What about built-up cutlery, moulded to his hand grip? Can occupational therapy help?

Casebox 4.5

Trevor, aged 47, is suffering from depression. He barely has the energy to get himself out of bed in the mornings, is off sick from his work as a storeman and goes to group therapy once a week.

What is likely to be the effect of this on his eating pattern and weight?

■ Trevor will probably suffer from early morning wakening but his activity level will be very low.

■ If he eats as much as he used to before he went off sick, and/or eats for comfort, with a high level of refined carbohydrate and fat, Trevor may put on weight.

■ It is also possible that he could lose interest in food, have no appetite and not bother to shop or cook for himself, ending up with weight loss, some of which will be loss of muscle mass from inactivity (see Chapter 8).

school meals has not helped those families with children who most need this support to supplement their often meagre diets, and changing benefit patterns do not appear to allow these families to catch up. It thus seems that the main factors in food deprivation are a low income or pension, inadequate benefits, the high cost of appropriate food and its availability. As well as affecting children's growth and development, a poor diet may contribute to dental disease, anaemia, obesity, low bone mass, coronary heart disease and cerebrovascular disease (stroke).

Cultural Issues – Ethnic and Religious Practices

Activity 21

Consider why the fish and chip shop is busier on Fridays.

Identify the food ideology of a client who comes from a different cultural, ethnic or religious group.

Activity 22

Imagine celebrating a friendly gathering without food or drink.

Identify one food that you regard as 'good' and one you regard as 'bad'. Why have these foods come to mean this to you? What is the basis for this belief? Is it rational?

Cultural factors inform food ideology, that is, the collection of customs, attitudes, beliefs and taboos that affect the diet of a particular group. Some people, for example, may feel that their diet is incomplete without a hot meal at least once a day. For centuries, Roman Catholics consumed no meat on Fridays, and Mormons do not consume caffeine or alcohol.

Clients' food ideology is important because it influences their behaviour as well as their motivation to alter their food habits across time. These food habits are acquired as part of primary socialisation in childhood and may be difficult to change, which reinforces the necessity of initially developing good food habits (Fieldhouse, 1995). Secondary socialisation takes place through the school and workplace, and may contradict food habits learned at home. The attempts of health professionals to change people's eating habits in more healthy directions can be termed 'resocialisation'. This process can be helped or hindered by influences at local, regional and national levels, including such factors as advertising. People may regard foods as 'good' or 'bad', Yin or Yang, 'hot' or 'cold', reward or punishment. The social meanings of food are bound up with notions and traditions of hospitality, expressions of love, friendship, affection and status (Fieldhouse, 1995).

Many world religions, such as Buddhism, Hinduism, Sikhism, Rastafarianism and spiritualism, advocate vegetarianism of varying strictness. Fruitarians eat only fruit, vegans eat no animal products, lactovegetarians eat no eggs, meat, fish or poultry, and lacto-ovovegetarians eat vegetables, pulses, nuts, milk, cheese and eggs. As vegetarianism seems to be on the increase, nurses need to be aware of how a diet can be balanced in the absence of meat, fish, cheese, eggs or dairy products. An alternative 'tilted plate' is outlined in Chart 4.3 and Figure 4.3 for guidance.

Religions and cultures that advocate fasting usually absolve the sick from participating, yet for many clients fasting before investigations, surgery or treatment or because of their illness is an unwelcome part of their lives.

Chart 4.3 ● Vegetarian tilted plate

1 serving of plant oil/margarine/butter

4–5 servings of fruit/vegetables

2–3 servings of pulses/nuts/seeds

3–4 servings of cereals/grains

2 servings of dairy products/soya

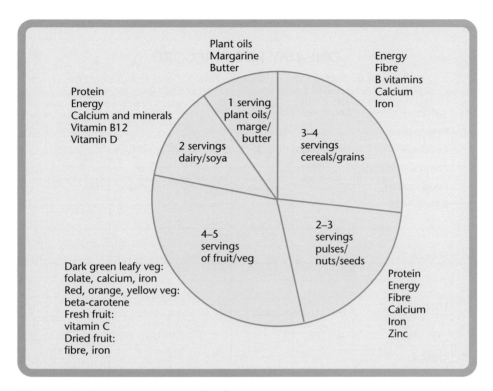

Figure 4.3 ● The vegetarian tilted plate

■ Monitoring Eating and Drinking

Some clients will need close monitoring to ensure that their nutrition and hydration needs are adequately met. Nutritional assessment should be a continuous process, particularly when clients have been identified as being at risk of malnutrition. Simple indicators, such as regular weighing, may be enough if the equipment is available and accurate (Micklewright and Todorovic, 1997), although short-term weight gains and losses over a day will reflect only body fluid changes. The client's mood may well be affected by nutrition level; the malnourished patient tends to be apathetic and have poor grip strength and very little motivation to participate in his or her own care.

Information can also be gained about the client's progress from the blood albumin level. Albumin is synthesised in the liver and transports small molecules including medications, hormones and vitamins. The normal blood level in adults is 34–50 g/l, and albumin has a **half-life** of 20 days. In very ill and malnourished patients, the level will lie below 35 g/l and will decline further if their condition deteriorates. This means that their ability to transport drugs around the body may be compromised (McPherson, 1993). Although the albumin level is not a

half-life

the time required by the body to metabolise half of a particular substance

ONE-DAY FOOD RECORD

List below all the food you ate and drank yesterday. For each item check (✓) the appropriate food group. Be sure to total the number of foods eaten for each group.

Self	33% 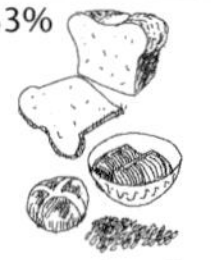 Bread and cereals	33% 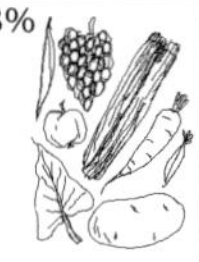 Fruit and vegetables	14% 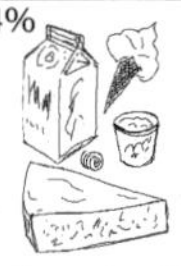 Milk and milk products	12% 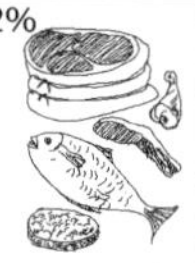 Meat and alternatives	8% 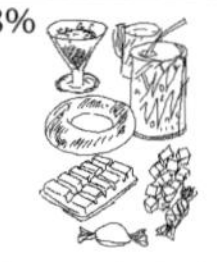 Sugar, alcohol, fatty foods
Elderly person					
Child age					
Pregnant woman					
Foods eaten					
BREAKFAST					
SNACK					
LUNCH					
SNACK					
DINNER					
SNACK					
Total fluid volume					
Total number of foods eaten from each group					
Percentage					

Height: Weight: BMI:

Figure 4.4 ● One-day food record

nutritional indicator on its own, it nevertheless gives some idea of the client's condition, and the trend of the readings is significant.

Food charts (Figure 4.4) can be useful provided they are added up and the findings acted upon. The severely compromised patient may well need referral to a specialist such as a clinical nutrition nurse or dietitian. The key features to check are the calorie and protein intakes. For example, is a male client aged between 19 and 50 achieving 10.60 MJ (2550 kcal) and 55.5 g of protein, and is a female client of this same age eating 8.10 MJ (1940 kcal) and 45g of protein?

Fluid charts also need to be checked for balance. The record must be an accurate one, reflecting the volume consumed rather than amount dispensed (Morrison, 2000). If patients have excessive losses, are being fasted, are vomiting or are being given any form of artificial nutrition or hydration, a careful check is absolutely essential to ensure that they are not over- or under-hydrated. Some clinicians pinch the skin on the back of the hand to check **skin turgor,** or monitor the central venous pressure or arterial blood pressure and pulse. The presence or absence of oedema may be relevant.

'Low-tech' rehydration techniques are theoretically possible, but rectal infusion, for example, is not currently in widespread use in the UK (Abdulla and Keast, 1997). Subcutaneous rehydration (**hypodermoclysis**) is gaining in popularity in many units as it is easy to set up and can be used in nursing homes, with older people and in palliative care (Donnelly, 1999) when large amounts of fluid are not needed in a short space of time (Iggulden, 1999). A rate of less than 125 ml per hour is suggested.

◾ Nutritional Support

The mainstay of nutritional support is to use the gastrointestinal tract if it is working (enteral feeding) and to use the intravenous (parenteral) route only if the gut is unavailable, for example as a result of complete intestinal obstruction. Parenteral support is beyond the scope of this text.

It must be stressed that the best route for feeding is via the mouth, anything else being a poor substitute. Tube feeding has psychological and social implications for the client, and complications may occur. It may be used to provide all the client's requirements or simply be supplemental feeding in those who find it difficult to take enough in orally.

The most straightforward route for gut access is the nasogastric route. A fine-bore polyurethane nasogastric tube (size 12 French gauge [Fr] for an adult, down to size 5 Fr for a very small baby) is inserted for the delivery of liquid feeds. The smallest possible tube is used to reduce the discomfort of leaving it in place and minimise the risk of nasal mucosal ulceration. Contraindications to enteral feeding include clients with:

- Persistent vomiting
- Delayed gastric emptying
- An oesophago-gastric fistula
- Oesophageal reflux

CONNECTIONS

Chapter 6 identifies the relevance of fluid balance to circulation and renal function.

skin turgor

the resistance of the skin to deformation when pinched between the fingers, related mainly to age but also to the level of hydration

hypodermoclysis

the introduction of fluid subcutaneously

CONNECTIONS

Chapter 5 mentions the importance of record-keeping to detect dehydration, also describing, in Activity 7, a kinder way to detect skin turgor.

- Complex fluid management problems
- **Paralytic ileus**.

paralytic ileus

paralysis of the intestinal
muscle

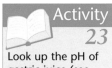

Look up the pH of
gastric juice (see,
for example,
Rutishauser,
1994, pp.133,
225).

CONNECTIONS

*Chapter 3 describes
checking the site of
a nasogastric tube in
relation to giving
medication via this
route.*

CONNECTIONS

*Chapter 3 describes
food hygiene
precautions.*

Insertion, by a trained nurse or doctor depending on local policy and
expertise, is facilitated by using the tube's own guidewire. It is essential to check
the position of the tip of the tube in the stomach before feeding begins. Once the
tube has been inserted, the exit site on the tube is marked to monitor for slip-
page: this is needed because the tube can migrate. One way of checking that the
tube is in position is to inject air through it and listen over the epigastrium with
a stethoscope (auscultation), but this is not a totally reliable method. Second,
every time the tube is disconnected, the fluid can be aspirated and tested for
acidity. This is best achieved after a period of rest from feeding, when the pH of
the gastric contents may be approaching normal. If these techniques fail, an
X-ray may be needed. A combination of methods is safest, and local policies and
procedures should be consulted. Feeding can usually begin immediately after
confirmation that the nasogastric tube is positioned in the stomach.

The main complications of nasogastric tube placement are:

- Malposition at insertion
- Displacement after insertion
- Subsequent occlusion.

Malpositioning of the tube in the trachea or bronchus may cause the accidental intrapulmonary administration of feed, or pulmonary or oesophageal
perforation.

Food hygiene is paramount, as these patients are often immunocompromised
by their malnutrition. The feeding tube must be rinsed through between feeds,
with sterile water (clinical settings) or cooled, boiled water (at home). Fizzy
water is sometimes used to dislodge particles and keep the tube clear. The giving
set tubing should be changed with each new bottle of feed, according to local
policy and procedure.

The response to feeds is monitored by:

- Recording the amount given against the client's prescription
- Checking nutritional values gained against the client's requirements
- Noting any side-effects, for example diarrhoea
- Checking the client's weight at agreed intervals.

Complications may include:

- Pulmonary aspiration of the feed
- Nasopharyngeal discomfort

- Nasal erosions
- Oesophagitis
- Oesophageal ulceration
- Otitis media (inflammation of the middle ear).

Activity

24

Why is otitis media a complication of nasogastric tube placement? Look at Rutishauser, 1994, pp. 437, 438 and 497 if you do not understand.

Gastrostomy tube feeding

For clients who need enteral feeding for a long period (more than 4 weeks), a tube is inserted directly into the stomach through the skin. This is performed by specially trained personnel, the client usually receiving local anaesthetic and sedation, in the X-ray department, endoscopy unit or operating theatre. Some tubes may remain in position for as long as 2 years.

Client problems requiring gastrostomy feeding via a gastrostomy tube include cerebrovascular accident (stroke), head injury with brain damage, motorneurone disease, multiple sclerosis and learning disability with multiple physical handicaps. Contraindications to the insertion of gastrostomy feeding tubes include gross ascites, severe obesity, blood clotting abnormalities, oesophageal or gastric varices (varicose veins), gastric ulceration and gastric malignancy.

ascites

excess fluid in the peritoneal cavity

New designs and types of gastrostomy feeding tube become available all the time. Current designs include those with an internal and an external retention

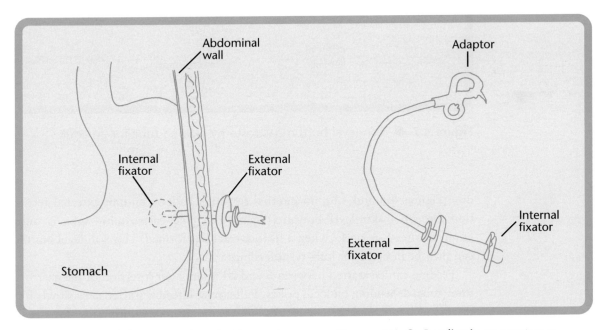

Figure 4.5 ● Adult gastrostomy feeding tube with internal and external retention discs

Figure 4.6 ● Paediatric gastrostomy feeding tube

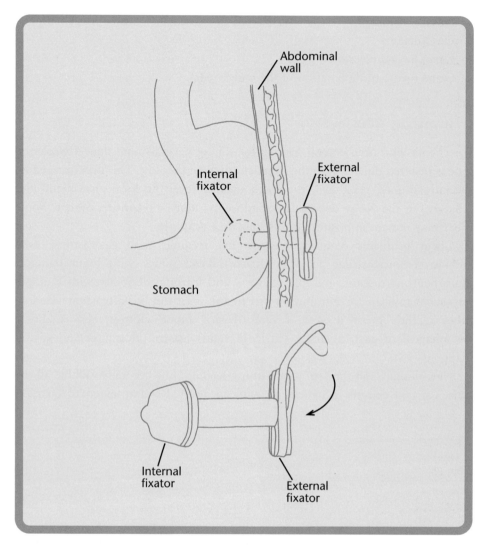

Figure 4.7 ● Skin-level button gastrostomy feeding tube for an adult

disc (Figures 4.5 and 4.6), an internal retaining balloon and an external retention disc or a skin-level button (Figure 4.7). The gastrostomy tube is only
removed after 5–6 weeks when a fibrous tract has formed. The skin-level button
can then be inserted for long-term feeding.

Feeding can be started between 6 and 24 hours after insertion of the gastrostomy tube, depending on local policy. Full-strength feed is started very slowly for
the first 4 hours, and the client's response is monitored. Continuous slow feeds
are recommended to aid gastric absorption, and metoclopramide may be
prescribed to enhance gastric emptying.

The residual volume in the stomach is aspirated and measured 1 hour after a feed has been completed in order to determine progress. If the adult's residual volume is more than 100 ml, the start of the next feed should be delayed for 1 hour. The residual volume is then rechecked; it must be less than 100 ml before starting the next feed.

The gastrostomy tube must be rinsed through between feeds with sterile water (immunocompromised patients in clinical settings) or cooled, boiled water (at home). The gastrostomy site must be observed for gastric acid leakage and infection. If necessary, it is usually cleaned aseptically with normal saline (sodium chloride 0.9 per cent) immediately after insertion.

Complications of gastrostomy feeding tube insertion include:

- Peritonitis (inflammation of the peritoneal cavity)
- Pulmonary aspiration of the feed
- Peristomal (around the hole) infection
- Ischaemic pressure necrosis (tissue death from a lack of blood supply as a result of pressure)
- Gastrocolic fistula (an abnormal passage between the stomach and the colon)
- Haemorrhage
- A blocked tube.

When the gasrostomy feeding tube is no longer required, endoscopy may be needed to remove the internal retaining disc. The balloon is simply deflated.

Clients who are tube-fed miss out on the social and emotional bonds that can be part of eating together with family and friends. It is also important to encourage oral stimulation to maintain chewing and swallowing skills (Townley and Robinson, 1997), which can be fundamentally important in children with disabilities who have never been orally fed. The client must be given the opportunity to see, hear, smell and taste the food before being fed via the tube as the sensory stimulation enables the client's body to prepare for the meal. Oral stimulation is not the same as oral intake, which may be unsafe because of the client's inability to swallow (Townley and Robinson, 1997).

■ Obesity

For many clients, obesity is more of a problem than undernutrition. The equation is deceptively simple: the energy expended must be balanced by the energy gained. The body's metabolism slows over time so, as people become less active because of age, illness or labour-saving devices, they need to adjust their intake downward and try to keep their activity level up. Nearly half of Britain's population is overweight (a BMI of over 25), and one in five is clinically obese (with a

BMI of over 30). Obesity can reduce a person's life expectancy, the increased weight relating to conditions such as coronary heart disease, **diabetes**, **gallstones**, hypertension (Field et al., 2001), blood lipid abnormalities, osteoarthritis and respiratory disease, not to mention endometrial and large bowel malignancies. There is also some suggestion that obesity is linked to childhood asthma (Von Mutius et al., 2001). The obese client may well experience psychological and social problems too (Thomas, 1998).

The role of the nurse is to help obese clients to identify the sources and causes of excess energy in their diet (usually fat, although it may be alcohol) and help them make their intake healthier. The distribution of food across the day may affect how many calories are absorbed. Breakfast 'kick-starts' the metabolism; the main meal of the day should be lunch, and the evening meal should be a light one.

Any changes made should be part of lifestyle modification rather than just 'going on a diet': diets do not work, eating sensibly does. 'Yo-yo' dieting tends to replace fat removed from the hips with fat around the waist, transforming the person from a 'pear' to an 'apple' shape, which increases the risk of coronary heart disease. Lean et al. (1995, 1998) showed that men with a waist size of greater than 102 cm (approximately 40 inches), and women with a greater than 88 cm (about 34 ⅔ inches) waist were more at risk, as this parameter appears to be a good measure of intra-abdominal fat. Waist circumference is hardly influenced by age or height, and reducing it improves cardiovascular risk factors (Lean et al., 1995, 1998).The best weight loss is a slow one, no more than 1 kg (2.2 lb) per week. If the activity level is being markedly increased, the weight loss could and should be slower, as muscle is heavier than fat, a pound of muscle being the size of a bar of soap, and a pound of fat the size of a football. Muscle is more metabolically active tissue and more useful to general health, rendering its owner more resilient. The role of exercise cannot be ignored in terms of the enhancement of mood as well as the burning of more energy. It is possible to slightly restrict the energy intake of sick clients without detrimentally affecting their condition (Sikora and Jensen, 1997).

The role of the nurse is to make sure that any strategies are thought through with the whole team, including a dietitian.

■ Chapter Summary

This chapter has reviewed the basic essentials of nutrition and hydration, and has made suggestions on how to enhance the health-giving benefits of food and fluid in both the short and the long term. Macronutrients, micronutrients and current recommendations on intake have been described. The assessment of clients' nutritional status is the basis for intervention, and ideas have been offered to assist clients in achieving optimum nutrition and hydration. A range of helpful strategies for feeding and hydrating clients, including artificial nutritional support, is outlined to extend your skills in promoting effective nutrition and hydration.

Throughout this process, it must be remembered that securing the well-being and dignity of the client is paramount. Thus, the education of readers, clients, carers and colleagues in terms of the objectives of care and monitoring the effectiveness of interventions is part of an ongoing process.

● Test Yourself!

1. Put the following into a league table according to their energy density in terms of kilojoules (or kilocalories):

   - alcohol
   - carbohydrate
   - fat
   - protein.

2. List at least two functions of fibre in the diet.

3. Name three sources of fibre in the diet.

4. Work out your fluid volume requirement per 24 hours.

5. What is an antioxidant?

6. Which are the antioxidant vitamins, minerals and trace elements?

7. Calculate your BMI, and do the same for one of your clients.

Further Reading

Ahmad, W.I.U. (ed.) (1993) *Race and Health in Contemporary Britain* (Black Report). Open University Press, Milton Keynes.

Blythman, J. (1996) *The Food We Eat*. Michael Joseph, London.

Bond, S. (1997) *Eating Matters*. Centre for Health Services Research, University of Newcastle, Newcastle upon Tyne.

British Nutrition Foundation (1995) *Vegetarianism: Briefing Paper*. British Nutrition Foundation, London.

Campbell, J. (1993) The mechanics of eating and drinking. *Nursing Times* **89**(21): 32–3.

Carlisle, D. (1997) Formula baby milk: what are the facts? *Nursing Times* **93**(24): 60–2.

Further Reading continued

Davies, J. and Dickerson, J.W.T. (1991) *Nutrient Content of Food Portions*. Royal Society of Chemistry, London.

Hamilton-Smith, S. (1972) *Nil by Mouth?* RCN, London.

Holmes, S. (1993) Building blocks. *Nursing Times* **89**(21): 28–31.

Jones, D.C. (1975) *Food for Thought*. RCN, London.

King's Fund Report (1992) *A Positive Approach to Nutrition as Treatment*. King's Fund Centre, London.

Orbach, S. (1986) *Fat is a Feminist Issue*. Arrow Books, London.

Paul, A.A. and Southgate, D.A.T. (1991) *McCance and Widdowson's The Composition of Foods*, 5th edn. HMSO, London.

Rogers, J. (2000) Maintaining fluid balance in children. *NTPlus* **96**(31): s7.

Saunders, T. and Bazalgette, P. (1991) *The Food Revolution*. Transworld Publishers, London.

Thompson, S.B.N. (1993) *Eating Disorders: A Guide for Health Professionals*. Chapman & Hall, London.

Tolonen, M. (1990) *Vitamins and Minerals in Health and Nutrition*. Ellis Horwood, Chichester.

Townsend, P. and Davidson, N. (eds) *Inequalities in Health. The Black Report*. Open University Press, Milton Keynes.

UKCC (2001) Disguising medication. *Register* **37**: 7.

Webb, G.P. and Copeman, J. (1996) *The Nutrition of Older Adults*. Edward Arnold, London.

Whitehead, M. (1992) *Health Divide*. Penguin, Harmondsworth.

Wilson, A.C., Stewart Forsyth, J., Greene, S.A. et al. (1998) Relation of infant diet to childhood health: seven year follow up cohort of children in Dundee infant feeding study. *British Medical Journal* **316**(7124): 21–5.

Wolf, N. (1991) *The Beauty Myth*. Vintage, London.

Wykes, R. (1997) The nutritional and nursing benefits of social mealtimes. *Nursing Times* **93**(4): 32–4.

■ References

Abdulla, A. and Keast, J. (1997) Hypodermoclysis as a means of rehydration. *Nursing Times* **93**(29): 54–5.

Barasi, M.E. (1997) *Human Nutrition: A Health Perspective*. Edward Arnold, London.

Bender, D.A. (1993) *Introduction to Nutrition and Metabolism*. UCL Press, London.

Bender, D.A. (1997) *Introduction to Nutrition and Metabolism*, 2nd edn. UCL Press, London.

Bonner, A. and Waterhouse, J. (eds) (1996) *Addictive Behaviour: Molecules to Mankind*. Macmillan – now Palgrave Macmillan, Basingstoke.

Coghlan, A. (1997) A cheeky little powder and it travels well. *New Scientist* **153**(2070): 4.

COMA (Committee on Medical Aspects of Food Policy) (1989). *Dietary Sugars and Human Disease*. Report on Health and Social Subjects No. 37. HMSO, London.

DoH (Department of Health) (1991) *Dietary Reference Values for Food Energy and Nutrients for the United Kingdom. Report of the Panel on Dietary Reference Values of the Committee on Medical Aspects of Food Policy*. HMSO, London.

DoH (Department of Health) (1992) *The Health of the Nation: A Strategy for Health in England*. HMSO, London.

DoH (Department of Health) (1995) *Sensible Drinking: The Report of an Inter-department Working Group*. DoH, London.

DoH (Department of Health) (1998) *Saving Lives: Our Healthier Nation*. HMSO, London.

Donnelly, M. (1999) The benefits of hypodermoclysis. *Nursing Standard* **13**(52): 44–5.

Field, A.E., Coakley, E.H., Must, A. et al. (2001) Impact of overweight on the risk of developing chronic diseases during a 10-year period. *Archives of Internal Medicine* **161**(13): 1581–6.

Fieldhouse, P. (1995) *Food and Nutrition. Customs and Culture*, 2nd edn. Chapman & Hall, London.

Higgins, C. (1997) Measurement of cholesterol and triglyceride. *Nursing Times* **93**(15): 54–5.

Iggulden, H. (1999) Dehydration and electrolyte disturbance. *Nursing Standard* **13**(19): 48–56.

Johnson, R. (2001) Burn rate: is it your metabolism or your eating habits? *American Vogue* April, 276–80.

Lean, M.E.J., Han, T.S. and Morrison, C.E. (1995) Waist circumference as a measure for indicating need for weight management. *British Medical Journal* **311**: 158–61.

Lean, M.E.J., Han, T.S. and Seidall, J.C. (1998) Impairment of health and quality of life in people with large waist circumference. *Lancet* **351**: 853–6.

Lyman, B. (1989) *A Psychology of Food: More than a Matter of Taste*. Van Nostrand Reinhold, New York.

McPherson, G. (1993) Absorbing effects: drug interactions. *Nursing Times* **91**(23): 30–2.

Marmot, M. (1995) A not-so-sensible drinks policy. *Lancet* **346**(8992): 1643–4 (letter).

Micklewright, A. and Todorovic, V. (1997) Good old home cooking. *Nursing Times* **93**(49): 58–9.

Milne, D.B. (2001) Too much soda pop takes the fizz out of your bones. Grand Forks Human Nutrition Research Center. http://www.gfhnrc.ars.usda.gov/News [accessed 8 March 2002].

Morrison, C. (2000) Helping patients to maintain a healthy fluid balance. *NTPlus* **96**(31): s3.

Nicholls, J. (2001) Should nurses give medication without the patient's consent? Yes. *Nursing Times*, **97**(41): 17.

Rollins, H. (1997) Nutrition and wound healing. *Nursing Standard* **11**(51): 49–52.

Rutishauser, S. (1994) *Physiology and Anatomy*. Churchill Livingstone, Edinburgh.

Sakurai, Y., Kono, S., Honjo, S. et al. (1995) Relation of waist-hip ratio to glucose tolerance, blood pressure, and serum lipids in middle-aged Japanese males. *International Journal of Obesity* **19**: 632–7.

Sanders, T. (1994) *Dietary Fats: Nutrition Briefing Paper.* Health Education Authority, London.

Shepheard, J. (1998) Learning disability: empowerment. *Nursing Standard* **12**(17): 49–55.

Sikora, S.A. and Jensen, G.L. (1997) Hypoenergetic nutrition support in hospitalized obese patients. *American Journal of Clinical Nutrition* **66**(3): 546–50 (editorial comment).

Simpson, P.M. (1992) Alcohol consumption in the elderly. *Nutrition Research Reviews* **5**: 153–66.

Thomas, D. (1998) Managing obesity: the nutritional aspects. *Nursing Standard* **12**(18): 49–55.

Townley, R. and Robinson, C. (1997) Comfort eating. *Nursing Times* **93**(34): 74.

UKCC (United Kingdom Central Council for Nursing, Midwifery and Health Visiting) (1997) Feeding of Patients (letter). UKCC, London.

Von Mutius, E., Schwartz, J., Neas, L.M., Dockery, D. and Weiss, S.T. (2001) Relation of body mass index to asthma and atopy in children: the National Health and Nutrition Examination Study III. *Thorax* **56**(11): 835–8.

■ Acknowledgement

Many thanks to Dr Sue Green for her rigorous review and helpful suggestions and support.

BARBARA MARJORAM

Chapter

Elimination

5

Contents

- Faecal Elimination
- Urinary Elimination
- Chapter Summary
- Test Yourself!
- Further Reading
- References

Learning outcomes

The purpose of this chapter is to explore the urinary and faecal elements of elimination, explaining the normal and abnormal processes and influences on it. At the end of the chapter, you should be able to:

- Explain the development of elimination that an individual experiences throughout the life span

- Identify specimens that may be collected and common abnormalities that may be found

- Understand the causes of constipation and diarrhoea, and the nursing care of clients experiencing these

- Outline the types of urinary and faecal incontinence and the possible treatments and interventions available

- Introduce the different types of stoma and the specific care that clients with them require.

The chapter provides an opportunity for you to undertake activities that will assist you in your understanding of some aspects of client care. It also includes case study scenarios to illustrate points made in the text.

Elimination of excess water and wastes is a basic need for all forms of life. (Lewis and Timby, 1993)

Successful elimination in humans depends on the individual having an intact and fully functioning gastrointestinal tract, urinary tract and nervous system.

■ Faecal Elimination

The lower gastrointestinal tract (Figure 5.1) includes the small and large intestines. The small intestine (duodenum, jejunum and ileum) is approximately 610 cm (20 feet) long and 2.5 cm (1 inch) in diameter in an adult. The partially

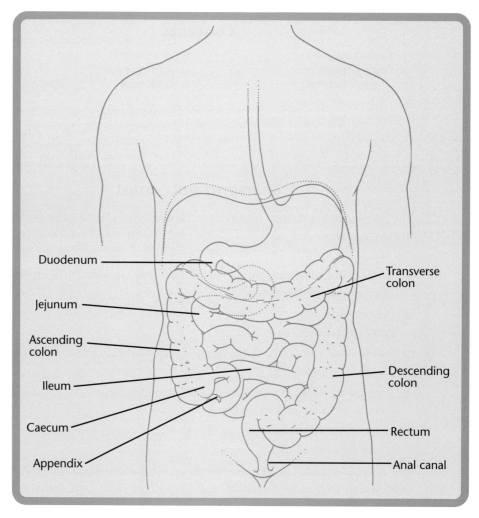

Figure 5.1 ● The main structures of the lower gastrointestinal tract

digested food (chyme) leaving the stomach is moved along the small intestine by **peristalsis**. The large intestine (caecum, colon, rectum and anus) is approximately 152 cm (5 feet) long and 6 cm (2.5 inches) in diameter. The faeces – the waste material of digestion that is passed out of the body via the anus or any other opening (stoma) designed for this purpose following surgery (see below) – are moved along the length of the large intestine in response to food entering the stomach. This **gastrocolic reflex,** which propels the faeces by mass peristalsis and is associated with eating, usually occurs three or four times a day, during or immediately after a meal.

The defaecation reflex is initiated by the response to faeces entering the rectum. This reflex encourages the internal anal sphincter to relax, the need to defaecate being conveyed to the brain and interpreted by the individual as an awareness of the requirement to eliminate faeces.

The 'normal' defaecation pattern varies from one individual to another, some defaecating three times a day, others only once a week.

Development of faecal elimination

Infant

At birth, the muscles of the infant's intestines are poorly developed and control by the nervous system is immature. The intestines contain some simple digestive enzymes but are unable to break down complex carbohydrates or proteins, so the infant can, therefore, digest only simple foods (Cox et al., 1993).

The infant's first bowel movement usually occurs within the first 24 hours of birth and comprises **meconium**, which contains salts, amniotic fluid, mucus, bile and epithelial cells. It is greenish-black to light brown in colour, almost odourless and of a tarry consistency. With the introduction of milk feeding, the characteristics of the infant's faeces change. The infant who is breastfed will have a stool that is bright yellow, soft and semiliquid, whereas the bottle-fed infant's stool will be light yellow to brown in colour and more formed (Cox et al., 1993). During the first 4 weeks of life, the infant will have up to 4–8 soft bowel movements per day. This number gradually decreases so that, by the fourth week, the number of bowel movements is 2–4 per day. By 4 months of age, the infant has gradually developed a predictable pattern of faecal elimination.

Toddler to preschool

The nervous and gastrointestinal systems gradually mature and are, by the age of 2–3 years, ready to control the function of faecal elimination. The infant develops patterns of defaecation so the parents can identify when their child will have success on the potty. Eating stimulates peristaltic activity and defaecation

---

peristalsis

the co-ordinated serial contraction of smooth muscle propelling food through the digestive tract

gastrocolic reflex

a mass peristaltic movement of the large intestine occurring shortly after food enters the stomach

---

CONNECTIONS

Chapter 4 suggests how to make use of the gastrocolic reflex in clients with communication difficulties.

---

meconium

the thick, sticky material that accumulates in the fetus' intestines and forms the newborn's first stools (see above), and this can be used as a sign to take the child to the toilet. As elimination is a natural process, it is important that the child does not feel that it is a dirty or unnatural procedure.

The child, even though toilet trained, can still have 'accidents', often when the urge to defaecate is allowed to progress inappropriately. If the child becomes so engrossed in what he is doing, he may ignore the need for defaecation and become constipated.

Activity 1

For further information, read Rutishauser 1994, pp. 114–36; Seeley et al., 1995, pp. 808–34; or Marieb, 1995, pp. 813–926.

School-aged child

During the school years, the gastrointestinal system attains adult functional maturity. Individuals with learning disabilities may not reach the indicated maturation milestones because of their disability or lack of perception.

Adolescent

Adolescence is important as the developing bowel habits will take them through their adult life. Adolescents often find it difficult to talk about any elimination problem as they develop sexually.

Activity 2

Make a list of all the words you have heard or read that describe bowel habit. You may like to discuss this list with your colleagues. This will help you to understand some of the 'language' your clients may use.

Adult

A healthy adult usually eliminates 100–150 g of faeces per day, 30–50 g being solids and the remaining 70–100 g water. The solids are made up of cellulose, epithelial cells shed from the lining of the gastrointestinal tract, bacteria, some salts and the brown pigment stercobilin. The brown-coloured faeces occur as a result of the breakdown of bile by the intestinal bacteria. If bile is unable to enter the intestines as a result of obstruction of the bile ducts (which transport bile from the gallbladder to the duodenum), the faeces are white.

irritable bowel syndrome

abnormally increased motility of the bowel, often associated with emotional stress

Crohn's disease

a chronic, often patchy, inflammatory bowel disease of unknown origin, usually affecting the ileum

There may be an increasing incidence of intestinal disorders (colonic and rectal carcinoma, and other gastrointestinal conditions such as **irritable bowel syndrome** and **Crohn's disease**) in adulthood. These can be caused by a decrease in the excretion of digestive enzymes (pepsin, ptyalin and pancreatic enzymes) and gastric acid. Elimination patterns are affected by changing lifestyle, for example marriage, having children and changes in employment, which may precipitate stress and anxiety.

Ageing adult

The decrease in the excretion of digestive enzymes continues with age. The elimination process may be affected by changing dietary intake caused by a reduced

Chart 5.1 ● Why do we collect specimens?

- To identify the nature of any disease or for diagnosis
- To assess the effect of treatment
- To confirm or eliminate a specific site of the body as a focus of infection or colonisation
- To determine whether a client who has had an infection is still harbouring the pathogen responsible for it. Clients who have *Salmonella* food poisoning may, for example, still harbour the bacteria in their stools even though their signs and symptoms have disappeared

production of saliva, fewer taste buds and the loss of natural teeth, which are replaced by dentures, caps, crowns and bridges.

Specimen collection

Specimens are samples of tissue, body fluids, secretions or excretions (Chart 5.1). Nurses often have responsibility for the collection, labelling and timely, safe transport of samples to the laboratory. The validity of test results therefore depends on good practice.

specimens
samples of tissue, body fluids, secretions or excretions

The most common observations the nurse will be required to make of the patient and the specimen are:

- Colour (see above)
- Frequency/time
- Amount
- Consistency
- Odour
- Foreign substances (presence or absence)
- Any pain/discomfort expressed by the client on eliminating.

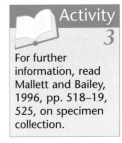

Activity
3
For further information, read Mallett and Bailey, 1996, pp. 518–19, 525, on specimen collection.

Using these observations, it is important that the nurse makes a clear, accurate and concise report in the client's records.

Faecal specimens

Faeces may be analysed to detect abnormal characteristics or contents, for example blood, parasites, parasite eggs and pathogens.

It is essential that the faecal specimen is not contaminated, so the client is asked to void urine separately into a toilet, bedpan or urinal; urine can interfere with the examination of the faeces, for example destroying some parasites. The client is then asked to pass the faeces into a bedpan. The nurse transfers approximately 15 g (3 teaspoons) of the faeces into the specimen collection container. Care should be taken not to contaminate the outside of the specimen container with the faeces (containers usually having a built-in spatula to assist with this).

Altered faecal elimination

Constipation

constipation

the abnormally difficult, infrequent or incomplete passage of hard faeces

Constipation refers to the abnormally difficult or infrequent passage of hard faeces and is caused by a decreased motility of the intestines. Some elderly individuals find it difficult to pass soft, bulky faeces. The longer the faeces remain in the intestine, the more water is absorbed from them, which makes them become harder and dryer.

Many individuals wrongly regard themselves as being constipated if they do not defaecate every day. Some individuals who are constipated have episodes of diarrhoea that can be the result of the hard faeces irritating the colon (often termed constipation with overflow). It is, therefore, essential that a note of the normal bowel habits of clients is included in the admission procedure and recorded.

Causes of constipation

Causes of constipation include the following:

Activity 4

List all the factors that may predispose the individual to constipation.

diverticular disease

a condition in which pouch-like extensions develop through the muscular layer of the colon, affecting the passage of faeces

paraplegia

paralysis or sensory loss of the lower limbs, usually including the bladder and rectum

- *Drugs:* tranquillisers, narcotics, anticholinergics and antacids containing aluminium as these reduce the motility of the intestines
- *Laxatives:* the abuse of laxatives or frequent enemas. The normal reflexes then diminish, causing the abuser to need more laxative to provide a result and thus become dependent on laxatives
- *Pregnancy:* limits the space for the faeces to pass through the intestine. Peristalsis slows because progesterone causes an excessive absorption of water from the faeces
- *Disease:* obstruction from outside or within the intestine, for example from an abdominal or intestinal tumour, interfering with the passage of faeces. Other causes include irritable bowel syndrome, **diverticular disease** and neurological deficiencies such as **paraplegia** and multiple sclerosis
- *Pain:* for example, from an anal fissure (a longitudinal ulcer in the anal canal) or external haemorrhoids (varicose veins in the anal canal, colloquially known as piles)

Casebox 5.1

Mary, aged 32, uses the mental health services for depression and takes her antidepressants as prescribed. She has found it difficult to hold down a job and is at present unemployed, living on benefit payments in her bedsit.

What is the probable impact of depression on Mary's elimination status?

Identify the associated symptoms and signs that

Mary may experience as a result of her elimination problems?

■ A lack of interest in her surroundings and diet, as well as her medication, may cause Mary to become constipated.

■ The symptoms and signs that Mary may experience are:
  – Altered bowel habit, with a lower than usual frequency
  – Straining on defaecation

– Abdominal and/or back pain
– Changing shape of the faeces
– Hard, formed faeces
– A palpable abdominal mass
– Halitosis
– Headache (because of possible dehydration and the build-up of toxins)
– Impairment of appetite
– Increased frequency of micturition (as a result of pressure from the faecal mass).

Casebox 5.2

Zandra, aged 5, was upset by her father's drinking and her parents' subsequent divorce. She has become chronically constipated.

Define constipation.

How would you relieve Zandra's constipation? (See Chapter 4.)

■ Constipation refers to the abnormally difficult or infrequent passage of hard faeces and is caused by the decreased motility of the intestines.

■ To relieve Zandra's constipation, first assess her diet and fluid intake, and advise accordingly. Try to

assess whether she is depressed because of the divorce, with a view to referring her for counselling if necessary.

● *Psychiatric reasons:* depression, leading to a lack of interest in the surroundings and diet, chronic psychoses and anorexia nervosa, which can cause an imbalanced or inappropriate dietary intake and therefore a low fibre and fluid intake
● *Diet:* food low in fibre or an inadequate food intake
● *Lack of fluid:* either an insufficient intake of fluid or, rarely, an excessive loss of fluid through vomiting and/or sweating
● *Immobility:* any disease that predisposes to immobility or any enforced immobility from bedrest reducing the motility of the gastrointestinal tract

CONNECTIONS

Chapter 4 explains the different types of fibre and how they affect elimination.

- *Ignoring the call to defaecate:* which allows more fluid to be absorbed from the faeces, thus making them harder and more difficult to eliminate
- *Psychological factors:* unfavourable lavatory conditions, poor hygiene or having to use commodes and bedpans, which may result in the client delaying the defaecation process.

Care of client with constipation

With his or her help, a history must be taken of the patient's normal elimination pattern. If a diagnosis of constipation is made, an assessment can be undertaken to aid the planning of the client's care.

It is the nurse's responsibility to promote an understanding of the measures available to overcome constipation. The client needs to be educated in the signs and symptoms that are associated with constipation, for example:

Activity 5

Calculate your fluid intake over 24 hours and compare it with the recommendation of 30–35 ml/kg per day.

- Altered bowel habit, with a lower than usual frequency
- Straining on defaecation
- Abdominal and/or back pain
- Changing shape of the faeces
- Hard, formed faeces
- A palpable abdominal mass
- Halitosis (bad breath)
- Headache (owing to possible dehydration and the build-up of toxins)
- Impaired appetite
- An increased frequency of **micturition** because of increased pressure on the bladder from an increased mass in the large intestines.

micturition

the voiding of urine

Clients may require advice on:

CONNECTIONS

Chapter 4 provides details of requirements for and sources of fibre, and the effects of various fluids.

- *Dietary intake:* increasing the proportion of fibre
- *Fluid intake:* increasing fluids and avoiding excess alcohol as this acts as a diuretic. The client should be advised to drink 30–35 ml/kg per day (unless other medical conditions restrict this)
- *Mobility:* doing more exercise, if other medical conditions allow, to aid in increasing the motility of the gastrointestinal tract.

Although laxatives should be avoided, they may be used only as a short-term measure as prolonged use can lead to dependency, which may result in faecal impaction at a future date.

Other measures to treat constipation include the use of enemas and suppositories. Suppositories are bullet shaped and are designed to melt once they have been inserted into the rectum. Some suppositories soften the faeces and some

Casebox 5.3

Mrs Ghosh is 89 and has been living in a residential care home for 3 years. She used to walk in the garden each day but now finds it difficult, requiring a helping hand for safety.

Mrs Ghosh spends most of her day sitting in either the lounge or her bedroom. Her gums are very sore as her dentures are not fitting properly, so she will only eat 'sloppy' food.

Why does Mrs Ghosh have a potential risk of suffering from constipation (see Chapters 4 and 8)?

What drugs can treat constipation but when abused can cause it?

■ There is a risk of constipation because of immobility, ignoring the call to defaecate, possible depression, leading to a lack of interest in her surroundings and diet, a lack of fibre and, because of her immobiliy, drinking only the amount of fluid on offer, which may not be sufficient.

■ Laxatives can both treat and predispose to constipation.

Casebox 5.4

Adam, aged 50, has learning disabilities and multiple physical disabilities. He has just moved to a group home in the community. He suffers from chronic constipation as a result of long-term care in an institution where he had a poor diet (lacking in fruit and vegetables), restricted access to fluids and little exercise. Previous care to relieve his constipation included enemas and laxatives.

Adam's new GP has advised the discontinuation of the enemas and laxatives in order to treat his constipation.

What changes to Adam's lifestyle would you consider to improve his elimination problems (see also Chapters 4 and 7)?

■ Adam needs to increase his mobility. His diet should be assessed and relevant advice given, emphasising an increase in the amount of fruit and vegetables. Fluid intake should also be assessed, the target being an intake of 30–35 ml/kg per day. Discourage Adam from ignoring the call to defaecate, and gradually reduce his enemas and laxatives.

lubricate the anal canal, whereas others use chemicals to stimulate peristalsis. Other types of suppository that the nurse may use do not promote elimination but are treatments for other conditions, for example infections and pain; these include antibiotic and analgesic preparations. Enemas are solutions that are instilled into the large intestine, the most common being a type of cleansing solution used to empty the lower intestinal tract of faeces.

To insert or introduce a suppository or enema, the client is asked to lie on his left side with his knees bent and drawn up gently towards his abdomen (Figure

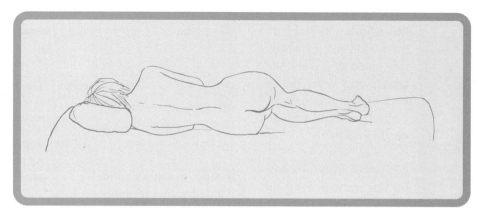

Figure 5.2 ● Left lateral position

5.2). The left side is the preferred side for lying on as the bowel will be angled downward, which will aid the retention of the suppository or enema and help to prevent trauma to the rectum. The suppository or enema is gently introduced into the rectum and the client is asked to retain it for approximately 15 minutes to allow the chemicals to stimulate defaecation. Clients often feel that they wish to defaecate as soon as the suppository or enema has been introduced into the rectum because of stimulation caused by the insertion: the anus and rectum react to the stretching of the muscle by sending the information to the brain that the rectum is full.

For some clients, for example those who are paraplegic/quadriplegic or grossly constipated, the only method of faecal elimination available to them is manual evacuation. The client is required to lie on the left side, and the nurse will remove the impacted faeces by hooking them out of the rectum using a gloved finger or two fingers to break them up. This should be used only in exceptional circumstances and not as a routine alternative to other methods of aiding faecal elimination. **Do not employ the procedure without specific instruction** as there is an associated danger of perforation of the lower gastrointestinal tract.

Diarrhoea

diarrhoea

the frequent passage of loose, watery stools

Diarrhoea results when movements of the intestine occur too rapidly for water to be absorbed. Faeces are therefore produced in large amounts and may range from being 'loose' to being entirely liquid. If the diarrhoea is severe, large amounts of fluid, consisting of ingested fluids and digestive juices together with sodium and potassium, are lost in the faeces; this can rapidly result in dehydration and electrolyte imbalance.

Causes of diarrhoea

Causes of diarrhoea include:

- *Lack of hygiene:* poor hygiene when preparing food after elimination, causing the contamination of ingested food
- *Laxatives:* laxative abuse
- *Infected food: Staphylococcus pyogenes, Salmonella, Escherichia coli* and *Campylobacter*
- *Stress:* excitement, stress and anxiety, causing an increased rate of peristalsis so that the faecal material moves faster through the intestines and less water is absorbed
- *Diet:* excessive fibre-rich foods, drinks high in caffeine, which stimulates intestinal motility, and allergy to some foodstuffs, causing irritation of the intestine
- *Disease:* diseases such as ulcerative colitis, Crohn's disease, diverticular disease and irritable bowel syndrome can result in swings between diarrhoea and constipation. Malabsorption syndrome can cause fatty diarrhoea (steatorrhoea).

Care of the patient with diarrhoea

It is essential that fluid balance is maintained as the client can quickly become dehydrated. The nurse must therefore assess the client for signs of dehydration (tachycardia and decreased skin turgor), and the client's input and output of fluid must be accurately recorded. Oral fluid should be high in added potassium and sodium, for example commercially prepared drinks such as Dioralyte or flat cola with a pinch of salt. In severe cases, an intravenous infusion may be required. Some herbal teas, for example rosehip, orange and rhubarb, should be avoided as they exacerbate diarrhoea (Newell et al., 1996).

A careful and thorough history must be taken from the client to ascertain the possible cause of the diarrhoea. All clients suffering from diarrhoea must be treated as potentially infectious until proved otherwise by laboratory examination of the faeces.

Skin care of the perianal region must be maintained as faeces contain digestive enzymes that cause local irritation. Barrier creams may be applied to the area once it has been thoroughly cleaned and dried.

Faecal incontinence

Faecal incontinence is very distressing for the individual as it is difficult to disguise expelled faeces. It is essential that a complete history is taken from the client as it may identify possible causes of the incontinence. These include:

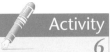

Activity 6

List all the factors that may predispose an individual to diarrhoea.

CONNECTIONS

Chapter 3 looks at food poisoning and food hygiene regulations that aim to reduce the risk of this.

ulcerative colitis

a chronic but inflammatory disease of the large bowel

steatorrhoea

fatty diarrhoea

CONNECTIONS

Chapter 3 identifies another method of assessing skin turgor.

Activity 7

Try the following exercise to assess skin turgor. Pinch the supraclavicular skin (above the collar bone). If a person is dehydrated, the skin fold will remain. In normal hydration, the skin will return to its normal position almost immediately. Older skin reacts more slowly than younger.

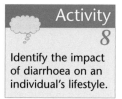

- Disease or injury: permanent or progressive conditions such as spinal cord damage, cerebrovascular accident (stroke) or multiple sclerosis: 50 per cent of patients with multiple sclerosis and 61 per cent of those with spinal injuries suffer from faecal incontinence (Kamm, 1998)
- Impacted faeces with overflow (spurious diarrhoea)
- Temporary loss of control caused by diarrhoea
- Laxative abuse
- Pudendal nerve damage after childbirth
- Infection
- Ulcerative colitis or Crohn's disease, which can lead to faecal urge incontinence
- Stress incontinence caused by chronic straining, trauma or a congenital defect, or arising post-partum
- Congenital malformation, for example anal atresia
- Rectal prolapse.

Management of faecal incontinence

The management will depend on the cause but will include:

- Administering suppositories or an enema every 2–3 days if the condition has been caused by faecal impaction, and then instigating a regimen to prevent recurrence
- Advice on changing the diet to one that is well balanced and high in fibre with an increased fluid intake (if other medical conditions allow)
- The treatment of any diarrhoea
- Controlling and trying to eliminate laxative intake if the condition has been caused by laxative abuse
- Advising clients to attend to their elimination needs after a meal to take advantage of the body's normal gastrocolic reflex
- The use of incontinence aids, such as pads, pants and bed protection
- Pelvic floor exercises (see below). For severe cases of stress incontinence, surgery is indicated, for example post-anal repair or repair after **rectoplexy** for rectal prolapse
- An artifical bowel sphincter (Ness 2000)
- When caring for clients with learning disabilities, a behavioural programme that involves prompt sitting on the toilet and other measures such as increased fluid intake and the use of fibre supplements or bulking agents to help normal bowel function (Smith et al., 1994).

rectoplexy

the fixation of the rectum by suturing to surrounding tissue

Stoma care

The word 'stoma' is derived from Greek meaning mouth or opening. A stoma is formed following surgical intervention for a disease process, its full name being determined by its site. A stoma for elimination purposes is therefore an opening on to the surface of the abdomen through which faecal elimination from either the small or large intestine (or urinary elimination; see below) takes place.

The formation of either a temporary or permanent stoma may be the result of elective surgery or an emergency procedure.

Colostomy

A **colostomy** is an opening from the colon, which may be temporary or permanent and is indicated for the treatment of the following conditions:

colostomy
an opening of the colon on to the abdominal wall

- Malignancy of the colon or rectum, Black (2000) reporting that colorectal cancer is the second most common malignancy in the Western world
- Diverticular disease
- Inflammatory disease of the intestine (for example Crohn's disease or ulcerative colitis)
- Trauma to the large intestine
- The relief of acute intestinal obstruction or perforation
- The protection of a distal **anastomosis**, the stoma being formed in a position higher in the gastrointestinal tract than the join between the two ends of intestine that remain after a section of bowel has been removed.

anastomosis
the joining of two hollow structures

A permanent colostomy is required when the distal segment of the large intestine has been removed, for example when the rectum has been excised because of cancer. The stoma is created by bringing the proximal end of the colon out through an opening on to the anterior wall of the abdomen.

A temporary colostomy is usually necessary to divert the flow of faeces away from the distal part of the large intestine. The surgical technique permits the stoma to be closed once the condition requiring the surgery has been resolved.

The faecal material eliminated from a colostomy, especially if it is on the transverse or descending colon, will be semisolid once the initial postoperative period is complete and the client returns to a 'normal' diet.

Ileostomy

An **ileostomy** is an opening into the ileum and can be indicated for the treatment of the following conditions:

ileostomy
an opening of the ileum on to the abdominal wall

Chart 5.2 ● Faecal consistency

- *Ileostomy:* fluid faeces (of a porridge-like consistency), normally 500–800 ml every 24 hours
- *Transverse colostomy:* unformed faeces, semiliquid
- *Descending colostomy:* more formed faeces, near to the normal output for that patient

- Inflammatory disease of the intestine (for example Crohn's disease or ulcerative colitis)
- As a temporary measure to rest the large intestine after major large bowel surgery.

An ileostomy can be a permanent stoma when the colon has been removed (panproctocolectomy) or temporary to allow the disease process to resolve. A temporary stoma can be closed by anastomosis at a later date and the intestine returned to normal functioning.

The faecal material eliminated through an ileostomy (Chart 5.2) is liquid in consistency, containing digestive enzymes that can cause excoriation and erosion of the skin if it is not well protected.

excoriation

injury to the skin caused by trauma such as scratching, rubbing or chemicals, for example the combination of urine and/or faeces and air

Management of a client with a stoma

Preoperative care

The client will require a rigorous preoperative assessment, particularly if presenting with a history of chronic disease, weight loss or anorexia. Such clients may be debilitated, so malnutrition and electrolyte imbalances must be corrected to ensure optimum recovery as a state of catabolism can be detrimental to a client undergoing surgery (Torrance, 1991). Clients also require psychological preparation to prepare them for the change in body image, to reduce anxiety and for reassurance that they can return to their previous place in society.

The stoma nurse should ensure that the client is offered counselling prior to surgery. She, or the consultant if no stoma nurse is available, should mark appropriate sites for the stoma so that the surgery does not interfere postoperatively with normal activities of living (Chart 5.3). The client should be shown and allowed to discuss the appliances available (Figure 5.3).

Postoperative care

Up to 20 per cent of clients who have a stoma experience significant psychological problems postoperatively (White, 1998; Black, 2000) and will therefore

Chart 5.3 ● Sites to be avoided to facilitate the easy management of a stoma

● Old scars
● Bony prominences
● The umbilicus
● The pubic area
● Skin folds
● Where the clothing may interfere, for example around the waistband area

require a great deal of support, especially in the initial days, weeks and months after its formation. The elimination process of the body has changed, as has body image. Clients therefore have to be helped to adapt to the changes: preoperative counselling may help them to make a full recovery, returning home to a 'normal' life. Patients may initially demonstrate evidence of withdrawal and depression. Overcoming this is an important part of nursing care; if nurses can show that they accept the clients, this will give their clients confidence.

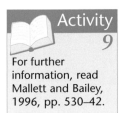

Activity 9

For further information, read Mallett and Bailey, 1996, pp. 530–42.

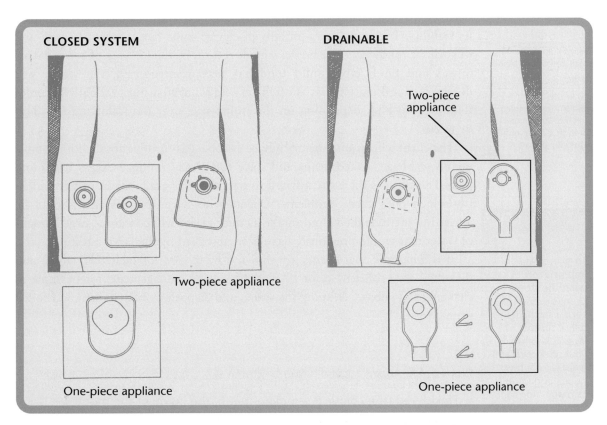

Figure 5.3 ● Stoma bags

CONNECTIONS

Chapter 7 mentions
the impact of stoma
surgery on body
image.

dyspareunia

the occurrence of pain
in the labial, vaginal or
pelvic region during or
after sexual intercourse

The formation of the stoma concerns not only clients, but also their partners, one reason being that the change in body image may cause their partners psychological difficulties from an inability to accept it. Clients who have an ileostomy or colostomy may experience sexual dysfunction (impotence in males and dyspareunia in females), but even if they suffer no problems, clients may not be able to return to their normal activities, including sexual activity until 2–3 months after the operation. This may be because of the trauma and oedema at the site of the surgery, or sometimes because of nerve damage.

Within our multicultural society, care must be provided that is appropriate to the health practices, values and beliefs of the client. As an example, clients who practise the Muslim religion of Islam are required to pray five times a day, before which they are required to perform a washing ritual called *al-wadhu* to signify the body's cleanliness inside and out. The client will need to apply a clean stoma appliance at each prayer time, so a two-piece appliance may be most suitable (Black, 2000).

Care specific to the stoma

haemoserous fluid

serous fluid containing
small amount of blood

flatus

gas in the
gastrointestinal tract,
which is often expelled
through a body orifice,
especially the anus

Postoperatively, the stoma must be checked regularly – its colour and size, whether it is retracting or prolapsing (Chart 5.4) and its function – to ensure its viability. The stoma may initially discharge some haemoserous fluid, and this will be followed, once bowel sounds return, by the passage of some flatus, mucus and fluid. Once solid food has been reintroduced, the stoma will discharge faecal matter that is often very liquid at first but gradually becomes fluid or semisolid, depending on the stoma site, over the following few days or weeks.

The client will require dietary advice as some gas-forming foods (for example onions, cabbage, baked beans and spicy food) may produce excess flatus and pain. The client is therefore advised to try out foods gradually in order to identify which ones cause problems. Clients who have an ileostomy should be advised to increase their fluid intake as their faeces will contain a large amount of water that would previously have been absorbed by the large intestine.

It is important that clients are shown how to care for their own stoma and that they are proficient prior to discharge in its management, for example in changing stoma bags, cleaning the stoma and disposing of equipment and soiled stoma bags.

Activity
10

To gain some
appreciation of
what the stoma
client experiences,
stick a stoma bag
full of slushy
Weetabix on to
your abdomen and
wear it for a few
hours, engaging in
as many 'normal'
activities as
possible.

Chart 5.4 ● Appearance of a normal stoma

- Pinkish red (the colour resembling that of the inside of the mouth)
- Initially postoperatively, the stoma is oedematous

Urinary Elimination

The normal anatomy of the urinary system is shown in Figure 5.4.

Development of urinary elimination

Infant

At birth, both nervous system control and renal function are immature, so there is an inability to concentrate the urine and urinary elimination is involuntary. Urinary output is affected by fluid intake, the amount of activity and the environmental temperature. If the infant is more active or the temperature is raised, more fluid will be excreted through the skin and more water vapour via exhaled air.

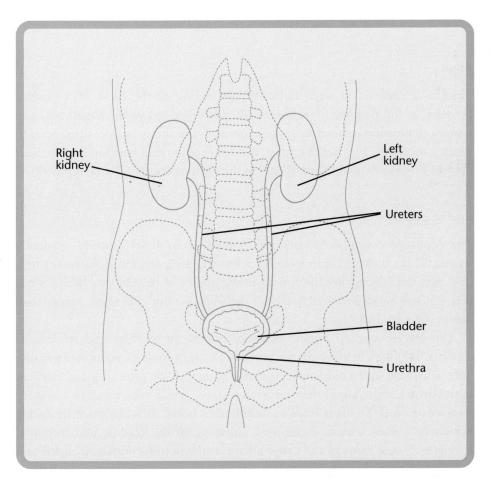

Figure 5.4 ● The main structures of the urinary system

Toddler to preschool

The bladder increases in size with the growth of the child and is now able to hold more urine. By 2 years of age, the kidneys are maturing and can conserve water and concentrate urine almost as well as those of the adult. The nervous system is mature enough for the toddler to control bladder functioning. Day-time bladder control is attained first, followed by night-time control. Even when toilet training has been achieved, however, there may be times of regression and 'accidents'.

School-aged child

The urinary system has now reached maturity.

Adolescent and young adult

There are no noticeable changes in urinary elimination during this time.

Adult

There is a decrease in renal function with ageing as the result of a gradual decrease in the number of nephrons. Bladder tone gradually diminishes, and urinary elimination is therefore more frequent as the ability to store urine prior to voiding decreases. In a healthy adult, the decrease in renal function is so gradual that the effects are minimal until later in the ageing process (Cox et al., 1993).

Ageing adult

sclerosis
―――――
hardening or induration
of an organ or tissue

The nephrons continue to decrease in number so renal function gradually lessens. This, combined with vascular **sclerosis**, decreases the glomerular filtration rate, thus decreasing the concentrating ability of the kidneys. Waste products are still processed effectively by the kidneys, but this takes longer than before (Cox et al., 1993).

urethritis
―――――
inflammation of the
urethra

The loss of smooth muscle elasticity affects the bladder and reduces its capacity. Inhibited bladder contraction can result in frequency and a premature urge to urinate. In the older male, the enlargement of the prostate gland can lead to **urethritis**, especially if there is urinary stasis, which may result in a urinary tract infection (UTI). This leads to dribbling of urine, difficulty in commencing urination, a poor stream, incomplete emptying of the bladder and increased frequency. These changes can cause nocturia (the need to urinate at night) and therefore disturbed sleep. The decrease in oestrogen level in females can predispose to stress incontinence.

Specimen collection

Urine specimens commonly collected are:

- Urine test for *routine screening*, for example on admission or as an outpatient screening procedure
- *Early morning urine* (EMU): because of **diurnal** variation, the first voided urine of the day is usually the most concentrated and is the preferred specimen when testing for substances present in a low concentration, for example hormones in a pregnancy test
- *24 hour urine collection*: used to assess the amount of a substance that is lost in the urine. Depending on the substance to be measured, a preservative may be required in the collection bottle, as in the creatinine clearance test (an increased amount of creatinine being found in the urine in the advanced stages of renal disease)
- *Midstream specimen of urine* (MSU), the object of collection being to obtain a specimen of urine uncontaminated by bacteria that may be present on the:
  - skin
  - external genital tract
  - perianal region
  - distal third of the urethra.

When a UTI is suspected, macroscopic and microscopic examination of an MSU will identify changes in the urine.

1. *Macroscopic examination:* although this is by no means diagnostic, the appearance of the urine can provide evidence of infection. Urinary infection, like any other bacterial infection, is associated with an increased number of white cells at the site of the infection and an inflammatory response that results in the production of pus. Pus in the urine (**pyuria**) renders it cloudy, so the majority of infected urine is cloudy and some is foul-smelling.
2. *Microscopic examination:* the number of white and red cells per mm^3 of urine is routinely counted. In good health, urine often contains a small number of these cells along with the occasional epithelial cell shed from the lining of the urinary tract. Fewer than 10 white cells/mm^3 is generally considered to be normal. Counts of between 20 and 50/mm^3 are most probably caused by infection but are also a feature of renal disease, so further tests may be requested to confirm the diagnosis. A count greater than 50/mm^3 indicates acute bacterial infection. Infected urine and urinary stasis can lead to crystallisation of the urine; both this and foreign bodies can cause urinary tract stones (Chart 5.5).

diurnal

occurring over a 24 hour period

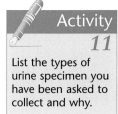

Activity 11

List the types of urine specimen you have been asked to collect and why.

pyuria

pus in the urine

Chart 5.5 ● Factors predisposing to urinary stone formation

idiopathic
_____

of unknown or
spontaneous origin

● Dehydration
● **Idiopathic** (most common)
● Urinary stasis
● Chronic urinary infection
● Foreign bodies (for example fragments of catheter tubing)
● Disease processes (for example gout and hyperparathyroidism)
● Immobility

Source: Burkitt et al. (1990).

Chart 5.6 ● Collection of a midstream specimen of urine

Protocol for women

meatus
_____

a passage or opening

1. The client should thoroughly wash her hands with soap and water
2. The area around the urinary **meatus** must be cleaned from front to back with soap and water
3. With one hand, the client should spread her labia, keeping them apart until the specimen has been collected
4. The client voids approximately the first 20 ml into the toilet and then passes a portion of the remaining urine into a sterile container. The remaining urine is passed into the toilet
5. The client's fingers should be kept away from the rim and inner surface of the container
6. The specimen is then labelled and, along with the investigation request slip, is forwarded to the laboratory for testing

Protocol for men

1. The client should thoroughly wash his hands with soap and water
2. The foreskin (if present) is retracted and the urinary meatus cleansed
3. The client voids approximately the first 20 ml into the toilet and then passes a portion of the remaining urine into a sterile container. The remaining urine is passed into the toilet
4. The client's fingers should be kept away from the rim and inner surface of the container
5. The client's foreskin (if present) should be returned to its normal position
6. The specimen is then labelled and, along with the investigation request slip, is forwarded to the laboratory for testing

Principles of collecting an MSU

Any bacteria present in the urethra are washed away in the first portion of urine voided, which is not collected. An avoidance of contamination by other bacteria is achieved by thorough cleansing and a good clean technique (Chart 5.6).

Catheter specimen of urine

A catheter specimen of urine (CSU) is taken using an aseptic technique. The catheter bag tubing is clamped (taking care not to damage the tubing) above the specimen portal and left for approximately 1 hour. The specimen portal is cleaned using an injection/alcohol swab and allowed to dry. A sterile needle (21 G × 1½ inches) is inserted into the portal, and a specimen of approximately 10–20 ml of urine is withdrawn into the syringe, the needle then being removed and the catheter bag tubing unclamped. The specimen should then be transferred to a sterile container, ensuring that the container is not contaminated. It is important that specimens are taken only from the portal that has been designed for this procedure as using any other site may cause the catheter, catheter bag or tube to leak. Urine taken from the catheter bag is too old and possibly too contaminated for an accurate test result.

Urine specimens should, if possible, be taken before antibiotics are commenced as any treatment may affect the result.

Urine testing for screening

It is important to remember that urine is a body fluid, so all precautions (as identified in a care setting's control of infection procedure book) must be taken for the nurse's safety.

All clients being admitted to hospital should have a urine test. This is one of the few times that urine is screened, and it can highlight any previously undiagnosed medical conditions, for example diabetes mellitus. It will also give baseline information on the client and may precipitate further investigations.

The client is asked to void a specimen of urine into a urinal, bedpan, jug or other clean receptacle.

The urine must be observed for its colour and odour before being tested with a reagent stick. Normal urine is pale and straw coloured, but the urine may be darker because of a loss of extra fluid through perspiration during hot weather, or from a limited fluid intake. Normal urine, when fresh, has little smell, but if left it may develop an odour of ammonia. Infected urine may be foul-smelling immediately after voiding and become worse on standing. The normal 'straw' colour may alter because of substances present in the urine (Figure 5.5).

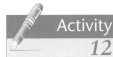

Activity 12

List the observations that may be made on a specimen of urine without using a test.

CONNECTIONS

Chapter 3 describes universal precautions.

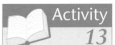

Activity 13

For exact details on how to test urine during routine screening, read the guidelines that are enclosed with all containers of urine test strips; these will be stocked in your clinical area.

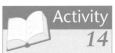

Activity 14

For further information, read Mallett and Bailey, 1996, pp. 525–6.

Casebox 5.5

Mrs MacDonnell, aged 72, has visited her GP complaining that her urine has been red.

What urinary test will the GP perform, and what do you expect the result to be?

What foods could Mrs MacDonnell have been eating that would turn her urine red?

■ A routine urine test and an MSU will be taken. These findings may be positive for haematuria, or negative if the problem is diet related. Even though Mrs MacDonnell is aged 72, vaginal bleeding (which could be disease related) should not be ruled out.

■ Beetroot or rhubarb could have this effect on her urine.

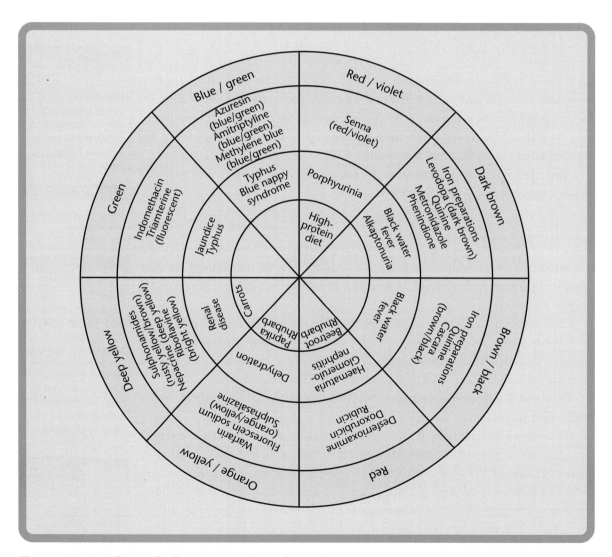

Figure 5.5 ● Effects of substances on the colour of urine (adapted from Ford, 1992)

Altered urinary elimination

Incontinence

Incontinence can be either permanent or temporary. It can be defined as the involuntary loss of urine and/or faeces at an inappropriate time or in an inappropriate place. This is a 'silent problem', many individuals being thought not to seek medical help because of embarrassment. The most recent figures report that 5–7 per cent of 15–44-year-olds, 8–15 per cent of 45–64-year-olds and 10–20 per cent of over-65-year-olds experience incontinence, 20 per cent of women aged over 40 years being affected by urinary incontinence (Thakar and Stanton, 2000). As well as causing clients considerable distress and discomfort, urinary incontinence costs the NHS approximately £424m per year (Continence Foundation, 2000).

Incontinence is not a disease but a symptom of an underlying disorder that can be mental, physical, social or environmental and affects both sexes at all ages. It may be primary, as in childhood **enuresis** or learning disability, or secondary to another cause such as prostatic enlargement, obesity or constipation. It can also result from a combination of these; that is, the cause can be multifactorial. As Cheater (1995) has identified, 'incontinence can have an adverse physical, psychological, social and economic consequence for the sufferer, family and carers'.

When assessing clients, their oral fluid intake should be reviewed as some herbal teas, for example elderberry, strawberry, rose, wild blackberry and nettle, act as diuretics (Newell et al., 1996).

There are four main types of urinary incontinence:

- Stress incontinence
- Urge incontinence
- Reflex incontinence
- Overflow incontinence.

The male and female urethras are shown in Figures 5.6 and 5.7 respectively (see also Chart 5.7).

incontinence

the involuntary loss of urine and/or faeces at an inappropriate time or in an inappropriate place

enuresis

an involuntary discharge of urine after the age by which bladder control should have been established. In children, a voluntary control of urination is usually established by the age of 5 years. Nocturnal enuresis is, however, present in about 10 per cent of otherwise healthy children at age 5 years, and 1 per cent at age 15

Stress incontinence

This type of incontinence is more common in females than males. A small amount of urine is leaked on physical exertion, coughing, sneezing or laughing. This results from an incompetent urethral sphincter, which is caused by a weakness of the supporting pelvic floor muscles. Predisposing factors include childbirth, hormonal changes owing to the menopause, vaginal prolapse, obesity, inactivity and constipation; in men, stress incontinence can occur after prostatectomy.

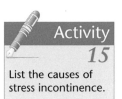

Activity
15

List the causes of stress incontinence.

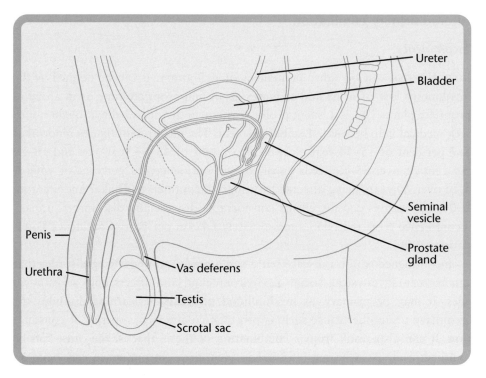

Figure 5.6 ● The position of the urethra in a male

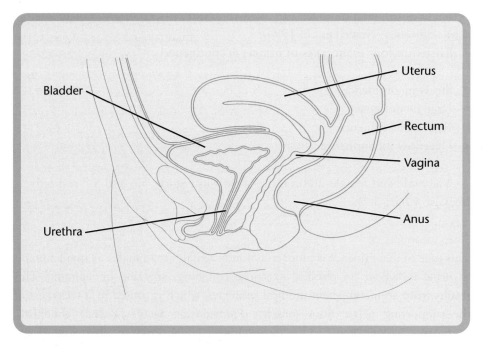

Figure 5.7 ● The position and angle of the urethra in a female

Chart 5.7 ● The female urethra

- The urethra is embedded in the anterior wall of the vagina
- It runs downwards and forwards behind the symphysis pubis and opens at the external urethral orifice, which lies just in front of the opening of the vagina
- Its diameter is approximately 0.7 mm
- It is approximately 4 cm long
- The urethra is 'slit-shaped' rather than cylindrical
- If there is a weakness of the pelvic floor muscles and the urethra becomes more vertical, it is easier for urine to leak out (incontinence)

Source: Haslam (1997).

Treatment includes pelvic floor exercises, weighted vaginal cones, electrical therapy that stimulates the nerves, causing the muscles to contract, special tampons, vaginal sponges and, in the case of postmenopausal women, hormone replacement therapy (Pomfret, 1993). Surgical intervention may include **vaginal repair**.

vaginal repair
following prolapse of the vagina and uterus, surgical repair is performed to return the structures to their normal position

Urge incontinence

Urge incontinence causes the loss of a variable amount of urine and is caused by **detrusor muscle** instability (an unstable bladder), neuropathic conditions and outflow obstruction. The individual often complains that he has little or no warning of a need to micturate and is often incontinent on the way to the toilet. Causes include urinary tract infection, bladder stones, an enlarged prostate gland, a urethral stricture, faecal impaction, Alzheimer's disease, cerebrovascular accident, spinal cord lesions and Parkinson's disease. Residual volumes of urine, left in the bladder after micturition, may occur causing urinary stasis and a subsequent UTI.

detrusor muscle
the external longitudinal layer of the muscular coat of the bladder

Treatment rarely involves surgery but does include bladder retraining exercises, **antimuscarinic** drug therapy and relaxation exercises.

There is a high level of mixed stress and urge incontinence, especially in the elderly.

antimuscarinic
opposing the action of muscarine or agents that mimic it, for example atropine and scopolamine

Reflex incontinence

This type of incontinence manifests itself as the individual's failure to recognise the need to micturate and is usually caused by damage of the peripheral nerves to the bladder or of the spinal cord. The bladder fills and empties on a reflex cycle, and the condition may be combined with incomplete voiding and a high residual urinary volume.

Treatment may involve surgery, for example urinary diversion or urostomy (see below). In addition, catheterisation (indwelling urethral, suprapubic or intermittent self-catheterisation) and other techniques, such as the Valsalva or Credé manoeuvre (Chart 5.8), may be used.

Overflow incontinence

Overflow incontinence is caused by urinary retention with overflow caused by:

- *Obstruction* from an enlarged prostate, prostatic cancer, urethral stricture or faecal impaction; treatment includes prostatectomy, urethrotomy and the clearance of any faecal impaction
- *Hypotonic bladder* (ineffective contraction of the bladder when voiding urine) caused by neuropathy (as in diabetes) or anticholinergic medication (such as imipramine); treatment includes intermittent self-catheterisation, drug therapy (for example carbachol) to enhance detrusor contractility and a review of drug regimens to ensure that other medication is not the cause of the hypotonia
- *Detrusor–sphincter dyssynergia* (uncoordinated muscle activity) caused by neuropathic conditions, for example paraplegia and multiple sclerosis; treatment includes intermittent self-catheterisation and **biofeedback** to teach co-ordination.

An indwelling catheter should be used only as a last resort for clients with voiding difficulties.

biofeedback

a training programme designed to develop one's ability to control the autonomic (involuntary) nervous system

Cystitis

Cystitis is inflammation of the bladder usually occurring secondary to an ascending UTI. It is more common in sexually active females because of the close

cystitis

inflammation of the bladder, usually secondary to an ascending UTI

Chart 5.8 ● Valsalva and Credé manoeuvres

Valsalva manoeuvre
The client is asked to inhale and then to attempt to forcibly exhale with the glottis (vocal cords), nose and mouth closed. This causes the diaphragm to flatten, thus increasing the intra-abdominal pressure. Unless the urethral sphincter is in complete spasm, the increased pressure forces urine to be voided. Clients with cardiac problems should not attempt this procedure

Credé manoeuvre
The client is asked to apply pressure over the symphysis pubis. The pressure may be enough to produce spasm of the bladder or cause voiding of the urine

proximity of the urethra and the vagina. In the acute stage, clients complain of frequent and painful micturition; in the chronic stage, it is secondary to a lesion that may have pyuria as its only symptom. Antibiotics are used to treat the infection, and the client should be encouraged to drink 2–3 litres of fluid per day (if the medical condition allows) to dilute the urine and decrease the pain on micturition.

Pelvic floor exercises

Pelvic floor exercises (Chart 5.9) are primarily intended to increase the strength of the levator ani muscles. In women, pelvic floor exercises involve the contraction and relaxation of the muscles that surround the vagina and anus, thus improving their tone. This helps to restore the normal anatomical relationships of the surrounding structures as well as the function of the urethral sphincter.

In males, pelvic floor exercises should be taught before prostatectomy so that they can help to stop post-micturition dribbling following prostatectomy by improving urethral sphincter function.

Urinary catheterisation

A urinary catheter is designed to remove fluid from or instil fluid into the bladder. Urinary catheterisation is a common procedure, 12 per cent of hospital clients (Crow et al., 1996) and 4 per cent of clients in the community (Getliffe, 1990) being catheterised at any one time.

Indications for catheterisation are:

● Pre- and postoperatively to empty the bladder before or after abdominal, rectal or pelvic surgery

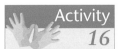

Activity 16

If you do not already practise pelvic floor exercises regularly, you should start now by following the instructions in Chart 5.9.

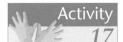

Activity 17

To perceive what clients experience when they are incontinent, wet a pad with water and wear it next to your skin in the perineal area. Undertake as many everyday activities as possible.

Chart 5.9 ● Pelvic floor exercises

The client needs to sit, stand or lie in a comfortable position and tighten the pelvic floor for approximately 10 seconds. (There should be feeling of tightening the anus but not the buttocks, abdomen or legs.) This should be repeated 10 times. Clients need to imagine that they are stopping a flow of urine. For females learning this exercise, a finger can be inserted into the vagina and 'squeezed'. Clients should progress so that, when passing urine, they can stop and start mid-flow; this should be carried out once a week to check the progress of the exercise regimen. Pelvic floor exercises should be performed at least twice daily

- The acute or chronic retention of urine
- To introduce drugs, for example antibiotics and **cytotoxic** drugs
- To irrigate the bladder in order to remove sediment and/or blood clots
- Trauma, for example any trauma to the pelvis or lower urinary tract (as any oedema resulting from the trauma may cause obstruction), in order to monitor for blood, and following burns to monitor urinary output
- The accurate measurement of urinary output
- Diagnostic investigations of bladder function
- Incontinence, when all other methods have failed.

cytotoxic

toxic to cells; the term is usually applied to drugs used in the treatment of cancer

Catheters

The nurse should assess the client prior to catheterisation and identify the reason for undertaking the procedure, the length of time the catheter is to remain in situ and the sex of the client. This will help to determine the type of catheter required. The size of catheter will depend upon whether clear urine or haematuria is to be drained (Chart 5.10). Catheters designed for women are shorter than those designed for men because the adult urethra is approximately 4 cm long in a woman and 20–23 cm in a man.

In the majority of cases, a retaining balloon 5 ml in volume will be sufficient. The catheter will require 10 ml of sterile water for its insertion: 5 ml to fill the balloon and 5 ml the balloon's inlet tubing. A balloon size of 30 ml volume should be discouraged, its main use being for clients following urological surgery, in particular prostatic surgery.

Common types of catheter

- *Teflon:* the latex is teflon coated to reduce urethral irritation; such catheters can be used for clients requiring short- or medium-term, up to 1 month, catheterisation
- *Silicone:* these catheters are very soft, are less irritating and cause less crystal formation than the latex variety. They should be used for clients who require catheterising for more than 2 weeks, the catheters having a life span of approximately 3 months

Chart 5.10 ● Catheter size (for an adult)

- Clients with clear urine: 12–16 Fr (Ch)
- Clients with haematuria: 18–22 Fr (Ch)

1 Fr (Ch) is equivalent to 0.3 mm, catheters being measured across their external diameter

- *Hydrogel:* these catheters absorb water to produce a slippery surface and therefore decrease friction to the urethra. They are more resistant to encrustation and adherent bacteria, and have a life span of up to 14 weeks
- *Conformable catheter:* these are designed to conform to the shape of the female urethra (slit-shaped) and allow partial filling of the bladder. They are approximately 3 cm longer than conventional female catheters.

Types of catheterisation

There are three types of catheterisation. The most common and probably the best known is indwelling catheterisation, the other two being intermittent self-catheterisation and suprapubic catheterisation.

Indwelling catheters

The insertion of a urethral catheter requires an aseptic technique, and it is preferable for the client to have a shower or bath prior to catheterisation to ensure good hygiene. The balloon size, the type of material and the size of the catheter used will depend on the reason for catheterisation.

Once the catheter is in situ, meatal and perineal hygiene should be performed. Soap and water are sufficient to clean the meatal and perineal areas, but the nurse or client must ensure that the area is thoroughly dried afterwards (Brown, 1992).

The type of urinary drainage bag will be determined by whether the client is mobile (for example clients able to continue normal mobility activities or clients in wheelchairs) or has limited mobility (for example after surgery or with a medical condition reducing mobility). Clients who are normally mobile may benefit from wearing a leg bag during the day, changing to a full-size drainage bag at night. Clients with limited mobility will wear a full-size bag until the catheter has been removed or 'normal' mobility restored.

To empty a urinary drainage bag, the nurse must wash her hands prior to and after carrying out the procedure, as well as wear gloves during the procedure. The outlet tap of the catheter system should be opened and the urine allowed to drain into a single-use receptacle, the outlet tap being closed after emptying. The urinary drainage bag must hang below the level of the bladder to ensure that urine does not seep back into the bladder; the bag can be supported by attaching it either to the side of the bed or to a stand specially designed for this purpose. If a leg bag is worn, it must be secured to the client's leg without causing traction to the catheter and therefore trauma to the urethra and bladder neck. The tap of the urinary drainage bag must not touch the floor as this will result in contamination and a possible UTI (Figure 5.8).

CONNECTIONS

Chapter 3 describes universal precautions.

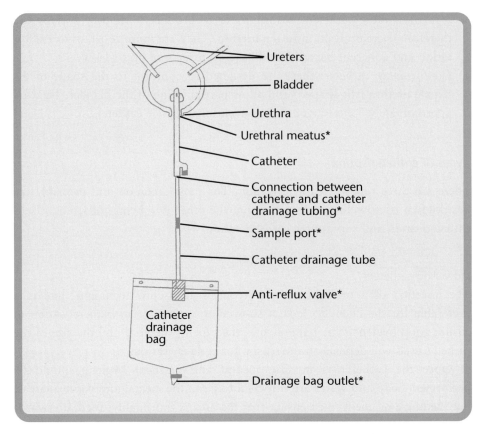

Figure 5.8 ● Points at which pathogens can enter a closed urinary drainage system (*)

It is important that meatal and perineal hygiene is maintained to reduce the risk of encrustation around the catheter and meatus. The client should, unless medically contraindicated, be encouraged to drink 2–3 litres of fluid every 24 hours in order to reduce the risk of UTI, constipation (as this may cause pressure on the bladder and urethra) and the irritant effect of concentrated urine on the bladder (Getliffe, 1993). Constipation should also be avoided as it can contribute towards leakage around the catheter. There is evidence that there is a very high incidence of UTI associated with the use of urinary catheters (Gould, 1994). The principles of care of the patient with a urinary catheter are shown in Chart 5.11.

Intermittent self-catheterisation

Intermittent self-catheterisation is the periodic drainage of urine from the bladder. A catheter is inserted into the bladder via the urethra by the nurse,

Chart 5.11 ● Principles of care for the client with a urinary catheter in situ

- Meatal hygiene – to minimise encrustation
- Fluid intake – adequate intake to reduce the risk of concentrated urine irritating the bladder and to lessen the risk of constipation
- Catheter selection – the appropriate size of catheter and balloon, in a material appropriate to the time proposed in situ, and of a length appropriate to gender; a shorter length for women can, for example, prevent accidental trauma from traction
- Catheter drainage bag – positioned lower than the level of the client's bladder and with effective support
- Catheter drainage bag tubing – ensuring that this is not kinked
- Catheter bag drainage outlet – not to touch the floor as this can cause contamination leading to UTI
- Having a catheter in situ affects body image and sexual activity in the long term. Therefore psychological support and understanding for the client and partner are essential

> CONNECTIONS
>
> *Chapter 7 investigates issues of body image.*

Source: Adapted from Britton and Wright (1990).

client or carer, and the bladder is emptied; the catheter is then removed until the next time voiding needs to take place. This method of emptying the bladder is particularly useful for clients who have difficulties in passing urine, for example clients with neurological problems and those who suffer from urinary incontinence, thus allowing them to gain control of their bladder. Prior to instruction, clients and/or carers should be assessed in terms of whether they are suitable to undertake this procedure (Chart 5.12).

The catheter's length will be determined by the client's gender. For a man, the catheter should be 38 cm long, and for a woman 20 cm as the female urethra is shorter than the male.

Chart 5.12 ● Criteria for clients undertaking intermittent self-catheterisation

Clients should:
- be incontinent of urine (overflow incontinence)
- have good manual dexterity and mobility
- have the mental ability to learn and understand
- show good motivation
- possess an intact urethra
- have a bladder capacity of 100 ml or more

The actual principles and procedure of intermittent self-catheterisation are the same as for the insertion of an indwelling catheter, but this is a 'clean' procedure rather than an aseptic one. Catheters may be used more than once and may be self-lubricating. Urinary tract infections are lower in incidence in this group than in clients with indwelling catheters.

Suprapubic bladder drainage

A self-retaining catheter is inserted through a suprapubic incision or puncture into the bladder (Figure 5.9). This is a temporary measure to divert the flow of urine from the urethra when the urethral route is impassable or impossible because of, for example:

Activity

18

For further information, refer to Mallett and Bailey, 1996, pp. 590–606.

- Trauma
- Stricture
- Prostatic obstruction
- Pelvic fractures
- Gynaecological operations: vaginal hysterectomy and vaginal repair.

Drainage can be maintained for several months.

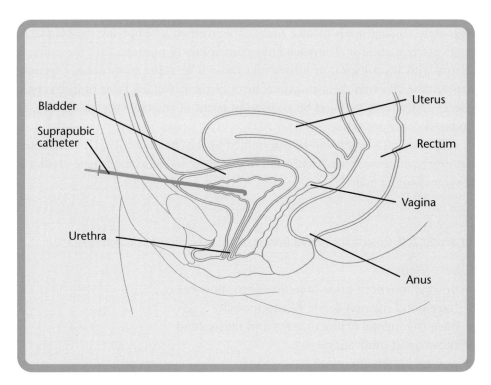

Figure 5.9 ● A suprapubic catheter in situ

Chart 5.13 ● Indications for urostomy formation

- Malignant disease of the bladder
- Malignant disease of the pelvis
- Trauma
- Neurological damage
- Congenital disorders
- Intractable incontinence

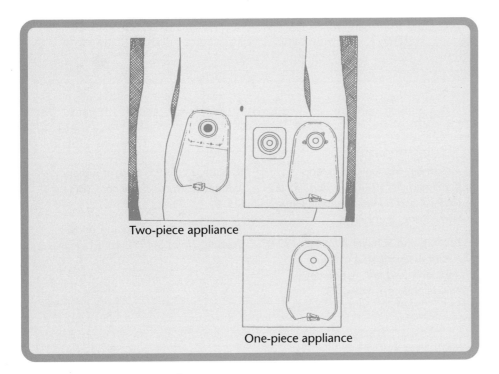

Activity
19

For further information, read Mallett and Bailey, 1996, pp. 530–2, 540–2.

Urostomy

A **urostomy** is performed when the bladder is being removed or is diseased (Chart 5.13). It is an opening from the ureters into a resected section of (usually) ileum, approximately 15 cm in length, which then channels the urine through a stoma that has been formed on the abdominal wall (known as an ileal conduit) and is fashioned into a spout to aid drainage.

Urine that is eliminated through a urostomy can excoriate the surrounding skin if it is not well protected. The urine will constantly 'dribble' from the stoma into a urostomy drainage bag (Figure 5.10). The management of a urostomy is the same as for stoma care.

urostomy

an opening in the abdominal wall to allow the diversion of urine

Two-piece appliance

One-piece appliance

Figure 5.10 ● Urostomy bags

■ Chapter Summary

This chapter has explored both the urinary and faecal elements of elimination. It explains the normal anatomy and physiology and then identifies the abnormal processes of and influences on elimination. It explores possible treatments, the advice available and nursing care for the conditions identified.

● Test Yourself!

1. What information do you need to obtain when making an assessment of your clients' elimination needs?

2. List and explain the factors that may cause a client to become constipated.

3. Identify four types of incontinence.

4. What is the difference between an ileostomy, a colostomy and a urostomy?

5. Identify the psychological factors that affect both urinary and faecal elimination.

6. How much fluid should a healthy individual weighing 65 kg drink in a day?

Further Reading

Alexander, M., Fawcett, J. and Runciman, P. (1994) *Nursing Practice Hospital and Home, the Adult.* Churchill Livingstone, Edinburgh.

Fuller, J. and Schaller-Ayres, J. (1994) *Health Assessment: A Nursing Approach,* 2nd edn. Lippincott, Philidelphia, pp. 185–223.

Getliffe, K. (1995) Care of urinary catheters. *Nursing Standard* **10**(1): 25–9.

Kelly, M. (1994) Mind and body. *Nursing Times* **50**(42): 48–51.

References

Black, P. (2000) Practical Stoma Care. *Nursing Standard* **14**(41): 47–53.

Britton, P.M. and Wright, E.S. (1990) Nursing care of catheterized patients. *Professional Nurse* **5**(5): 231–4.

Brown, M. (1992) Urinary catheters: patient management. *Nursing Standard* **6**(19): 29–31.

Burkitt, H., Quick, C. and Gatt, D. (1990) *Essential Surgery: Problems, Diagnosis and Management*. Churchill Livingstone, Edinburgh.

Cheater, F. (1995) Promoting urinary continence. *Nursing Standard* **9**(39): 33–9.

Continence Foundation (2000) Making the case for investment in an integral continence service: a source book for continence services. In Thakar, R. and Stanton, S. (2000) Management of urinary incontinence in women. *British Medical Journal* **321**: 1326-31.

Cox, H., Hinz, M., Lubno, M. et al. (1993) *Clinical Applications of Nursing Diagnosis: Adult, Child, Mental Health, Gerontic and Home Health Considerations*, 2nd edn. F.A. Davis, Philadelphia.

Crow, R., Chapman, R., Roe, B. and Wilson, J. (1996) *A Study of Patients with an Indwelling Urethral Catheter and Related Nursing Practice*. Nursing Practice Research Unit, University of Surrey, Guildford.

Ford, A. (1992) Feeling off-colour. *Nursing Times* **88**(5): 64–8.

Getliffe, K. (1990) Catheter blockage in community patients. *Nursing Standard* **5**(9): 33–6.

Getliffe, K. (1993) Care of urinary catheters. *Nursing Standard* **7**(44): 31–4.

Gould, D. (1994) A framework for the control of infection. *Nursing Standard* **8**(27): 32–4.

Haslam, J. (1997) Floor plan. *Nursing Times* **93**(15): 67–70.

Kamm, M.A. (1998) Faecal incontinence. *British Medical Journal* **316**: 528–32.

Lewis, L.W. and Timby, B.K. (1993) *Fundamental Skills and Concepts in Patient Care*. Chapman & Hall, London.

Mallett, J. and Bailey, C. (1996) *The Royal Marsden NHS Trust Manual of Clinical Nursing Procedures*, 4th edn. Blackwell Scientific, Oxford.

Marieb, E. (1995) *Human Anatomy and Physiology*, 3rd edn. Benjamin/Cummings, Redwood City, CA.

Ness, W. (2000) Living with an artificial bowel sphincter. *Nursing Times* **96**(19): 15–16.

Newell, C.A., Anderson, L.A. and Phillipson J.D. (1996) *Herbal Medicines. A Guide for Healthcare Professions*. Pharmaceutical Press, London.

Pomfret, I.J. (1993) Stress incontinence. *Practice Nursing* (15): 25.

Rutishauser, S. (1994) *Physiology and Anatomy: A Basis for Nursing and Health Care*. Churchill Livingstone, Edinburgh.

Seeley, R., Stephens, T. and Tate, P. (1995) *Anatomy and Physiology*, 3rd edn. C.V. Mosby, St Louis.

Smith, L.J., Franchetti, B., McCoull, K., Pattison, D. and Pickstock, J. (1994) A behavioural approach to retraining bowel function after long-standing constipation and faecal impact in people with learning disabilities. *Developmental Medicine and Child Psychology* **34**: 41–9.

Thakar, R. and Stanton, S. (2000) Management of urinary incontinence in women. *British Medical Journal* **321**: 1326–31.

Torrance, C. (1991) Pre-operative nutrition, fasting and the surgical patient. *Surgical Nurse* **4**(4): 4–8.

White, C. (1998) Psychological management of stoma related concerns. *Nursing Standard* **12**(36): 35–8.

RUTH SADIK AND DEBRA ELLIOTT

Chapter

Respiration and Circulation

6

Contents

Learning outcomes

The purpose of this chapter is to examine factors associated with respiratory and cardiac function. It will explore the nurse's role in relation to assessing and implementing care with clients who experience difficulties of maintaining breathing and circulation. At the end of the chapter, you should be able to:

- Monitor and interpret a client's respiratory and cardiac vital signs

- Rationalise common deviations from normal values

- Identify techniques for maintaining cardiorespiratory function

- Assist clients in maintaining effective cardiorespiratory function

- Recognise the signs of cardiorespiratory arrest

- Describe the appropriate response and initial management of a collapsed client.

Respiration

oxygen

a colourless, odourless gas that constitutes one-fifth of atmospheric air

carbon dioxide

the gaseous waste product of respiration that is excreted by the lungs

The purpose of respiration is to ensure that the cells of the body are provided with oxygen and that the waste products of their metabolism, carbon dioxide and water, are excreted. Effective respiration is achieved through the exchange of these two gases within the lungs, which in turn depends on the competence of the related structures of respiration. The regulation of respiration is, however, controlled by the brain in response to both neural and chemical factors.

Although brief overviews will be provided within this chapter, you should consult specialist texts on the subject in order fully to understand the anatomical and physiological principles of respiration, including the organs of respiration, pulmonary ventilation, lung volumes and capacities, gaseous exchange, the transport of gases and the control of respiration. Your lecturers may recommend alternative texts, but Martini's *Fundamentals of Anatomy and Physiology* (2001) has a valuable chapter entitled 'The Respiratory System' (pp. 797–840), which will give you the background to the relevant structures and their function in facilitating effective respiration. Whichever text you choose, it should be available for reference while working through this chapter.

Respiratory assessment

In order to make a comprehensive assessment, one first needs to understand the way in which air is taken into and expelled from the lungs, carried around the body and utilised by the cells.

Spontaneous respiration depends on regular neural impulses from groups of neurones in the medulla oblongata and pons. The medulla contains two areas of specialised nerves, known as the inspiratory and expiratory centres, whereas the pons contains nuclei referred to as the pneumotaxic and apneustic centres, which influence and modify the medullary neurones. These areas are required to work together to bring about effective respiration, both voluntary (under our conscious control) and involuntary (unconsciously). The voluntary mechanisms include actions that are non-gaseous in nature, for example coughing, swallowing, vomiting and speech. Involuntary or subconscious respiration, which is needed to sustain life, consists of inspiration, expiration and the fine-tuning of the system relating to increased need such as when exercising, and decreased need during sleep.

During inspiration, nerve impulses pass from the medulla to the diaphragm and intercostal muscles (Figure 6.1), causing them to contract and thus enlarge the thoracic cage, therefore lowering the intrapleural pressure. As the outside air pressure is greater than the air pressure inside the lungs, air flows into the alveoli until the intrapleural pressure is equal to atmospheric pressure.

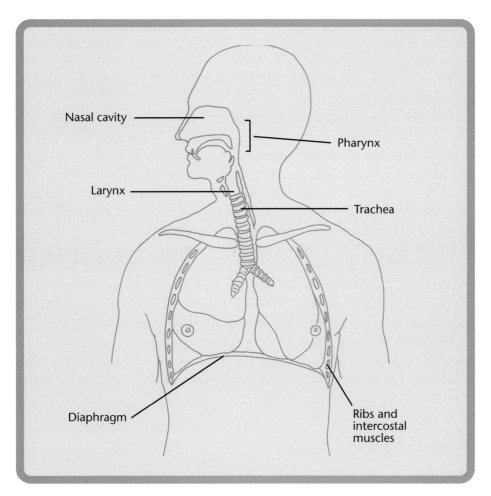

Figure 6.1 ● The respiratory system

As the lungs expand, stretch receptors within the lung tissue convey nerve impulses to the pneumotaxic centre, which further inhibits inspiration. When muscle contraction ceases and relaxation commences, the stretched muscles recoil to their original length. The thoracic cage and lungs return to their normal sizes, and intrapleural air pressure exceeds atmospheric pressure, forcing air out of the airways and into the atmosphere. Expiration is a passive process, dependent only on the inhibition of inspiration.

The chemical control of respiration is attained by groups of specialised cells in the walls of the aorta and carotid arteries known as **chemoreceptors**. Their function is to monitor and respond to changes in the **partial pressure** (denoted by the letter P, see below) of either carbon dioxide (CO_2) or oxygen (O_2) in the

chemoreceptors

nerve endings or groups of cells that are stimulated by chemicals

partial pressure

the pressure of a gas in a mixture of gases, related to its concentration

blood. Any increase in P_{CO_2} is transmitted to the respiratory centre, where inspiration is initiated. A small drop in P_{O_2} acts as a similar trigger, although a substantial decrease in level can have the effect of depressing respiration. The body can normally maintain the balance between blood P_{CO_2} and P_{O_2} through quiet respiration.

The notion of partial pressure is explained by the fact that all gases in a mixture exert their own pressure as if the other gases did not exist. If we take air as an example, this is a mixture primarily of oxygen (two molecules of oxygen), carbon dioxide (one molecule of carbon and two oxygen), nitrogen (two molecules of nitrogen) and water vapour (two molecules of hydrogen and one of oxygen). The pressure that these gases exert allows them to move across membranes from an area of high concentration to one of a lower concentration.

Increases in respiratory rate occur in relation to the demands of body tissues for oxygen. Factors that increase the demand for oxygen in healthy individuals are exercise, increased body temperature and emotional responses such as laughing or crying. Ineffective breathing patterns occur when the individual 'experiences actual or potential loss of ventilation' (Carpenito, 2001).

The health worker's role as part of the multidisciplinary team approach lies in the accurate assessment and diagnosis of factors affecting clients' breathing, in planning and carrying out effective interventions and in evaluating the degree of success.

Physical assessment

Nursing assessment can be made by collecting data from:

- The client, significant others and previous notes
- Observation of the client
- Physical examination
- Laboratory investigations.

The following paragraphs will cover assessment in terms of the quality, rate, pattern and depth of breathing, the colour of the mucous membranes and skin, the presence of any cough, the shape of the chest, the equality of movement on both sides of the chest and the use of any **accessory muscles of respiration**.

accessory muscles of respiration

muscle groups in the neck, back and abdomen that aid respiration by moving the rib cage

Respiratory rate

This is the number of inspirations and expirations recorded in 1 minute without the client's knowledge while he is at rest (Chart 6.1). The normal respiratory

Chart 6.1 ● Hints for assessing the respiration rate

Sitting at the client's right side, reach across and take the pulse in his left wrist while laying his hand on his upper abdominal area. When you have completed this observation, keep hold of the wrist as if you were still counting the pulse; you can then feel the chest or abdomen moving against your hand. Count the frequency of movement for 1 minute and then make the other necessary observations

Chart 6.2 ● Effects of exercise on respiration

During exercise, the muscles of the body utilise oxygen and provide carbon dioxide in higher concentrations than when resting. This reduction in Po_2 is identified by the aortic and carotid bodies, and stimulates the respiratory centre to increase the rate of inspiration. This consequently increases oxygen intake and carbon dioxide output

Table 6.1 Resting respiratory rates by age

Age	Rate (breaths/minute)	Age	Rate (breaths/minute)
Newborn	50	4 years	23
3 months	40	6 years	21
6 months	35	8 years	20
1 year	30	10–12 years	18
2 years	25	13–adult	12–16

Source: Ramsey (1989) with permission.

rates for adults and children are shown in Table 6.1, and the effects of exercise on respiration are described in Chart 6.2.

In certain conditions, abnormalities of the rate of breathing may occur:

- *Bradypnoea:* slow but regular breathing as a result of depression of the respiratory centre. It is a normal phenomenon during sleep but in ill-health may indicate oversedation, opiate poisoning or the presence of a cerebral lesion
- *Tachypnoea:* an increased respiratory rate caused by the body's demands for extra oxygen or by a decreased amount of oxygen being available when the

bradypnoea

slow but regular breathing as a result of depression of the respiratory centre

tachypnoea

an increased respiratory rate caused by a lack of oxygen or a need for extra oxygen

circulation is diminished or respiration impeded. Tachypnoea may be present in **anaemia**, **shock**, **cardiac failure** or **alkalosis**. It may also indicate infections such as meningitis or pneumonia.

- *Apnoea:* cessation of breathing, although short periods of apnoea may be normal in neonates.

Respiratory rhythm

Normal breathing is effortless, regular and quiet. Each breath takes approximately as long as five heart beats, so for an adult with a pulse rate of 80 beats per minute, one would anticipate a respiratory rate of 16 breaths per minute.

As the regulatory centres in their brains are immature, the respiratory pattern of newborn babies is more erratic, periods of bradypnoea and tachypnoea being interspersed with periods of apnoea of up to 10 seconds in duration. A typical pattern is represented in Figure 6.2.

Changes from the normal pattern of respiration are known as:

- *Dyspnoea:* difficult, laboured breathing, present when the airways are obstructed, as in chronic obstructive airways disease or **pulmonary oedema**
- *Orthopnoea:* the ability to breathe without difficulty only when sitting upright. It may be a result of heart failure with pulmonary oedema, or occur in an infant or small child when abdominal pressure is exerted on the diaphragm.
- *Cheyne–Stokes respiration:* breathing cycles of gradually decreasing rate and depth, followed by cycles of increasing rate and depth. This alternating pattern is repeated at intervals of between 45 seconds and 3 minutes, and there may be periods of apnoea during the cycles. Cheyne–Stokes respiration frequently indicates impending death

anaemia

a deficiency of haemoglobin in the blood

shock

inadequate blood flow to the tissues

cardiac failure

occurs when the heart muscle is unable to pump blood effectively around the body

alkalosis

an increase in the amount of alkali in the blood

apnoea

cessation of breathing

dyspnoea

difficult, laboured breathing

pulmonary oedema

fluid in the alveoli and lung tissue

orthopnoea

the ability to breathe without difficulty only when sitting upright

Cheyne–Stokes respiration

breathing cycles of gradually decreasing rate and depth, followed by cycles of increasing rate and depth

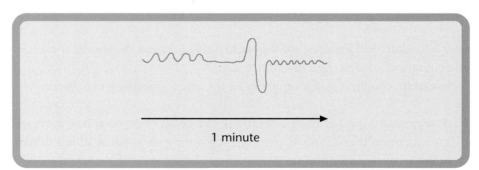

1 minute

Figure 6.2 ● Normal respiratory pattern of the newborn

- *Biot's respiration:* periods of rapid, deep breathing interspersed with periods of apnoea, which may indicate fear or metabolic **acidosis**
- *Kussmaul's respiration:* an increased rate and depth of breathing associated with metabolic acidosis
- *Asthmatic breathing:* prolonged expiration (greater than 2 seconds) accompanied by a wheeze.

acidosis

a loss of alkali from or an increase in acid in the blood

Respiratory depth

Respiratory depth is assessed by observing the degree of movement in the abdominal wall in children under the age of 7 years and in the chest wall in older children and adults (Hazinski, 1999). The total amount of air inspired and expired in one normal breath is known as the **tidal volume** and can be assessed using a spirometer. Its value differs depending on the gender, age, height and weight of the client, but an approximate figure of 6–7 cm^3/kg can be used if required.

Hyperpnoea is shallow, rapid breathing, usually in an attempt to avoid pain of either a thoracic or an abdominal nature.

tidal volume

the total amount of air inspired and expired in one normal breath

hyperpnoea

shallow, rapid breathing

Respiratory sounds

Whereas normal respiration is soundless, there are a variety of sounds associated with respiratory assessment that indicate respiratory disease:

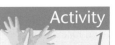

Activity

1

Observe a colleague laughing, excited or upset and assess their respiratory rate, depth and rhythm without their knowledge. Describe the event and behaviour; for example, was the laugh a giggle or a 'belly' laugh?

Did you notice that there were changes in all three aspects of the respiratory pattern? In what ways were the rate, depth and rhythm affected?

- *Stridor:* a harsh sound heard on inspiration, indicating obstruction of the larynx
- *Snoring:* a noise that occurs on inspiration through the nose, usually during sleep. It is indicative of partial obstruction of the upper airway. Causes include inflammation of the nasal mucosa, deviation of the nasal septum, the tongue relaxing into the airway, or enlarged tonsils or adenoids. In severe cases, short stoppages in respiration, known as sleep apnoea, may occur
- *Wheeze:* a melodic whistling or rasping noise heard on expiration; it is indicative of an obstruction to the airflow in the lower respiratory tract
- *Grunting:* the noise heard on expiration in infants with severe respiratory difficulty; it is a compensatory mechanism to keep the alveoli from collapsing
- *Rattle:* audible to the ear on inspiration or expiration and associated with excessive mucus secretion or retention. If a hand is placed on the mid-sternum, rattles can be felt as a 'fluttering' on forced expiration.
- *Râles and crepitations:* audible with a stethoscope, these are associated with excess fluid in the lungs.

Colour

In health, the skin is warm and well perfused, with pink mucous membranes and nail beds. If, however, tissue oxygenation is low (hypoxia) or unusually high, there may be noticeable changes in the client's colour. The palms of the hands and feet, the nail beds and the mucous membranes of the mouth and eyes are good places to look for possible changes in clients of all nationalities:

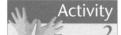

Activity 2

To help you to identify some respiratory sounds, use a stethoscope to listen to the chest of a colleague or client, preferably one with a smoker's cough or respiratory infection.

Is there any difficulty differentiating between the noises made on inspiration and those on expiration? Can you hear the heart beat as well?

- *Cyanosis:* blue tinging of the skin with or without involvement of the mucous membranes indicates that there is an abnormally high level of carbon dioxide in the blood. This may be observed in overdoses of drugs that depress the respiratory centre, for example opiates, or in cases where there is a mixing of oxygenated and deoxygenated blood, as in right-to-left intracardiac shunts.
  – peripheral cyanosis: a blue tinge to the hands and feet
  – central cyanosis: blueness of the mucous membranes of the mouth, lips and conjunctivae
- *Cyanosis with dyspnoea:* laboured breathing and blue extremities may be indicative of damage to the chest wall or lung tissue.

Cough

This is part of a response group that defends the bronchi, trachea and lungs against irritation from a foreign body or excessive secretions. A cough is a sudden, violent expulsion of air from the lungs, which may contain a mix of mucus, cell debris, pus and micro-organisms.

There are numerous types of sputum, amounts varying from 100 to 500 ml (Law, 2000), that are indicative of differing disease processes:

- *Mucoid:* has the appearance of raw egg white and occurs in chronic bronchitis
- *Tenacious mucoid:* as above but is sticky and difficult to expel; this occurs in asthma
- *Mucopurulent:* thick, sticky and green/yellow in colour, indicating the presence of infection in the lungs; also occurs in smokers and asthmatics
- *Purulent:* slimy and green or yellow in colour, produced during bronchopneumonial infection
- *Frothy:* a bubbly, white secretion that may appear pink if tinged with blood, which is produced when the client has pulmonary oedema
- *Haemoptysis:* indicates that the client is bleeding into the lungs. The expectorate, that is, the secretions coughed up from the lungs, is bright red and

haemoptysis
_____

coughing up blood from the respiratory tract

frothy. Haemoptysis may indicate that the client is suffering from tuberculosis, carcinoma of the lung or **pulmonary embolism**.

To enable an accurate diagnosis to be made, the nurse may be asked to collect a sputum specimen to be sent to the laboratory. It may be easier to collect the specimen in the morning when the client awakens, prior to breakfast (Middleton et al., 1998). This is because, while the client is recumbent overnight and respiration is shallow, a high volume of secretions may have accumulated, which will be expectorated as the respiratory depth increases. If the client has eaten, food particles may be present in the specimen, making analysis difficult. The principles of collection are outlined below:

- Explain to the client, using methods appropriate to her understanding, that the substance you want to collect is mucus from the lungs rather than saliva from the mouth
- If the client is able to comply with self-collection, give her a covered wide-necked sterile collecting pot to expectorate into the next time she coughs
- Explain to the client that accidental contamination of the inside of the container by her fingers should be avoided as the laboratory staff need to be certain that any organisms found in the specimen have come from the client's lungs
- If coughing is difficult or the client is exhausted, there are a variety of techniques that the nurse can utilise to ease expectoration. A warm drink or a eucalyptus inhalation may be beneficial.

Once the client has provided a specimen, and you are happy that it is sputum, the pot should be labelled with the client's name, the ward and the date and time of collection, and be dispatched to the laboratory within the hour along with the doctor's request form.

The client needs the opportunity to clean her teeth or rinse her mouth after providing the sputum specimen as it may taste unpleasant.

Chest shape

The thoracic cage is circular in infants, whereas in the older child and adult, the chest becomes wider from side to side than it is from front to back. Deviations from these shapes are indicative of chronic disease processes. The classical 'barrel' chest that occurs in asthma or chronic bronchitis is probably the most common abnormality.

---

pulmonary embolism

blockage of the pulmonary artery or one of its branches by foreign matter, usually a thrombus originating somewhere in the venous system

CONNECTIONS

Chapter 8 explains pulmonary embolism in more detail.

Activity 3

Ask a physiotherapist to show you how he or she intervenes with clients who experience difficulty expectorating. Interventions may include postural drainage, percussion and vibration.

postural drainage

positioning the patient in a way that allows gravity to move fluid from one part of the body to another

percussion

tapping with the fingers on parts of the body

Chart 6.3 ● Causes of airway obstruction

- Anaphylaxis
- Foreign body
- Coma
- Trauma
- Chemical irritants
- Infection
- Near-drowning
- Neurogenic or cardiac causes of pulmonary oedema

anaphylaxis

a potentially fatal reaction occurring when a second exposure to a foreign protein occurs. It consists of breathing difficulty, a rapid pulse, sweating and collapse

hypoxia

a low oxygen concentration at the cellular level

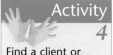

Activity 4

Find a client or colleague with a known respiratory infection or cough. Ask him or her to describe the type of cough and sputum produced.

What could be the cause of the cough? Did you review the text to help you determine a cause? Did you perform a respiratory assessment to provide more clues?

Nursing interventions

Airway maintenance

'Airway' is the generic term for those parts of the respiratory system through which atmospheric air containing oxygen is inspired to reach the lungs, and expired. If a loss of patency occurs in any part of the airway, the flow to the lungs of oxygen-containing air is impeded and a state of **hypoxia** results. Blockages to airflow may result from a disease process or from mechanical reasons – either a foreign body being inhaled or the tongue relaxing into the airway during periods of unconsciousness. The causes of airway obstruction are listed in Chart 6.3.

In either event, it is essential that the student is able to assist the client in maintaining an effective airway and thus sustaining oxygen delivery to the tissues. Airway maintenance can be achieved by the following methods.

Head tilt/chin lift

This is performed when the client experiences a loss of consciousness; it forces the tongue forward into the mouth and away from the airway. The head tilt can be accomplished in adults, children and infants by placing one hand on the client's forehead and applying a firm backward pressure. The fingers of the other hand are placed underneath the chin to support and lift the chin forward. The preferred degree of tilt is (a) neutral in infants, (b) sniffing in the child, and (c) hyperextension in the adult (Mackway-Jones et al., 2001), as shown in Figure 6.3.

Insertion of a Guedel's (oropharyngeal) airway

An artificial airway (Figure 6.4) is used when the client is unconscious, or the airway is occluded and she is unable to support respiration unaided.

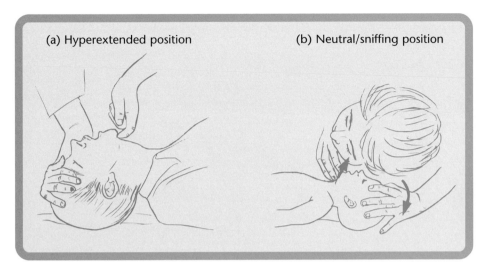

Figure 6.3 ● Airway opening manoeuvres

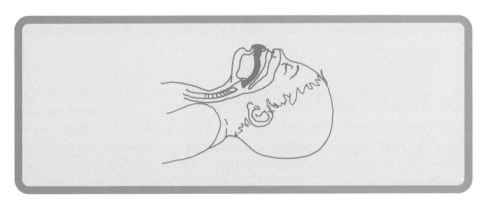

Figure 6.4 ● Guedel's (oropharyngeal) airway

The Guedel's airway extends from the teeth to the **oropharynx**, keeping the tongue in its normal anatomical position. The airway is a concave structure that fits over the tongue, although the insertion technique differs depending on the age of the client. If a gag reflex is present, an oropharyngeal airway is not used as it may cause vomiting, choking or **laryngospasm**.

Although you need to be aware of the technique, you are unlikely to participate in this procedure during your common foundation experience.

Heimlich manoeuvre

The Heimlich manoeuvre (Figure 6.5) may be applied if a foreign body has been aspirated into the airway and is obstructing the flow of air entry to the lungs. It

oropharynx

the area behind the mouth from the soft palate to the hyoid bone

laryngospasm

the prolonged contraction of the muscles controlling the vocal cords, which results in the airway being blocked off

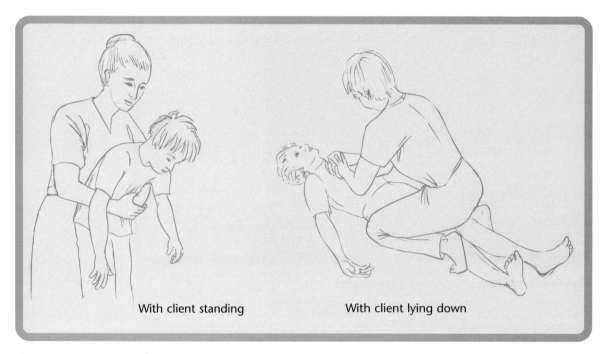

With client standing   With client lying down

Figure 6.5 ● Heimlich manoeuvre

is an alternating series of mouth-to-mouth ventilations, abdominal or chest thrusts and interscapular back blows. The full manoeuvre is performed only on clients who have stopped breathing as it can prove hazardous for young children and pregnant women if executed while they are still breathing. In infants and children under school age, the rib cage does not protect the liver or spleen, which may be vulnerable to trauma; thus, back blows should be the alternative technique of choice for this age group. If used, back blows should be administered with the child lying prone across your thigh, his head hanging over your knee in a head-down position. Using the flat of your hand, administer five sharp slaps between the shoulder blades. If this fails to dislodge the foreign body, turn the child over and compress his chest five times.

Abdominal thrusts can be achieved by standing behind the client with your hands around his waist. With one fist under the xiphoid process, clench the other fist and pull your arms sharply upwards. This action increases the intra-thoracic pressure, forcing the foreign body out of the airway.

Cardiac/respiratory arrest

Clinical death is characterised by respiratory and cardiac arrest. This is in some cases reversible by the prompt application of resuscitative measures, the aim of resuscitation being to 'prevent or reverse premature death in patients with severely compromised or arrested respiration and circulation' (Baskett and Chamberlain, 1997). There are, however, also times when the order to resuscitate is withheld. This is frequently applied on moral grounds, if resuscitation will deny the client the right to a dignified death, each case being considered individually. In most instances, the client who is not for resuscitation is known to be going to die or might potentially die from their injuries or disease, and as there can be no generic rules applied to the 'Do not resuscitate' (DNR) or 'Not for resuscitation' (NFR) order, each establishment should have published guidelines relating to this policy. In all cases where a DNR or NFR order is not in place, full resuscitation measures should be employed.

The arrest will, in many instances, be unwitnessed, and the rescuer will have no idea of either the cause or any underlying disease. Assessment should therefore follow a methodical process to establish whether the client has airway obstruction, respiratory arrest or cardiopulmonary arrest. This process of assessment is known as 'ABC', which denotes the sequence of checking the airway, breathing and circulation. Only a preliminary assessment of the environment and client is required before resuscitator action is commenced. First aid principles should be followed at all times, including the principle that the rescuer will come to no harm by undertaking resuscitation.

Once an initial assessment has been made, stimulate the client by shaking his shoulder gently and asking him whether he is OK. If the client responds, leave him where he is, place him in the recovery position and get help if necessary.

If he does not respond and is not breathing, summon help. If you are alone at this point in a non-hospital setting, leave the client and ensure that the emergency services are alerted by phoning 999. If you are alone in a medical setting, leave the client and call for the 'crash' team: you will be taught the specific procedure for your clinical setting. If you are within earshot of other staff, shout for help.

Open the client's airway using the chin lift or jaw thrust and look, listen and feel for signs of breathing. In the event that opening the client's airway fails to restore ventilation, he requires someone to do it for him. In an emergency situation this is achieved artificially through mouth-to-mouth resuscitation or, in the infant, mouth-to-nose resuscitation and mouth insufflation:

- With the client lying supine (on his back), open the airway using the chin lift, or the jaw thrust shown in Figure 6.6
- If using the mouth-to-mouth technique, close off the client's nostrils with one hand while supporting the chin with the other (Figure 6.7). In the infant, this is not required

Activity 5

Find out the policy in your clinical area for clients who suddenly collapse or are expected to die. Does the policy include boundaries related to age or mental or physical competence?

If there is no policy, do all staff share a common understanding of what to do in such an event?

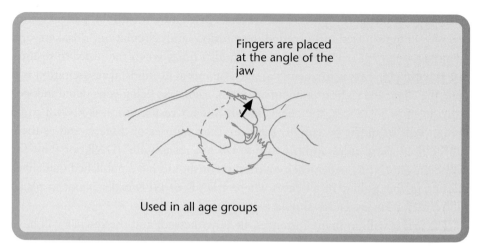

Fingers are placed at the angle of the jaw

Used in all age groups

Figure 6.6 ● Jaw thrust

- The rescuer takes a normal breath, seals his lips over the client's mouth, or in the case of an infant the nose and mouth, and exhales over the next 1.5–2.0 seconds until the chest rises as with a normal breath
- Once the client's chest has risen, the rescuer removes his own mouth and observes exhalation over the next 1–2 seconds. This should be repeated up to five times until two effective rescue breaths have been achieved. Over 1 minute, the rate should equate to the normal value for the appropriately aged client. This means 10–12 breaths for the adult, 20 for the infant aged 6 months to 2 years and 30 for the younger infant

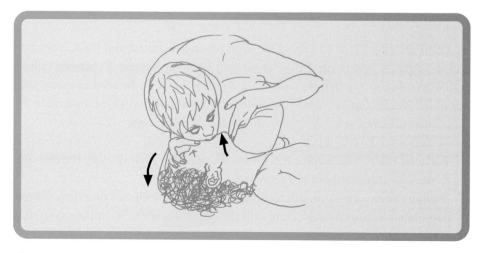

Figure 6.7 ● Mouth-to-mouth seal

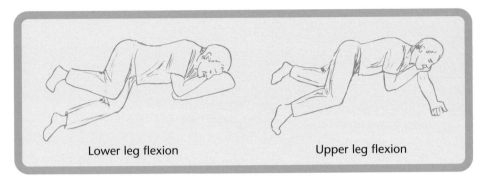

Lower leg flexion   Upper leg flexion

Figure 6.8 ● Recovery positions

● The client should then be assessed for signs of circulation. In the infant, this is achieved by feeling the brachial pulse, and in all other age groups by palpating the carotid pulse for 10 seconds. If you are confident that you have identified signs of circulation and adequate oxygenation, including an appropriate pulse rate, place the client in a recovery position (Figure 6.8). If signs of adequate circulation appear to be absent, commence chest compression.

If the client has a pulse but is not breathing, continue to ventilate until help arrives.

Compression of the heart is needed when the client's heart abruptly stops circulating blood, and therefore oxygen, around the body. To reinstate the cardiac output, the rescuer must perform these compressions at the same rate per minute as the client's normal pulse rate. To perform this on an older child and adult:

● Ensure that the client is lying on his back and that his chest area is resting on a firm surface
● Kneel at the side of the client and locate the site for compression by placing two fingers on the xiphoid process with the heel of the other hand immediately above them on the sternum (Figure 6.9)
● Remove your fingers from the xiphisternum and place this hand over the other one, either grasping the wrist with the thumb or intertwining the fingers. Raise your fingers away from the chest wall, leaving just the heels of the hands in contact (Figure 6.10). This manoeuvre decreases the risk of fracturing the ribs
● Position yourself vertically above the client's chest and, with your elbows straight, press down on the sternum to depress it by one-third of the depth of the chest
● Release the pressure and repeat at a rate of approximately 100 beats per minute.

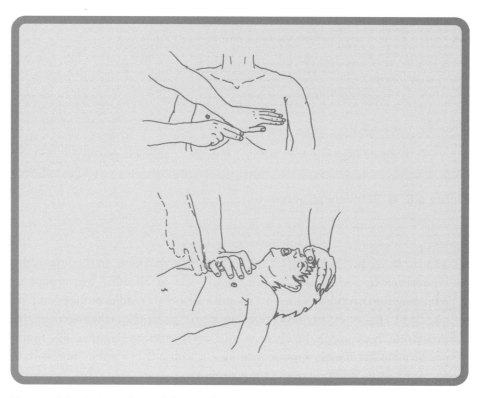

Figure 6.9 ● Location of the cardiac compression site in an older child and adult

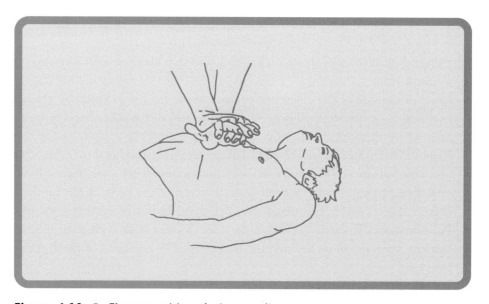

Figure 6.10 ● Finger position during cardiac compression

For children (aged 1–8 years), the process is the same but the rescuer should use only one finger on the xiphoid process and one hand to compress the chest.

If an infant's heart has stopped or is beating at 60 beats per minute or less, cardiac compression should be commenced. As the heart lies more centrally in the thorax in an infant than in any other age group, the compression position differs:

- Ensure that the infant's chest area is resting on a firm surface
- Locate the correct site for compression by imagining a line joining the infant's nipples. As can be seen in Figure 6.11, the tips of two fingers are placed on the sternum, one finger's breadth below the intermamillary line. Cardiac compression is then administered
- Press downwards on the chest until the thorax has been compressed by one-third of its depth five times. This is repeated in cycles of five, at a rate of 100 per minute, until medical help arrives.

The above procedures of artificial respiration and cardiac compression are frequently carried out in combination to maintain effective oxygen delivery to the major organs. The ratio for a one-person resuscitation with an infant is 1 respiratory insufflation to 5 cardiac compressions, whereas with an adult or older child it is 2 insufflations to 15 compressions.

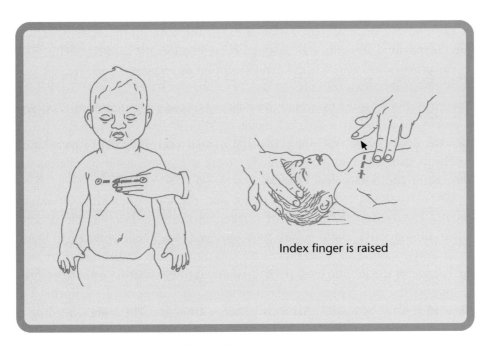

Index finger is raised

Figure 6.11 ● Location of the cardiac compression site in the infant

Now do Activity 6 and then read on. Did you ascertain that acute hospital wards tend to have a 'crash' trolley where all the equipment and drugs are kept together? On less acute wards and in community areas, minimal resuscitation equipment, such as a back board, oxygen, ventilatory equipment and suction, is available. If the ward has its own trolley, a nurse will usually be first on the scene to fetch it. If, however, a group of wards or areas share equipment, a porter may be delegated. Equipment and drugs should be checked, and replaced if necessary, immediately following use. If emergencies occur regularly, a first-level nurse usually checks the 'crash' trolley every day, whereas in less acute settings, this may be done once a week or even monthly.

Have you asked your assessor or a senior colleague to show you how the equipment works and connects?

Volume measurements

The common units for recording measurements of lung function are volumes and capacities, one capacity comprising two or more volumes (Figure 6.12). In healthy individuals, these values are reliant upon age, height, gender and nationality (Kendrick and Smith, 1992). During one normal respiration, the amount of air inhaled and exhaled is known as the tidal volume. The amount of air remaining in the lung on completion of normal expiration is the functional residual capacity (FRC), which is in turn made up of the expiratory reserve volume (ERV) and the residual volume (RV). The total amount of air in the lungs following maximal inspiration is called the **total lung capacity** (TLC), and the maximal amount of air inspired is the **inspiratory capacity** (IC).

As airflow obstruction is the main symptom of respiratory disease, the two most important measurements are the TLC and the RV. The **peak expiratory flow rate** (PEFR) is the maximum flow during forced expiration from TLC and is usually measured by a Wright's meter or Mini-Wright's meter (Figure 6.13), the latter device being available in low and standard versions. The former is used for clients with severe dyspnoea, elderly clients and young children, whereas the latter is for adults and older children.

When recording a PEFR, any drugs that the client is taking should be known. Ensure that the pointer or marker on the flow meter is set at zero. When all restrictive clothing has been loosened, the client is asked to stand or sit upright and take a deep breath in. With her lips sealed tightly around the outside of the mouthpiece, she is then asked to breathe out as hard and for as long as she can. Three sequential readings should be made, allowing the client to rest for at least 30 seconds between attempts. The highest reading is then recorded.

total lung capacity
the total amount of air in the lungs following maximal inspiration

inspiratory capacity
the maximal amount of air inspired

peak expiratory flow rate
the maximum flow during forced expiration from full capacity

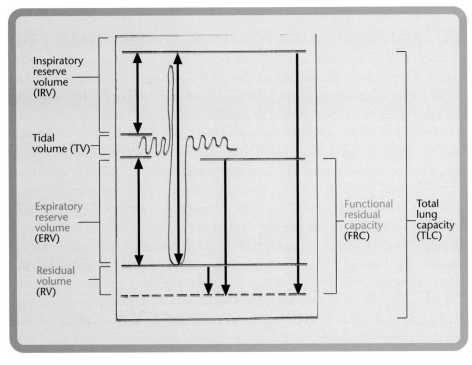

Figure 6.12 ● Lung volumes and capacities

expiratory reserve volume

the maximum volume of air that can be expired from the resting level

residual volume

the amount of air remaining in the lungs after a maximum expiration

functional residual capacity

the amount of air remaining in the lung on completion of normal expiration

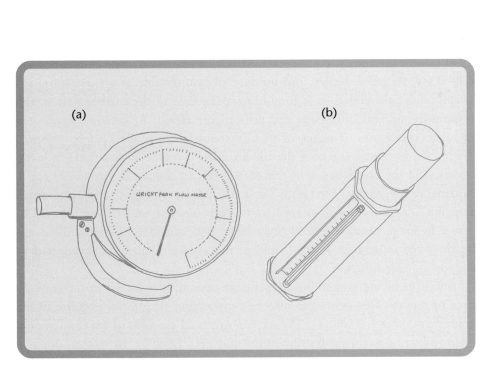

Figure 6.13 ● (a) Wright's meter   (b) Mini-Wright's meter

Pulse oximetry

Pulse oximetry is a non-invasive way of providing constant information about the client's cardiovascular and respiratory systems by measuring the level of oxygen saturation in the peripheral blood. It combines a light-emitting diode (sensor) that transmits red and infra-red light waves through the peripheral vascular bed to be received by a light-sensitive photodiode (detector). As arterial blood is red, it filters out infra-red light but allows red light to pass through, whereas venous blood is blue, which filters out red and allows infra-red light to pass. The photodiode records the intensity of both infra-red and red light transmitted through the haemoglobin. To work accurately, the sensor and detector must lie opposite each other. The pulse oximeter has various types of sensor depending on the site of use, usually a finger or toe, an ear lobe or the bridge of the nose. When a sensor is in place, the skin underneath it should be checked regularly for signs of abrasion or circulatory impairment. Normal values for pulse oximetry are 97–99 per cent. Document the date, time and site in the notes.

vasoconstriction

contraction of the blood vessel wall, causing the lumen to narrow

Pulse oximetry may prove inaccurate in cases in which the client has severe anaemia, is in shock or is experiencing **vasoconstriction**. Cautious use should also be made of oximetry if the client smokes heavily or is suffering from carbon monoxide poisoning, as these factors can compromise the accuracy of the reading. Identify the parameters to inform the medical staff.

Oxygen delivery

Most cells in the body need oxygen to survive and carry out their functions. As cells work, they use oxygen and produce carbon dioxide as a waste product, which must be excreted. It is the ultimate function of the cardiovascular and respiratory systems, alongside red cells in the blood, to deliver oxygenated blood to the tissues. If either of these systems becomes diseased or compromised, the level of oxygen in the tissues falls. Hypoxia (a low oxygen level) occurs, and the continuance of this state leads to cellular death as oxygen is essential to life. Many of the body's cells are able to regenerate and/or compensate, but brain cells lack this capacity and their function may be lost for ever. In severe hypoxia, brain cell death may be so widespread as to bring about the death of the individual. Extra (supplemental) oxygen can be administered to support cellular function.

Atmospheric air, containing 21 per cent oxygen, is breathed in through the nose or mouth. This figure can also be expressed as the partial pressure of the constituent gases (see above). The oxygen exerts 21 per cent of the total atmospheric pressure, so the proportion of the pressure caused by the oxygen can also be stated as 21 kPa. Some of the oxygen, however, is lost during the journey to the alveolar air sacs, which at this point contain just 13.2 per cent or kPa of oxygen. Whereas the blood in the capillaries surrounding the air sacs already contains some oxygen (5.3 kPa), this value is less than that encountered in the alveolus. Gases diffuse from an area of high to one of low concentration, so oxygen moves from the alveoli into the blood until equilibrium has been reached. Carbon dioxide leaves the blood in the same way, diffusing from a high concentration in the blood (6 kPa) to a lower concentration in the alveoli (5.3 kPa). Once in the blood, a small amount of the oxygen dissolves directly, but the majority combines with haemoglobin in the red cells to become oxyhaemoglobin and be conveyed around the body to the cells. The situation with carbon dioxide is more complex, the gas being carried in several forms – carbonic acid, hydrogen carbonate ions and bound to protein elements, where it becomes known as a carbamino compound.

Tissues differ in their requirement for oxygen, three main areas accounting for 60 per cent of oxygen consumption:

- The brain
- The liver
- Skeletal muscle.

Once in the tissues, oxygen is used to produce adenosine triphosphate (ATP), the fuel for cell maintenance and survival.

Hypoxia can arise when the control mechanisms that ensure an adequate oxygen delivery to the cells fail. This may be due to:

1. Deficient oxygenation of the blood through being in a low-oxygen environment, for example during strangulation, suffocation, drowning, inadequate ventilation of the lungs following major abdominal surgery, chest injury, prematurity or paralysis of the respiratory muscles, shunts between the right and left heart (as in infant ventricular septal defect and persistent patent ductus arteriosus) and inflammatory lung disease such as asthma and bronchitis.
2. Inadequate transport of oxygen by haemoglobin as a result of anaemia, a sudden loss of blood or carbon monoxide poisoning.
3. Circulatory inadequacy due to low blood pressure or heart failure.
4. Inability of the cells to use oxygen, which is usually an indication of cyanide poisoning.

ventricular septal defect

an abnormal opening in the septum between the right and left ventricles of the heart

persistent patent ductus arteriosus

a developmental defect leading to an abnormal connection between the pulmonary artery and the aorta

The consequences to the client may be that the cells' ability to produce ATP is lost, so, depending on which tissues are affected, the signs and symptoms observed by the nurse will vary:

- Disorientation and drowsiness if the brain is affected
- Decreased urine output if there is kidney damage
- Muscle weakness
- The skin appearing blue (peripheral cyanosis) or, in central cyanosis, the whites of the eyes, the lips, the tongue and the nails taking on a blue tinge
- Tachycardia (a rapid pulse rate)
- Changes in respiratory rate and depth
- The infant's skin becoming grey and mottled
- The hands and feet becoming cool or cold.

This list is not comprehensive and you may like to add any other observations you make.

Oxygen therapy is, according to Allan (1989), the provision of an atmosphere of increased oxygenation with or without the use of specialised equipment. It is used when the adult's blood oxygen saturation is less than 90 per cent (Thiagamoorthy et al., 2000) and the infant or young child's is 94 per cent or less (Hazinski, 1999). This difference in level is related to the young child's larger consumption of oxygen for cellular growth and function.

As a result of potential dangers, oxygen is treated in the same way as drugs and should as such be prescribed by a doctor. The prescription should include:

CONNECTIONS

Chapter 3 investigates safety issues related to medication.

- The percentage of oxygen to be administered
- The flow rate in litres per minute and mode of delivery
- Whether it is to be continuous or intermittent, or to be given immediately.

As oxygen may need to be administered in an emergency without a doctor present, the ward, hospital or unit should have an agreed written policy to cover this eventuality.

Each oxygen delivery system comprises five basic components:

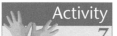

Activity

7

When on your clinical placement, find out whether there is a policy governing the use of oxygen, and if so, what it recommends.

What type of oxygen delivery system is available in your clinical area?

1. *An oxygen supply:* which may be piped to the ward or come from a portable cylinder that is universally coloured black with a white top and is marked 'Oxygen'. These come in a variety of sizes and are often confused with cylinders containing medical air; a careful check thus needs to be made for accuracy. A portable cylinder for home use holds 300 litres, whereas cylinders for use with adults in an acute setting hold 3400 litres.
2. *A flow meter:* a device that measures the flow of oxygen in litres per minute.
3. *Tubing:* usually green in colour, albeit found in different lengths and diameters, which connects the source to the patient or client.
4. *A delivery mechanism:* mask, cannula, hood, incubator and mechanical ventilator.

5. *A humidifier:* which may be used to warm and moisten the oxygen during delivery.

The choice of method of administration depends upon:

● The concentration of oxygen required
● The client's compliance.

For infants, oxygen is provided via a head hood or box that can provide up to 100 per cent oxygen, the flow rate being set at 7 litres per minute to prevent carbon dioxide accumulation inside the hood. The hood or box allows both good visibility of the patient's face and access to the infant or child's body without disrupting the flow of oxygen. If, however, humidification is used, visibility may be decreased and the child may become cold and wet, which can in turn lead to cold stress and skin irritation. There should be no impedance to the outflow of carbon dioxide, and an oxygen analyser must be used.

Oxygen delivery to newborn babies may be carried out inside an incubator, which allows for the control of environmental temperature and high visibility. The disadvantages are that the oxygen concentration is poorly controlled and that, in the humid environment, micro-organisms such as *Pseudomonas* may grow. The oxygen flow should normally be between 4 and 5 litres per minute; a concentration of up to 40 per cent can be consistently delivered if a head box is used.

A Derbyshire chair can be used optimally for infants and young children as the oxygen can be consistently administered while the child is sitting in an upright position, allowing for downward displacement of the diaphragm.

Several kinds of disposable face mask, similar to that illustrated in Figure 6.14, are available for both adults and children, these being capable of delivering a concentration of oxygen ranging from 24 per cent to 60 per cent. The nurse should ensure that the client's nose and mouth are just covered. Masks provide a rapid and accurate delivery to the client, with high visibility. The client may also move around within the confines of the length of oxygen tubing. Disadvantages are that clients cannot eat or speak with the mask on, and if they vomit, this may not be easily noticed.

If oxygen is being administered via a face mask, the nurse should ensure that the mask fits snugly around the client's nose, otherwise oxygen may blow into the eyes, causing discomfort and possible damage. As oxygen can cause mucous membranes to become dry, leading to inflammation and trauma, both eye and mouth care are required for clients wearing oxygen masks. When used for infants and children, it can help to position the mask upside down if the oxygen flow causes problems with the eyes.

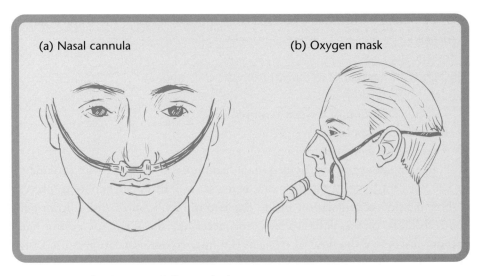

(a) Nasal cannula

(b) Oxygen mask

Figure 6.14 ● Oxygen delivery devices

Nasal cannulae are reserved for flows of less than 1 litre per minute or if an infant or child requires less than 24 per cent oxygen. Nasal prongs are usually more comfortable for children and infants, who can eat and vocalise while they are in situ. They are not advocated if the client is mouth-breathing.

Nasal catheters are not usually used for infants, who rely predominantly on nose breathing, because irritation to the airways on insertion and removal may cause further respiratory distress. They are advocated for adults and are positioned at the level of the uvula.

Thus, adults can be given nasal cannulae, catheters or face masks. The advantages and disadvantages are the same in adults and children for all three types of system, although an oxygen flow of more than 1 litre per minute is administered to adults, up to a maximum of 3 litres per minute. Fluid intake should also be closely monitored to ensure adequate hydration.

Oxygen may need to be humidified because:

● Oxygen from piped or cylinder sources is dry
● Dry gases lead to drying out of the mucous membrane lining the respiratory system
● Dry mucous membranes may become inflamed, causing excessive mucus production.

As a result, clients needing continuous oxygen therapy may be prescribed humidification. In this technique, oxygen is bubbled through sterile water at room temperature, picking up moisture and thus increasing its humidity. The humidifi-

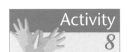

Activity
8

Find out whether your area's policy is routinely to humidify oxygen. If so, how long should a client be prescribed oxygen before it is humidified?

Is there any recent research linking respiratory infection and humidification? If there is, have you shared it with the staff in your clinical area?

cation of oxygen has, however, recently been linked to waterborne infections of the respiratory tract, so it appears to be losing favour as a routine procedure.

Oxygen concentration should be assessed at the point of delivery, but as a guide:

- 28 per cent oxygen can be achieved from a flow rate of 5–6 litres per minute
- 35 per cent from 6–9 litres per minute
- 40 per cent from 8–12 litres per minute
- 60 per cent from 10–14 litres per minute.

Dangers associated with oxygen administration are linked to the fact that it is a colourless, tasteless, odourless, transparent gas that is heavier than air and supports combustion. As such, there are various precautions that must be taken when caring for clients receiving oxygen therapy:

1. Avoid the use of grease or oil on any part of the system delivering oxygen to the client, as it may support combustion.
2. No electrical devices should be operated when the client is receiving oxygen. This includes battery-operated shaving equipment and battery-operated toys for children.
3. Volatile solutions should be used cautiously. Petroleum-based products, which may be inflammable, should not be used to moisten patients' lips.
4. Explain that the client or visitors should not smoke near oxygen supplies.
5. Make sure that you know where the fire extinguishers are positioned or accessed.

Complications of oxygen therapy arise because the prolonged breathing of a high level of inspired oxygen can cause changes in the brain and lung tissue, resulting in fibrosis and decreased efficiency of the relevant organ. In infants, it can also cause a type of blindness known as retrolental fibroplasia.

Clients of all ages with certain types of chronic respiratory disorder need to have a relatively low oxygen level to maintain their breathing. This is known as the 'hypoxic drive'. If oxygen is delivered without due consideration to the underlying disease, it can lead to the cessation of respiration.

Some clients complain of pain behind their breastbone, which is thought to be related to tracheitis (inflammation of the trachea) and may be an indication for humidification. Humidification during oxygen therapy has itself been linked to an increased risk of chest infection.

When caring for a client receiving oxygen therapy, the nurse should make regular checks (the patient care plan detailing the exact frequency and the observations to be made) on:

Activity 9

You are informed by the accident and emergency department that a client (of the age group appropriate to your area) with severe dyspnoea is to be admitted to your ward within the hour. The client has bilateral chest movement, an obvious use of accessory muscles and an oxygen saturation value of 87 per cent.

You are asked by a staff nurse to prepare a bed space for the new arrival. What do you need to do?

- Vital signs, such as respiratory rate, pulse rate, temperature and blood pressure
- The colour of the client's skin and mucous membranes
- The oxygen saturation level if a pulse oximeter is in use.

Now do Activity 9. Did you remember to prepare an upright position for the client, with a backrest and four pillows for an adult and a chair for an infant? The client should be easily observable from the nurses' station. You also need the appropriately sized oxygen equipment with humidity, suction and pulse oximetry. As the client is probably mouth-breathing, equipment for oral hygiene, a drink and, in the event of the client having a productive cough, a sputum pot and tissues will be needed. If breathlessness is severe, the older client may appreciate being close to a window or fan to give the impression of an airy environment.

Airway suctioning

Although it is unlikely that you will be asked to undertake this procedure, it is frequently performed on medical and surgical wards, and clients with severe physical disabilities often require airway clearance. As such, it is necessary to have some background knowledge on the rationale for airway suctioning. Suctioning is an essential skill for the nurse caring for the patient who has respiratory compromise. It is used to help maintain a patent airway in cases where the patient is unable to do this herself.

Ineffective airway clearance is the state in which the client experiences a real or potential threat to respiratory status related to an inability to cough effectively. Clients at risk of accumulating secretions in the airway may be diagnosed as demonstrating:

- An ineffective cough reflex
- The inability to remove secretions
- Abnormal breath sounds
- An abnormal respiratory rate, depth or rhythm
- An increased pulse rate
- Pallor or cyanosis of the skin.

chronic obstructive airways disease

a condition with a progressive loss of inspiratory and expiratory capacity of the lungs

This may be as the result of:

- An acute or chronic inflammatory response, such as pneumonia or **chronic obstructive airways disease**
- Burns or trauma to the face, chest or abdomen

- Having an endotracheal or tracheostomy tube in place, which may cause narrowing of the airway or increase the amount of secretion present
- Paralysis of the muscles of respiration because of medication or disease.

In episodes of unconsciousness or paralysis involving the muscles of respiration and the stomach, the patient may be at risk of vomiting and subsequently inhaling vomitus into the respiratory system. This is most acutely possible during, or immediately following, the reversal of anaesthetic agents within the operating department. An impaired level of consciousness through the ingestion of noxious substances, for example alcohol, or through head injury is a cause likely to be seen in the accident and emergency department.

Although the art of airway suctioning may appear somewhat barbaric and distressing because of the visual, auditory and aesthetic images it conveys, it is the most effective way of maintaining a clear airway and sustaining life. The nurse is placed in the position of observing a patient who is ineffectively ventilating and showing all the signs of respiratory distress, but knowing that the procedure she is about to perform could potentially either save the patient's life or cause untold damage. Both prior to and following the procedure, the patient's respiratory rate, rhythm, depth, effort and sounds should be reassessed.

> **Activity**
> **10**
>
> To acquaint yourself with the principles of airway suctioning, read Lewis and Timby, 1993, pp. 225–9 and Hazinski, 1999, pp. 262–3, making notes in your own words.

Inhaled drug delivery methods

Drugs administered directly into the lungs are rapidly absorbed through the alveolar–capillary network into the bloodstream, therefore avoiding many of the side-effects associated with oral forms of the drug. This method is known as 'inhalation' therapy and consists of drugs in either powder or liquid form being breathed into the lungs, thus penetrating the cells directly.

> **CONNECTIONS**
>
> *Chapter 3 identifies other methods of drug delivery.*

Metered-dose inhalers, which deliver a high dosage of drug locally to the lung tissues, rely on pressurised air passing over powder to force the drug deep into the lungs. This is the method frequently used to administer broncho-dilators or steroids to clients with asthma or chronic obstructive airways disease, but the effectiveness of this method is determined by the client's ability to combine activation of the inhaler with inhalation of the drug. Elderly clients, the very young and those with learning disabilities may be unable to achieve this degree of co-ordination.

The nebulisation of drugs involves compressed gas (either oxygen or air) passing through a quantity of liquid drug within a nebuliser attached to a face mask; this then forms an aerosol spray that is inhaled into the lungs. Little co-ordination is needed so there is a greater compliance of clients who may experience difficulty with a metered-dose inhaler. A number of machines are available that deliver nebulised drugs to the lungs through a process known as intermittent positive-pressure ventilation. The nurse should familiarise herself with the equipment in order to understand the nature of the therapy being given.

Teaching a client to use a metered-dose inhaler

Although there are a variety of devices on the market, the principles of action remain the same:

1. Remove the cover of the inhaler.
2. Load the inhaler as instructed by the manufacturer.
3. Ask the client to breathe out gently but not fully.
4. With the client's head tilted slightly backwards, place the mouthpiece between his lips and ask him to breathe in as deeply as possible.
5. Remove the inhaler from between his lips.
6. Tell the client to hold his breath for 10 seconds and then breathe out slowly.
7. Repeat the procedure if necessary.

Circulation

myocardium

the muscular layer of the heart

The purpose of circulation is to provide an adequate blood flow to vital organs such as the brain and **myocardium**. An adequate circulation ensures the delivery of oxygen and nutrients to the body tissues, the removal of carbon dioxide and waste products, and the dissipation of heat from active organs to ensure temperature regulation by redistribution around the body. Effective circulation is achieved via two separate circuits, the systemic and pulmonary circulations, both of which originate and terminate within the heart.

In order to understand the physiological and anatomical principles of circulation, including the cardiovascular system and its components, coronary and peripheral blood flow, the cardiac conduction system and the cardiac cycle, your lecturers may recommend specialist texts on the subject. Rutishauser (1994, pp. 77–107) and Hinchliff et al. (1996, Section 4) may, for example, be useful.

Circulatory assessment

CONNECTIONS

Chapter 1 gives examples of pain assessment techniques.

Inadequate circulation results in an ineffective delivery of oxygen to the tissues. The assessment of cardiovascular function includes a physical examination of the patient and an assessment of his heart rate, blood pressure, peripheral perfusion and fluid balance. A pain assessment should also be performed.

Davol Singh is a 62-year-old gentleman who has presented to the nurse at his general practice complaining of worsening shortness of breath over the past week. He is accompanied by his wife, who is extremely anxious and worried about his deterioration. Mr Singh is known to be a heavy smoker (35 a day) and suffers from chronic obstructive airways disease.

■ Prior to undertaking a full cardiovascular assessment, the nurse could observe the texture, temperature and colour of Mr Singh's skin, which may reveal signs of sweating (from cardiac strain), infection or cyanosis (from circulatory shutdown).

■ A simple question such as 'How are you feeling?' will also help to establish mental alertness and the degree of respiratory difficulty: can the client complete sentences or only gasp individual words?

Activity 11

Count your resting pulse and respiratory rate. Run up a flight of about 10 stairs five times. Count your pulse and respiratory rate now and again after 2 minutes. Chart these readings and note the correlation between the respiratory and pulse rates.

Consider what physiological changes have occurred. There is usually a 1:4 or 1:5 differential between the respiratory and pulse rates.

Physical examination

As discussed in Chapter 1, a physical examination will frequently commence with an initial rapid observation of the client. Consider the client in Casebox 6.1 and determine what general information could be obtained from a rapid initial assessment prior to a detailed cardiovascular assessment.

Heart rate

The heart rate is most commonly assessed by calculating the pulse rate. The **pulse** arises from the rhythmical wave of distension in an artery caused by contraction of the left ventricle of the heart, which results in a pressure change within the aorta that can be felt along the arterial wall, this being known as the pulse (Chart 6.4).

The pulse rate is the number of beats in a 60 second period. It is calculated most accurately by counting the number of beats felt within a full period of 60 seconds or, at a minimum, over a 30 second period, then doubling the result. Accuracy is particularly important and is most difficult in patients who have a fast or irregular heart rate. Normal heart rates for children and adults are shown in Table 6.2. These rates may vary as a result of age, exercise, posture, temperature, emotion or change in health status (Marieb, 2001).

An abnormally fast heart rate is known as a **tachycardia**. In adults, this is considered to occur at over 100 beats per minute, and in children at 20 per cent above the normal rate. Causes of an increased heart rate are exercise, stress, fear, excitement, pyrexia (fever), blood or fluid loss, certain drugs and heart conditions (for example **atrial fibrillation** and cardiac failure).

pulse

the regular expansion and contraction of an artery caused by pressure waves as the heart contracts

tachycardia

an abnormally fast heart rate

atrial fibrillation

an irregular and ineffective heart rhythm

Chart 6.4 ● Hints for pulse measurement

The pulse is detected by placing two fingers over an artery close to a bony or firm surface. The most common site used for pulse rate detection in adults and children over the age of 2 years is the radial pulse because it is one of most easily detected and accessible sites. This can be felt on the anterior aspect of the wrist (Figure 6.15). The arm should be supported and relaxed, and the palm rotated uppermost. The pulse should be felt with the index and middle fingers over the groove along the thumb side of the inner wrist. Toddlers may need distracting to ensure accurate counting of the pulse. Further sites available for pulse rate palpation are shown in Figure 6.16. In infants, the most common method used for calculating heart rate is taking the apical rate (see below). When assessing a person's pulse, three factors should be observed: its rate, its strength and its rhythm

Table 6.2 Normal resting heart rates for children and adults

Age	Beats per minute	Age	Beats per minute
Newborn	120–130	5–10 years	110–90
1 year	110	10–adult	90–60
2–5 years	115–110	Adult	80–50

Source: Adapted from Whaley and Wong (1995).

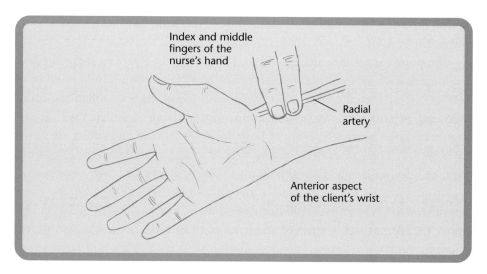

Figure 6.15 ● Locating the radial pulse

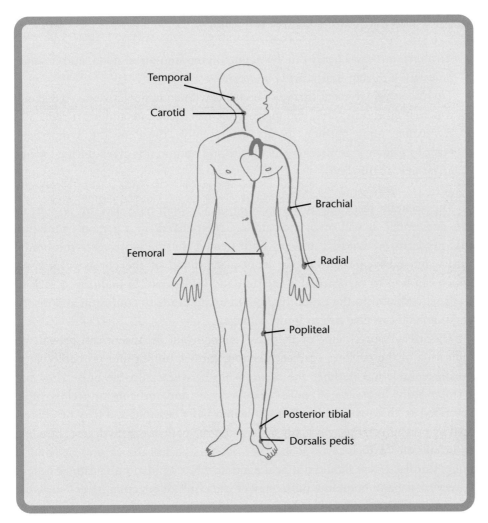

Temporal

Carotid

Brachial

Femoral

Radial

Popliteal

Posterior tibial

Dorsalis pedis

Figure 6.16 ● Common sites in the body for pulse rate palpation

An abnormally slow heart rate is known as a **bradycardia** and is regarded as one of less than 60 beats per minute in adults, and one 20 per cent below the normal rate in children. Causes of a low heart rate are hypothermia, certain drugs (for example **digoxin** and **beta-blockers**), activation of the parasympathetic nervous system (for example during sleep or rest), certain heart conditions (such as heart block, which results from a disorder of the conduction system) and cerebral oedema (excess fluid) following head trauma. A low heart rate may also result from athletic and endurance training.

bradycardia

an abnormally slow heart rate

digoxin

a drug that slows and strengthens the heart beat, and is used for cardiac irregularities

beta-blockers

drugs that slow the heart rate and reduce the blood pressure

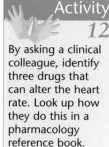

Activity 12

By asking a clinical colleague, identify three drugs that can alter the heart rate. Look up how they do this in a pharmacology reference book.

Now carry out Activity 12. Did you consider:

- *Atropine:* increases heart rate by acting on the sino-atrial node, and is sometimes given during bradycardia and cardiac arrest
- *Thyroxine:* replacement therapy for clients with an underactive thyroid gland, which, if taken in excess, will increase the metabolic rate and heart rate
- *Adrenaline* (epinephrine): its actions resemble those of the sympathetic nervous system so it increases heart rate and output; it is given during cardiac arrest and anaphylaxis.

The accurate recording and reporting of an abnormally fast or slow heart rate is essential. It will often indicate a sudden change in a person's condition that needs to be assessed and possibly treated. Furthermore, extreme bradycardia and tachycardia result in inadequate filling of the coronary arteries, which can lead to myocardial starvation and infarction. In addition, a lack of oxygenated blood to the brain (hypoxia) initially leads to confusion and disorientation, and can give rise to brain damage.

The strength or volume of the pulse is important because it can provide an indication of the person's cardiac function, cardiac output and probable blood pressure. Table 6.3 outlines the relationship between palpable pulse sites and systolic blood pressure. A pulse that is weak and difficult to feel is often described as 'thready'. A thready pulse will usually be rapid and may be obliterated by pressure on the artery, suggesting that the patient is dehydrated, bleeding or exhausted. In such cases, it may be necessary to feel the carotid or femoral pulse. Cardiac arrest should not be diagnosed when a radial pulse cannot be felt. A very strong and bounding pulse may be the result of infection, stress, anaemia or exercise. An inconsistent pulse pressure within each beat may indicate a Corrigan's or waterhammer pulse, found in children with aortic valve incompetence. The first half of the pulse is normal or full but, after reaching its peak, the wave suddenly recedes under the finger.

The rhythm of the pulse is the pattern in which the beats occur. In a healthy person, the pattern or rhythm is regular because the chambers of the heart are contracting in a co-ordinated manner, producing a regular pulse beat. In children,

infarction

the death of tissues (necrosis) due to the lack of an oxygenated blood supply

Table 6.3 Correlation between palpable pulse and systolic blood pressure

Palpable pulse site	Systolic blood pressure
Radial	>80 mmHg
Femoral	>70 mmHg
Carotid	>60 mmHg

the pulse is regular but there is a slight acceleration during inspiration and a slight deceleration during expiration, known as sinus arrhythmia. This may also be present in fit young adults and is not considered to be an important deviation.

Irregularity of pulse rhythm can be divided into three types: occasional irregularity, regular irregularity and irregular irregularity. An occasional irregularity may be perceived as a missed pulse or 'dropped beat' and is often the result of an occasional ventricular ectopic (an extra beat, followed by a compensatory pause). This should be reported but might not be treated. A regularly occurring irregularity may be detected as a cyclical event and could be the result of a heart block. Again, this should be reported as it may well compromise the circulation, sometimes with catastrophic effects. An irregularly irregular rhythm is often a result of atrial fibrillation, which is one of the most common irregular cardiac rhythms, occurring in 2–4 per cent of the adult population over the age of 60 years.

Apical pulse rate measurements (heard through a stethoscope placed over the apex of the patient's heart; Figure 6.17) are advocated in children from birth to 24 months of age because, during this period, the pulse rate is fairly labile and can be considerably influenced by crying, activity and feeding. Apical measurements are more accurate (Wong, 2000) and should be counted for 1 minute. The apical pulse rate is also incorporated into the assessment of adults who have an

sinus arrhythmia

an irregular heart rhythm following the pattern of respiration

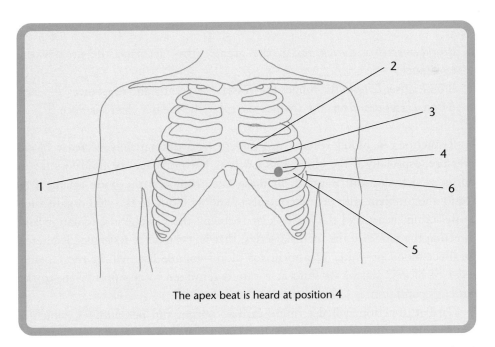

The apex beat is heard at position 4

Figure 6.17 ● Locating the apex beat. Numbers 1–6 relate to the positioning of the ECG V leads

pulse deficit

the difference between the apical heart rate and the peripheral pulse rate, indicative of a lack of peripheral perfusion

irregular heart rate and/or when a measurement of **pulse deficit**, the difference between the apical and peripheral pulse rates, is required. The procedure for obtaining these measurements is explained in Mallett and Dougherty (2000).

Blood pressure

Blood pressure is the pressure exerted by the blood on the walls of the blood vessel. Each blood vessel has its own pressure, the pressure in the vessels falling continuously from the aorta to the end of systemic circulation; this pressure gradient or fall needs to exist for blood to flow. During contraction of the ventricles of the heart, blood is ejected into the systemic and pulmonary circulations, causing a distension of the arteries and an increase in arterial pressure. When contraction ends, the arterial walls recoil passively and blood is driven further through the arterial circulation. Arterial pressure therefore rises and falls during the contraction and relaxation of the heart. The maximum pressure is known as the **systolic pressure**, the minimum pressure that occurs during relaxation of the heart being known as the **diastolic pressure**. For a more detailed explanation of the physiology of blood pressure, see Hinchliff et al. (1996), Mallett and Dougherty (2000) or Marieb (2001).

Factors determining blood pressure are **peripheral resistance**, blood volume and cardiac function. Peripheral resistance is the opposition to the blood flow and is determined by:

- *Blood viscosity ('stickiness'):* the greater the viscosity, the greater the resistance
- *Blood vessel length:* the longer the vessel, the greater the resistance
- *Blood vessel diameter:* the smaller the tube, the greater the resistance.

Reductions in blood volume can directly and dramatically decrease blood pressure, especially if the blood loss (such as haemorrhage) or fluid loss (as in burns or dehydration) is rapid. In these circumstances, the body attempts to rectify the problem with neural controls to supply blood to the vital organs such as the brain, heart and the kidneys by reducing the peripheral circulation and directing the blood to the major arteries; that is, peripheral resistance is altered to affect blood pressure. Treatment for blood volume loss will be the replacement of blood, plasma or fluid at a rate determined to be appropriate to the patient's condition.

Cardiac function will determine cardiac output (ml per minute), which is equal to the **stroke volume** (ml per beat) multiplied by the heart rate (beats per minute), normal cardiac output being about 5.5 litres per minute. Change in stroke volume is expressed by the Frank–Starling Law, which decrees that the

systolic pressure

the blood pressure recorded during contraction of the heart

diastolic pressure

the pressure occurring during relaxation of the heart

peripheral resistance

the opposition to blood flow

stroke volume

the amount of blood ejected from the ventricle during contraction

critical determinant of stroke volume is the degree of stretch of the cardiac muscle cells just before they contract. The most important factor determining this degree of stretch is the amount of blood returning to the heart (the venous return). Hence we can see that peripheral resistance, cardiac function and blood volume are all interlinked in determining blood pressure. For further details, see Marieb (2001) or Hinchliff et al. (1996).

The measurement and recording of blood pressure is routinely undertaken in adults and is advocated in children aged 8 years and over as part of a cardio-vascular assessment. The most frequent, non-invasive method of measuring arterial blood pressure employs a sphygmomanometer. The frequency of recording will depend on the patient's condition, the reason for admission and the results of the reading. It is therefore essential that the technique is performed accurately, on the same arm each time, and that the patient is prepared prior to the procedure (Chart 6.5, Figure 6.18). The patient will, ideally, not have exerted herself or smoked in the preceding 30 minutes as these activities can increase the reading. Anxiety also has this effect, and for the patient having a routine blood pressure recording as part of her admission assessment, it is best to allow her to settle into her new environment for at least half an hour prior to the procedure.

Chart 6.5 ● Hints for taking blood pressure

During the procedure, the patient should be comfortably seated, or lying if unable to sit, with his arm supported on a pillow at the level of the heart. An appropriately sized cuff (the bladder should encircle the arm) should be used and tight clothing removed. The rubber, inflatable cuff is then applied to the upper arm just above the elbow (over the brachial artery) and the cuff is inflated. Inflating the cuff compresses the brachial artery, and this is continued until no radial pulse can be felt (the artery at this point being collapsed with no blood flowing through it distally). The observer should be at eye level with the mercury manometer, the stethoscope being placed over the brachial artery (just below the cuff). The cuff is slowly released while listening for audible sounds that indicate flow of blood through the artery and the systolic and diastolic pressures.

The Russian surgeon Korotkoff classified these audible sounds into five phases that are now known as Korotkoff sounds (Table 6.4). Controversy exists over whether phase 4 or phase 5 is the best measure of diastolic pressure, but what is probably more important is that agreement exists within units and that either method is used consistently when recording blood pressure in the client population. It may also be useful to note, in the client's records, the phase used

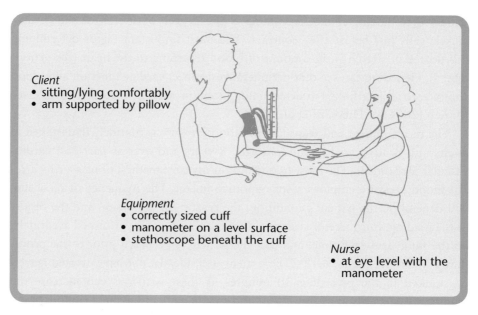

Figure 6.18 ● Preparation for blood pressure reading

Activity

13

Find out which Korotkoff sounds are used in your clinical area to determine systolic and diastolic readings. Have you consulted Table 6.4?

An inspection of patients' charts will frequently show the initial blood pressure to be higher if anxiety has not been allowed for. In an emergency admission, this will be inappropriate, and the blood pressure result will frequently be required as soon as possible, perhaps dictating the patient's treatment (Chart 6.5). For further information, see O'Brien (1997).

Normal blood pressure values are difficult to define, varying between individuals and in the same person in differing circumstances. Age, sex and race also affect blood pressure values, blood pressure increasing with age in Western society and being slightly higher in men and in individuals of Afro-Caribbean descent. The factors listed above that affect pulse rate can also alter blood pressure values within individuals. Average blood pressure values are shown in Table 6.5.

hypertension

persistently high blood pressure

A persistently high blood pressure reading is known as hypertension. Disagreement exists over whether this condition should be diagnosed from blood pressure readings or from an epidemiological viewpoint, but most authorities agree that a persistent resting diastolic pressure of over 90–95 mmHg indicates hypertension (Hinchliff et al., 1996). Clinicians are concerned with blood pressure readings because a significantly increased mortality exists for individuals who are hypertensive. This risk increases rapidly with increasing pressure, an individual then being most at risk of a cerebro-vascular accident or myocardial infarction.

Table 6.4 Korotkoff sounds with examples of pressure values

Phase	Sound	mmHg	Pressure
1	Tapping that is sharp and clear	120	Systolic
2	Blowing or swishing	110	
3	Sharp but softer than phase 1	100	
4	Muffled and fading	90	Diastolic
5	No sound	80	

A persistently low blood pressure reading, known as hypotension, is rare. Hypotension is usually transient and is the result of haemorrhage, shock or dehydration. If a patient has a low blood pressure, you may be asked to perform postural blood pressure recordings, these being performed on the same arm with the patient first lying and then standing. If a difference exists between the two systolic pressures, the patient is said to have a postural fall in blood pressure (postural hypotension); this is particularly significant if the difference is 20 mmHg or more and can indicate a large-volume fluid loss. Always be careful when undertaking this procedure as the patient may faint if the blood pressure is particularly low. If the patient is particularly shocked, never undertake a standing blood pressure without advice from a trained nurse. The alternative option for blood pressure recordings is to compare pressures in the left and right arms; this may indicate a dissecting aneurysm.

Peripheral perfusion

Peripheral perfusion is assessed by considering the colour, texture and temperature of the skin, the presence of peripheral pulses or oedema and the capillary refill time.

hypotension
persistently low blood pressure

Activity 14

Measure a colleague's resting blood pressure. Using guided imagery, conduct him or her on a fearful experience and measure the blood pressure again. Note the difference and consider the physiological changes that have occurred.

Try asking your colleague to have a warm bath and then measure the blood pressure again.

Table 6.5 Average blood pressure values

Age (years)	Systolic pressure (mmHg)	Diastolic pressure (mmHg)
Newborn	80	46
10	103	70
20	120	80
40	126	84
60	135	89

When assessing the colour of the skin, any pallor and/or cyanosis should be noted. Pallor may indicate shock, haemorrhage or poor perfusion and is obviously easier to detect in Caucasian skin. Darker skin may become grey or ashen if severe haemorrhage has occurred. The internal surface of the eyelids can also be inspected; a lack of their usual reddish colour indicates anaemia. Cyanosis, a bluish tinge to the skin or mucous membranes, can be central or peripheral. Central cyanosis is an indicator of poor gaseous exchange and is assessed in the mucous membranes of the mouth. Peripheral cyanosis is an indicator of poor blood flow and becomes apparent when the arterial oxygen saturation is less than 75 per cent (normal being 96–100 per cent). It is assessed in the extremities and the nail beds (see above for further information).

The texture and temperature of the skin will reveal any localised or generalised warmth or coolness and any signs of sweating. A localised heat reaction may occur following a bite or sting, whereas generalised heat may be present with an underlying pyrexia or sepsis. Patients who are sweating may also be pyrexial or may have severe pain or blood loss.

Palpation of the peripheral pulses will indicate the presence of arterial blood flow to the extremities (see Figure 6.16 above). If an area of tissue is not adequately perfused, it becomes **ischaemic**, the metabolic function of the tissue deteriorates and the damage eventually becomes irreversible (necrosis). During the process of increasing arterial insufficiency, the following signs may be observed: ulceration of skin, thickening and slow growth of the nails, and the skin becoming shiny, scaly and hairless. Oedema and pain may also be present in the limb. Characteristically, the patient will awake in pain at night and hang the limb over the edge of the bed to increase the blood supply, thus alleviating the pain. Doppler testing is a non-invasive continuous-wave ultrasonic investigation that can be used to determine blood flow if the pulses are undetectable (remembering that an inability to detect them does not necessarily indicate a lack of blood flow). Both limbs should always be checked for pulses or blood flow as this may vary considerably.

Capillary refill time can be assessed using the capillary refill test. The assessor applies cutaneous pressure on a fingertip for 5 seconds, which causes it to blanch (go pale owing to blood being squeezed out of the capillaries). The length of time taken for the skin to turn pink again indicates the speed of capillary refill: longer than 2 seconds usually indicates poor tissue perfusion (Smith, 2000).

Peripheral **oedema** usually occurs with congestive cardiac failure and indicates that the heart is unable to function effectively with its workload. Oedema is usually gravitational and may be observed in the feet or legs, or even in the genital area or sacral region if it is excessive. If patients present with these problems, it is essential to elevate their lower limbs to waist level to encourage reduc-

ischaemia

lack of blood supply to the tissues, usually resulting in acute pain and dysfunction

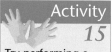

Activity 15

Try performing a capillary refill test on yourself and then on a colleague. Read the text to ascertain the normal values.

oedema

an effusion of fluid into the tissues

Casebox 6.2

Frances Riteur is an 80-year-old lady with known congestive cardiac failure. Her diuretic therapy has been altered, and the practice nurse is monitoring the effects of her new treatment.

What will the nurse be monitoring?

■ Frances will probably be weighed weekly. A maximum weight loss to reduce fluid retention should be no more than 1 kg per day, representing a loss of 1 litre of fluid per day.

■ Any reduction in peripheral oedema will be noted.

■ Any reduction in breathlessness will be noted.

■ Any improvement in exercise tolerance, appetite and bowel function will also be noted as it may indicate a lessening of her cardiac failure.

tion of the oedema. Patients may be taking diuretic therapy, so fluid balance or daily weight should be accurately ascertained to determine fluid loss. Pulmonary oedema is characterised by acute breathlessness, often with frothy sputum, and is caused by acute left ventricular failure. These patients are often seriously ill and are frequently unable to talk, feeling as if they are 'drowning'. Urgent medical assistance is necessary, and the patients will usually be prescribed oxygen and diuretics.

Fluid balance

A fluid balance record may be requested for clients who have circulatory compromise. An accurate recording of all forms of input and output is essential as it will compare total input and output and show whether these are optimal. Urinary ouput normally ranges from 1.5 to 2 litres per day (1 ml/kg per hour), but this depends on normally functioning kidneys, the kidneys receiving an adequate blood supply and a lack of obstruction to urinary flow (Smith, 2000). Problems with any of these three mechanisms therefore can affect urinary output. If, for example, a client has an acute circulatory complication, her cardiovascular output may be ineffective and urinary output will not be adequate. You may be asked to monitor this output on a fluid chart.

Similarly, your client may be started on medication to improve urinary output (diuretics), and a fluid chart will reveal the effect. You may also see clients who are weighed daily or twice weekly (instead of having fluid chart monitoring) as a method of assessing the weight/fluid balance. Total fluid balance figures are often transferred onto a cumulative fluid balance chart, which allows several days or weeks of recording to be easily viewed. Continuous fluid balance over a longer period of time is vital in some groups of patients, for

CONNECTIONS

Chapter 5 reviews urinary elimination in more detail.

oliguria
_____

inadequate production
of urine

example those with renal failure or cardiac failure. In an acute situation, a decrease in urinary output, oliguria, may be an early indicator that a patient is deteriorating, and you should certainly never allow a urinary output of less than 0.5 ml/kg per hour to go unreported (Smith, 2000).

Pain

CONNECTIONS

Chapter 1 gives further examples of pain assessment methods.

The ability to assess and effectively manage a patient's pain is an essential nursing skill. Pain was discussed in Chapter 1, this section referring specifically to the assessment, recording and monitoring of pain arising from circulatory problems. As part of the pain assessment, the nurse should identify the location, severity and description of a patient's pain, consider whether there are any precipitating or alleviating factors and ascertain the resulting effects on the patient's pain.

An individual may be able to state the location of his pain (for example central chest pain) or point to it, but a site may be difficult to establish in individuals who do not use English as their main language or who have learning disabilities. Anatomical diagrams and multilanguage tools may be helpful with such patients. Some departments use graphical tools to chart a patient's pain; these can be referred to again in subsequent reviews and evaluations.

It is important to establish the severity of the pain, three types of scale existing to assist with this process. The first main tool to assess pain severity is the verbal descriptor scale (Chart 6.6), in which an individual is asked to select

Chart 6.6 ● Verbal descriptor pain scale

- None
- Slight
- Moderate
- Severe
- Agony

Chart 6.7 ● Pain behaviour scale

- Verbal response
- Body language
- Facial expression
- Behavioural change
- Conscious level
- Physiological change

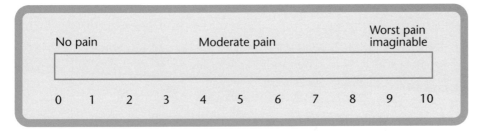

Figure 6.19 ● Visual analogue pain scale

a word that describes his pain. These scales are quick and easy to use but require an understanding of English or translation to other languages.

The second type, visual analogue scales (Figure 6.19), are usually straight lines with either numbers or describers along them. These are, again, quick to use, but they require abstract conceptualising by the patient, which may be difficult if learning disabilities exist.

The third type, pain behaviour tools, rely on the principle that patients who are in pain exhibit certain types of behaviour (Chart 6.7). These tools require observation of the patient for at least 10–15 minutes and are a subjective assessment of the patient, not including his own perception of his pain.

A pain assessment tool ideally allows for a quick but comprehensive pain assessment and provides for the individual interpretation of pain along with an assessment by the nurse of any change in the patient's functioning. The tool needs to facilitate the ongoing assessment and evaluation of pain and pain control; Figure 6.20 shows a pain ruler that meets these criteria. The Manchester Triage Group have also designed a pain ruler aimed at accident and emergency departments but with obvious uses outside these environments (Mackway-Jones, 1997). The Manchester tool combines the verbal descriptor, visual analogue and pain behaviour tools, which provides for both individual and practitioner assessment.

It is important to remember that patients frequently understate the amount of pain that they are in. This may especially be seen in the elderly client group, who may have become used to chronic pain and have therefore adapted to and are able to cope with pain. Children are also a client group who may understate pain, possibly because of fear of the consequences, for example an injection.

A description of the pain is necessary to clarify and confirm its location and severity; it may also indicate the probable cause. For example, a client who describes leg pain that is cramping and excruciating, being worse on walking, may have intermittent claudication. Investigations obviously need to be performed to confirm the initial suspicion, but the description helps the practitioner to prioritise the management of these patients.

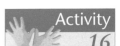

Activity

16

Identify the pain assessment tools used in your clinical area. Ascertain whether pain scores are linked to an analgesic protocol, for example a pain score of 8 to giving opiate analgesia.

Do nurses make their own judgements of what pain clients are experiencing? Do particular clients express more pain than others?

claudication
_____

pain in the lower limbs due to a lack of blood supply, which causes limping

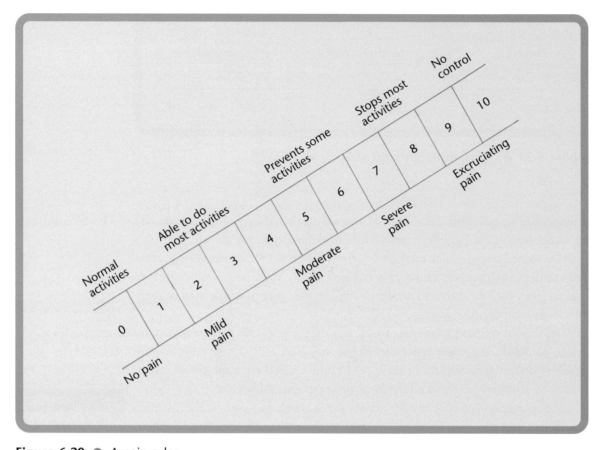

Figure 6.20 ● A pain ruler

Precipitating factors such as exercise, stress, movement, respiration, position, time and duration are helpful in determining the probable cause and possible effects of the pain. Chest pain on respiration, particularly inspiration, may, for example, arise from the pleura or **pericardium**.

Alleviating factors such as heat, cold, rest, analgesics, position and distraction may again indicate the cause of pain but may also help with pain management strategies. A patient with angina, for example, who complains of chest pain when walking in the cold can be advised to alter her walking habits or to try prophylactic vasodilators such as glyceryl trinitrate prior to exercise.

The effects of pain may be minimal or may cause profound physiological changes, for example extreme tachycardia or hyper- or hypotension. They may also curtail a patient's activities or lifestyle, so health education advice may be appropriate. For further information, see Macintyre and Ready (1996) or Park et al. (2000).

pericardium

the covering of the heart, comprising two layers – an outer fibrous and an inner serous layer

Nursing interventions

Cardiac monitoring

A cardiac monitor displays a graphical representation of the electrical activity occurring in the cardiac muscle fibres. It is a useful tool to assess a client's heart rhythm and also provides information about her condition and progress. Whereas cardiac monitors were once the domain of specialist units, they are now increasingly used in a variety of clinical settings. Chart 6.8 outlines hints on using cardiac monitors.

When a patient is being monitored, it is important to remember that the electrocardiograph (ECG) tracing is a tool to assist with the management of a patient and not the reason for managing a patient. It is essential always to consider the patient's condition and the effect of any cardiac rhythm on a patient's well-being. It is also important to note that, during some cardiac arrests, patients can have a normal ECG rhythm. This is known as **electromechanical dissociation** and occurs when the electrical activity is normal (hence the normal ECG rhythm) but there is no mechanical activity (and therefore no cardiac output), leading to an inability of the heart to propel blood around the body. There are various causes, for example **hypovolaemia** and pulmonary embolism, but the guiding principle is to look at the patient first and the monitor second.

The normal cardiac rhythm, or **sinus rhythm**, has characteristic waveforms (Figure 6.22), and an understanding of these, in addition to the physiology of normal cardiac conduction, will enable you to identify any deviations from the normal ECG. What follows is a basic introduction to ECG interpretation; for a more detailed approach, see Schamroth (1990).

electromechanical dissociation

normal electrical activity of the heart accompanied by a lack of mechanical activity

hypovolaemia

an abnormally low circulating blood volume

sinus rhythm

the normal rhythm of the heart

Chart 6.8 ● Hints on using a cardiac monitor

- Ensure that the cardiac monitor is situated in a safe and observable position
- Switch it on at the wall and on the monitor (if appropriate)
- Set the monitor to lead 2 unless told otherwise
- Attach the electrodes to the client's skin surface as shown in Figure 6.21
- The electrodes need to be firmly attached to the patient's skin. This may be difficult if the patient is shocked and sweating. If the leads do not adhere, the following may be useful: abrade the skin lightly (most electrodes have a rough edge to achieve this), dry the skin (iodine solutions are useful, providing no allergy is known) and shave the chest (in the area where the electrodes need placing)
- Ensure that the rhythm tracing is visible and observe it regularly

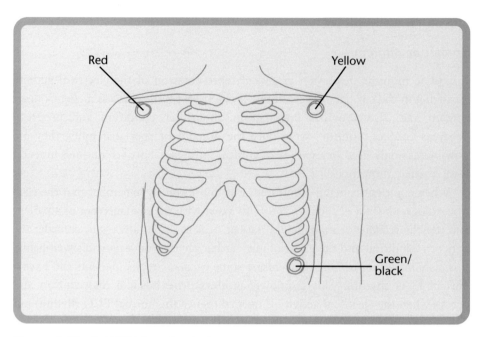

Figure 6.21 ● ECG chest lead placement

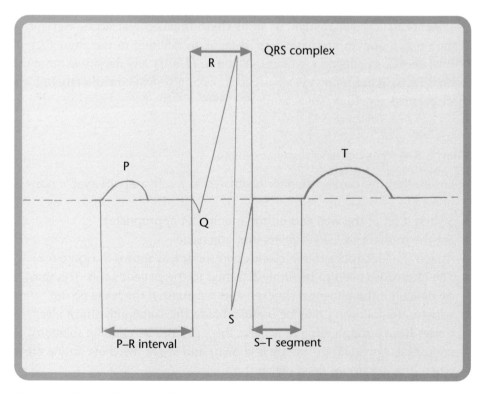

Figure 6.22 ● Normal ECG waveform

Casebox 6.3

Joan Hammett is a 52-year-old lady who is recovering from minor surgery that was carried out 2 days ago. She suddenly complains of central chest pain, which is making her feel dizzy and nauseated. She is known to suffer from ischaemic heart disease but says that this is not the pain she normally suffers.

What could you ask her about the description of pain to help you in your management?

- The site of the pain and any radiation, for example to the neck, arms or back.

- The intensity of the pain and whether anything relieves it.

- The onset and duration of the pain, for example sudden or gradual.

- The consequences of the pain. For example, when she says that she feels dizzy and nauseated, can she concentrate or has this pain taken control of her thoughts?

- Anyone presenting with chest pain potentially has a serious condition such as a myocardial infarction and you should always seek help.

The questions above will help the assessor to determine whether the pain is likely to be cardiac in origin.

The isoelectric line, or baseline, is seen as a straight line and signifies **polarisation** of the myocardium. The first wave of the ECG is the P wave, representing the **depolarisation** of the atrial myocardium. Following atrial depolarisation, atrial systole should occur, during which blood is expelled from the atria into the ventricles. The P wave is followed by the QRS complex, which represents the depolarisation of the ventricular muscle. The Q wave is the first downward (or negative) deflection after the P wave and may not be present in normal conduction. The R wave is the first upward (or positive) deflection after the P wave, and the S wave is the downward deflection that follows an R wave. Following ventricular depolarisation, ventricular systole should occur, resulting in blood being expelled into the systemic and pulmonary circulations. The next deflection on the ECG is the T wave, representing ventricular muscle repolarisation. During ventricular repolarisation, the heart refills with blood ready to commence the next cardiac cycle. Atrial repolarisation occurs during ventricular depolarisation, but the waveform is masked by the greater electrical activity occurring in the ventricles. A normal or sinus beat has a P wave, a QRS complex and a T wave, the S–T segment being isoelectric. Alterations to these waveforms indicate cardiac **arrhythmia**, disease or damage.

When analysing the ECG rhythm, various pieces of information are required to ascertain whether the rhythm is sinus in origin or whether there is an arrhythmia. What follows is a six-stage process that can be used for the basic analysis of an ECG rhythm:

polarisation

the resting state of the plasma membrane in which the inside of the cell is negative relative to the outside

depolarisation

loss of the polarised state of the plasma membrane, involving a loss or reduction of the negative membrane potential

arrhythmia

a deviation from the normal (sinus) heart rhythm

1. Heart rate.
2. Regularity of heart rhythm.
3. Presence/absence of P waves.
4. P–R interval.
5. QRS complex duration/width.
6. Rhythm interpretation.

Heart rate

The heart rate can be obtained in several ways. If the rhythm is regular, count the number of large squares between two consecutive R waves and divide the number into 300 to determine the heart rate. For example, 5 large squares between two R waves divided into 300 gives a heart rate of 60. If the heart rate is irregular, the number of large squares on a 6 second strip can be counted and multiplied by 10. Several types of ECG mark 6 second strips; alternatively, 30 large squares can be counted on ECG paper, which represents 6 seconds.

Regularity

The regularity of the rhythm should be noted. If this is not obvious, it can be ascertained using a ruler or ECG rule, or merely by marking a piece of paper at the top of two complexes and moving it along the rhythm strip to see whether the other complexes fall regularly. Irregular rhythms are unlikely to be sinus in origin except for sinus arrhythmia, in which acceleration and deceleration occur with respiration.

P waves

The presence of a P wave should be noted; it is an essential component of a sinus rhythm.

P–R interval

The P–R interval is measured from the beginning of the P wave to the beginning of the QRS complex. It can be measured in either time (0.12–0.20 seconds) or squares (3–5 small squares on the ECG paper). For the rhythm to be sinus rhythm, the P–R interval must fall within this duration. If the P–R interval is greater, it may indicate first-degree heart block.

QRS complex

The QRS duration is measured from the beginning to the end of the QRS complex. Again, it can be measured in time (0.08–0.12 seconds) or squares (2–3 small squares on the ECG paper). Beats that are sinus in origin and are conducted normally through the conduction system will fall within these parameters.

Rhythm interpretation

Having established the above, you should be able to decide whether or not the rhythm is sinus in origin. Further skills are necessary to determine which other rhythm it could be, but these are beyond the scope of this section.

Anti-embolic precautionary measures

Patients who are immobile or who have reduced mobility are at risk of venous **thrombosis**. Venous thrombi are most common in the deep veins of the calf (95 per cent) and result from coagulation in the pocket-like valves of the deep veins owing to venous stasis. Stasis occurs as a result of lying supine (possibly during prolonged surgery or following a major illness), which increases pressure in the leg veins, promoting the stagnation of the blood. The clinical signs of thrombosis include pain in the calf, especially on dorsiflexion of the foot (Homans' sign), inflammation and localised flushing of the affected limb, with associated warmth and swelling. The more serious risk from a venous thrombosis is pulmonary embolism, which results from the dislodging of a clot in the lower limbs. This produces acute dyspnoea and haemoptysis, and can in some instances result in sudden death.

thrombosis
an abnormal condition in which blood clots (thrombi) develop in the blood vessels

Virchow proposed that three factors, now known as Virchow's triad, are related to the development of venous thrombosis, these being blood flow changes, vessel wall damage and alterations in blood viscosity. Although it is recognised that all three are important, it is now believed that blood flow changes are the dominant component.

Although young, fit, mobile individuals can develop deep vein thromboses (DVTs), the most common cause is a precipitating illness, injury or operation. The greatest risk factors associated with venous thrombosis are a previous history of DVT, abnormal leg veins, possibly taking oestrogens, heavy smoking, paralysis, congestive cardiac failure, malignancy, pregnancy and **hypercoagulability**. Precautionary measures can be taken to minimise the risk.

hypercoagulability
a tendency towards excessive clotting of the blood

Anti-embolic stockings

Anti-embolic stockings, or graduated compression stockings as they are also known, are a non-invasive, inexpensive, easy-to-use prophylactic method of reducing stasis in the legs. *Bandolier*, the Anglia and Oxford Regional Health Authority magazine that seeks the results of research to provide evidence-based health care, conducted the following meta-analysis. It searched 122 articles, 12 of which were randomised trials with comparable methodology; these revealed that the risk of a DVT was reduced by 68 per cent when patients were using compression stockings. They concluded that, in moderate-risk patients, stockings were a highly effective method of prevention, whereas in high-risk patients, alternative or adjuvant treatment, for example heparin, might be required.

Activity 17

Consider clients of any age who are immobile and at risk of venous thrombosis. What precautionary measures can be adopted to prevent this?

Have you considered accompanying a physiotherapist or nurse specialist for the day?

Exercises

Passive/active exercises are an important measure to promote venous return and decrease venous stasis in order to prevent a DVT. Preoperative and bed-bound patients can be taught and encouraged to combine deep breathing techniques and active leg exercises to achieve this. Exercises can be performed passively for unconscious or immobile individuals. Further measures to encourage blood flow are regular changes of position, the use of bed cradles to relieve pressure on the limbs and ensuring that the top sheets are not tightly tucked in. In some units, intermittent pneumatic compression devices are applied to the calves to assist venous return.

Blood transfusion

A blood transfusion, the administration of either whole blood or one of its components, is a transfer of living tissue from one person to another, and it must therefore be remembered that problems can arise. The types of blood or blood product commonly used are whole blood, concentrated (packed) red cells, washed red cells, platelets, plasma and plasma substitutes.

Safety precautions prior to transfusion are as follows. Blood should be stored in a specific fridge (not a domestic fridge) whose temperature is constantly maintained between 2°C and 6°C to prevent bacterial contamination and be removed from the fridge no longer than 15 minutes prior to its use. Each hospital will have a local procedure for checking blood that usually involves two nurses, one of whom is a trained nurse, and includes confirming the patient's name, date of birth and hospital number, the expiry date of the blood, the blood groups of the donor and recipient, and the serial number of the unit of blood. Once checked, this information is recorded either in the patient's notes or on a prescription sheet or checklist. The unit should also be checked for signs of deterioration or damage. If there is any doubt, the blood should not be given but returned to the laboratory and advice requested (World Health Organization Regional Office for Europe, 1999). The transfusion should be prepared aseptically and the blood administered via a giving set with an in-line filter. Some units use additional filters, and local policies must be checked. Glucose solutions should not be given immediately prior to or following blood administration as they cause the formation of aggregates. You may therefore be asked to 'prime' the giving set with a saline solution before giving the blood.

Observations during transfusion are an integral and essential part of the client's care and should commence with a set of baseline observations prior to commencement of the transfusion. Local policies vary, but the patient should be constantly observed and regularly monitored for any signs of a transfusion reaction. Reactions can occur very rapidly and are most likely to occur during the initial administration of each unit. Most hospital policies include 15 minute observations during the first hour, followed by either half-hourly or hourly observations of pulse, temperature, blood pressure and respiration for the remainder of the unit. This pattern is repeated for all new units of blood.

Transfusion complications

Circulatory overload occurs from an excessive intravascular volume that usually results in pulmonary oedema. This is most likely to occur in chronically anaemic patients who require the additional oxygen-carrying capacity of red blood cells but not the volume. The problem is prevented by using packed cells and giving diuretics. If circulatory overload occurs, the patient should be seated upright and reassured, the transfusion should be discontinued immediately and medical advice should be sought.

Haemolytic mismatch is one of the most serious complications of a blood transfusion, and clinical problems can arise rapidly following as little as a 10–15 ml infusion of incompatible blood. Problems are caused by antigen–antibody reactions, leading to acute intravascular **agglutination** and **haemolysis**. Early symptoms include fever, shivering, tachycardia, wheeze, rash and hypotension. Further complications are chest tightness, loin pain and oppressive head fullness, which result from agglutination within the capillary beds. The degree of the reaction ranges from mild to severe, with shock and death in some instances. The transfusion should be stopped immediately and any remaining blood sent for analysis. Treatment is symptomatic and is aimed at maintaining a reasonable blood pressure and renal perfusion.

Allergic reactions are fairly common, ranging from mild irritation to anaphylactic shock. Symptoms include flushing, **urticarial hives**, wheezing, chest tightness, laryngeal oedema and peri-orbital oedema. Anaphylaxis is potentially fatal and requires urgent treatment. This may include intravenous adrenaline to maintain cardiac output, the antihistamine chlorpheniramine (Piriton) given intravenously, intravenous hydrocortisone acting as an anti-inflammatory agent, and salbutamol via a nebuliser as a bronchodilator.

Disease transmission is theoretically possible following transfusion and has occurred in the past, but today all blood in the UK is routinely screened for HIV and hepatitis. It is also extremely rare for blood to be contaminated with other microorganisms, although Gram-negative bacteria can reproduce at 4°C. Reactions include pyrexia, rigor, chest and abdominal pain and the development of **septicaemic shock**.

Pyrogenic reactions occur from agglutination following mismatch. They are

agglutination

the clumping of foreign cells due to an antigen–antibody reaction

haemolysis

the disintegration of red blood cells, causing severe anaemia and possibly jaundice

urticarial hives

a skin condition that manifests as red weals causing intense irritation; it is usually a result of hypersensitivity

septicaemic shock

a type of shock usually caused by bacterial endotoxins in the blood

pyrogenic reaction

a reaction that results in pyrexia (a raised temperature of above 37.5°C), caused by chemicals secreted from white blood cells and injured tissues

much rarer because of advances in screening techniques, but when they do occur, they result in pyrexia and urticaria.

Cold blood can cause ventricular fibrillation when given in large quantities. It is therefore advisable to use a blood-warming device to bring the blood to 37°C if a large volume is required in an emergency.

Intravenous fluid therapy

A client may receive intravenous fluid therapy when she is unable to maintain her fluid balance orally. Causes include dehydration because of a lack of oral intake, severe vomiting or dehydration, excess urine output or perspiration, severe burns, surgical procedures and unconsciousness. Intravenous fluid therapy is common in acute hospital settings, but it must be remembered that it is an invasive procedure with many potential complications. These include:

- Infection
- Inflammation
- **Thrombophlebitis**
- Extravasation (infiltration of fluid into the surrounding tissues)
- Septicaemia
- Air or particle embolism
- Circulatory overload
- Anaphylactic reaction.

thrombophlebitis

inflammation of the lining of the veins

The nurse's role is described in Chart 6.9.

▪ Chapter Summary

This chapter examined the key factors related to a client's respiratory and cardiac function. You have learnt how to monitor and interpret respiratory and cardiac vital signs and how to differentiate deviations from what is normal. You have considered how to assist and maintain respiratory function with supplemental oxygenation, physiotherapy and drugs delivered via inhaler devices. In addtion, you will have examined techniques to optimise cardiac function, for example pain assessment, cardiac monitoring, anti-embolic therapy, blood transfusion and intravenous therapy. Finally, you have learnt how to recognise and initially manage a cardiorespiratory arrest.

Chart 6.9 ● Hints for intravenous therapy

● Ensure that whoever sites the cannula selects an appropriate position and uses an aseptic procedure

● When sited, the cannula should be firmly secured

● The cannula should be regularly inspected (at least twice a day) for signs of infection and inflammation

● If fluids are being delivered via the cannula, it is essential to ensure that the right fluid is given to the right patient via the right route at the right time at the correct rate

● Most hospitals operate a policy whereby intravenous fluids need to be checked prior to delivery by two nurses, one of whom is a qualified nurse. To ensure that fluids are delivered at the correct rate, electronic pump devices are frequently used in many clinical settings. If these are not available, a formula for calculating the number of drips per minute is required. One such formula is described in Figure 6.23

● The system that is used for delivering the fluid must be inspected for damage and sterility

● It is essential to ensure that the system is free of air bubbles when primed with fluids and during the process of fluid delivery

● All contact with the intravenous system should be aseptic to reduce the risk of infection

● You may also see drugs added to the fluid system. The additives may be prepacked or require adding. In most hospitals, this is a procedure for a trained nurse

$$\frac{(\text{Number of ml} \times \text{drops/ml})}{(\text{Number of hours} \times 60)} = \text{drops/minute}$$

The following example represents a client who is prescribed 1000 ml (1 litre) of fluid over 4 hours. The giving set in use delivers 10 drops per ml. The figure 60 is a given constant representing 60 minutes in 1 hour.

Therefore:

$$\frac{(1000 \times 10)}{(4 \times 60)} = 41.7 \text{ or } 42 \text{ drops/minute}$$

Note: the giving set package must be carefully inspected for the number of drops per ml as this may vary

Figure 6.23 ● Formula for drip rate calculation

● Test Yourself!

1. What is the normal respiratory rate for a 2-year-old child?

2. What are Cheyne–Stokes respirations?

3. Describe four types of sputum and their causes.

4. Describe the jaw thrust manoeuvre and when it would be used.

5. List six effects of hypoxia.

6. Where do you assess signs of circulation in the infant and adult?

7. What are the five Korotkoff sounds?

8. How do you assess capillary refill time?

9. Describe the types of pain assessment tool available.

10. Describe five complications of a blood transfusion.

Further Reading

Chandler, T. (2000) Oxygen saturation monitoing. *Paediatric Nursing* 12(8): 37–43.

Peate, I. and Lancaster, J. (2000) Safe use of medical gases. *British Journal of Nursing* 9(4): 231–6.

Resuscitation Council (UK) (2000) *Advanced Life Support Course Provider Manual*, 4th edn. Resuscitation Council, London.

Woodrow, P. (1999) Pulse oximetry. *Nursing Standard* 13(42): 42–6.

References

Allan, D. (1989) Making sense of oxygen delivery. *Nursing Times* 85(18): 40–2.

Baskett, P.J.F. and Chamberlain, D. (eds) (1977) The ILCOR advisory statement. *Resuscitation* 34: 97–8.

British Medical Journal (1993) *Advanced Paediatric Life Support. The Practical Support.* BMJ Publishing, London.

Carpenito, L.J. (2001) *Nursing Diagnosis: Application to Practice*, 9th edn. J.B. Lippincott, Philadelphia.

Hazinski, M.F. (1999) *Manual of Nursing Care of the Critically Ill Child.* C.V. Mosby, St Louis.

Hinchliff, S.M., Montague, S.E. and Watson, R. (1996) *Physiology for Nursing Practice*, 2nd edn. Baillière Tindall, London.

Kendrick, A.H. and Smith, E.C. (1992) Simple measurements of lung function. *Professional Nurse* 7(6): 395–402.

Law, C. (2000) A guide to assessing sputum. *Nursing Times* 96(24): 7–10.

Lewis, L.W. and Timby, B.K. (1993) *Fundamental Skills and Concepts in Patient Care.* Chapman & Hall, London.

Macintyre, P.E. and Ready, L.B. (1996) *Acute Pain Management: A Practical Guide.* W.B. Saunders, London.

Mackway-Jones, K. (ed.) (1997) *Emergency Triage.* BMJ Publishing, London.

Mackway-Jones, K., Molyneux, E., Phillips, B. and Wieteska, C. (eds) (2001) *Advanced Paediatric Life Support.* BMJ Publishing, London.

Mallett, J. and Dougherty, L. (eds) (2000) *The Royal Marsden Hospital Manual of Clinical Nursing Procedures*, 5th edn. Blackwell Scientific, Oxford.

Marieb, E. (2001) *Human Anatomy and Physiology*, 5th edn. Benjamin Cummings, San Francisco.

Martini, F.H. (2001) *Fundamentals of Anatomy and Physiology*, 5th edn. C.V. Mosby, London.

Middleton, S. and Middleton, P.G. (1998) Assessment. In Pryor, J.A. and Webber, B.A. (eds) *Physiotherapy for Respiratory and Cardiac Problems.* Churchill Livingstone, Edinburgh.

O'Brien (1997) *Blood Pressure Measurement: Recommendations of the British Hypertension Society.* BMJ Publishing, London.

Park, G., Fulton, B. and Senthuran, S. (2000) *The Management of Acute Pain*, 2nd edn. Oxford University Press, Oxford.

Ramsey, J. (1989) *Nursing the Child with Respiratory Problems.* Chapman & Hall, London.

Rutishauser, S. (1994) *Physiology and Anatomy: A Basis for Nursing and Health Care.* Churchill Livingstone, London.

Schramroth, L. (1990) *An Introduction to Electrocardiography*, 7th edn. Blackwell Scientific, London.

Smith, G. (2000) *Alert: A Multi Professional Course in Care of the Acutely Ill Patient.* University of Portsmouth, Hampshire.

Thiagamoorthy, S., Merchant, S., Carter, M., Jarvis, D. and Bateman, N. (2000) An audit of oxygen therapy: is oxygen prescribed, administered, monitored and withdrawn according to guidelines? *Journal of Clinical Excellence* **2**(2): 127–9.

Whaley, L.F. and Wong, D.L. (1995) *Nursing Care of Infants and Children.* C.V. Mosby, St Louis.

World Health Organization Regional Office for Europe (1999) *Third Workshop on the Use and Abuse of Blood and Blood Products in Clinical Settings: A Report on a WHO Workshop.* WHO, Copenhagen.

Wong, D.L. (2000) *Wong and Whaley's Clinical Manual of Paediatric Nursing.* C.V. Mosby, St Louis.

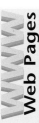
Web Pages

http://www.hospice-spc-council.org.uk

http://www.resus.org.uk

http://www.child-resuscitation.org.uk

7

Body Image and Sexuality

Contents

Learning outcomes

The expression of sexuality and body image appear to be interrelated, particularly when associated with physical or mental illness, disease or physical trauma. Sexuality, sexual health and body image can, when negatively affected, decrease a person's self-image and self-esteem. When individuals have contact with a health-care setting, their illness or disability will probably impact on their sexuality (RCN, 2000). There can be many adjustments to sexuality and body image, and with these can come changes to self-care (Salter, 1997). The nurse has a vital role to play here.

After reading this chapter, you will be in a better position to:

- Understand the interrelationship between sexuality and body image and your responsibility in understanding these two important aspects of a person

- Recognise the part you will play in helping patients and clients when body image and sexuality need to be addressed as an aspect of patient care

- Recognise your own feelings with respect to these areas

- Realise the importance of your own self-awareness when communicating with patients and clients who want support and guidance with their sexuality and altered body image needs.

What Is Self-image and Normal Body Image?

Over the past two decades, nursing has integrated holistic perspectives and approaches into the care of patients and clients: we now consider the psycho-social, cultural and spiritual wants and needs of patients and clients when we tend to their physical requirements. To perceive the patient and client as a 'whole' and not as components that need separate attention is an important ideal and can help the nurse to be more receptive to the patient's self-image and self-esteem. **Self-image** is, according to Price (1990), 'our own assessment of our social worth'. A positive self-image gives us confidence and increases our self-esteem.

An important element of self-image is **body image**, the mental picture each person has of his or her body. At birth, infants do not have a body image, but as they develop as babies their awareness expands and they begin to explore parts of their body. As they receive sensory stimulation through physical contact with others, they become aware of their own separateness (Sundeen et al., 1994).

Children have a relatively simple view of their own bodies. When they are asked to draw pictures of themselves and the different parts of their bodies, their view of the body and the way in which it functions will be represented using elementary shapes to represent organs. Once children go to school, these concepts are developed and become more sophisticated as they start to view body image within the context of gender identification (Price, 1998). Towards the end of primary education, children's concepts of themselves, their body and its functions are influenced by the attitude of their parental figures in terms of what they do and say and the things that are discussed or not discussed within the family context (Sundeen et al., 1994).

Adolescence, a time of rapid physical development, can bring with it feelings of awkwardness. Secondary sexual characteristics have to be incorporated into the individual's developing body image. With this go society's expectations of conforming to the social roles of being a man or woman, for example the different ways in which we groom and adorn ourselves when in the social arena.

If body image is affected, either positively or negatively, this will inevitably influence the person's self-image. McCrea et al. (1982) state that body image as a term:

> Refers to the body as a psychological experience and focuses on the individual's feelings and attitudes towards his own body.

Chilton (1984) demonstrates the links between self-esteem and body image when stating:

> Body image also plays an important part in self-understanding. How a person feels about himself is basically related to how he feels about his body.

CONNECTIONS

Chapter 9 briefly discusses spirituality and nursing care, and Chapter 2 looks at the spiritual needs of nurses.

self-image
our own assessment of our social worth

body image
the mental picture we have of our body and our feelings towards it

The body is a most visible and material part of one's self and occupies the central part in a person's perceptions. Body image is the sum of the conscious and unconscious attitudes that the individual has towards his body. Present and past perceptions and feelings about size, function, appearance and potential are included. A person with a high level of self-esteem will tend to have a much clearer understanding of himself.

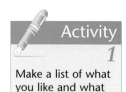

Activity 1

Make a list of what you like and what you dislike about your body.

Added to this complex concept of body image is the element of change. How the individual perceives him- or herself can alter depending on external and/or internal influences, which may be psychosocial, cultural or physiological or any combination of these. An example of this is menstruation and the hormonal changes that occur in the body in association with the menstrual cycle. These hormonal changes cause physiological alterations: for example, when the level of progesterone is at its lowest, menstruation occurs. This may affect the woman's mood and also influence how she perceives herself when menstruating. Added to this could be the woman's view of whether or not she wants to be pregnant and how she associates menstruation with being womanly and feminine. There are also cultural differences of opinion towards the menstruating woman: historically, the West has used terms like 'the curse' to describe the process of menstruating, which can affect how women view their menstrual blood and their bodies when menstruating (Kitzinger, 1985).

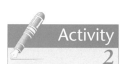

Activity 2

How do you perceive yourself in your later years? List the changes you envisage occurring as you age.

Your list could be influenced by how you view your body now and how it functions, your older family members and how they have changed and learned to adapt. Your list could also be affected by someone you know who has taken on new challenges as they have aged.

Ageing will also influence body image. As well as there being physiological changes, which may affect mobility and independent living, society's views on ageing are also an influence on the older person's body image (Price, 1990). Alterations in body function and appearance are a feature of health as well as illness and can usefully be viewed along an age continuum. It is important for nurses to understand how the body is affected by normal physiological change, illness, ageing and hospitalisation, and how this influences self-image. Nurses' self-awareness in relation to how they perceive their own bodies and the bodies of others is an important contribution to this process of understanding. Even admission to hospital, before any procedures are commenced, will affect a person's body image and self-image. Removing one's day clothes and getting into bed can bring about feelings of dependency, loss and passivity. Changes to or a loss of self-image caused by hospitalisation have been well documented and can be linked with the changes in or a loss of self-identity observed in people who spend more than a few days in hospital (Goffman, 1961; Sanderson, 1985; Savage, 1987).

Trying to understand individuals' feelings about their body image should also include how they value the different parts of their body. This is highly individualised, but the nurse can explore this with the patient when completing the initial assessment. If, for example, a jockey puts on weight, this will seriously affect his or her career. An orchestral conductor with a damaged shoulder will be unable to work without suffering pain.

Body reality, body ideal and body presentation

Price (1990) defines body image using three fundamental and interrelated concepts: body reality, body ideal and body presentation.

Body reality

Body reality refers to the body, as it is, an objective representation, for example stating someone's height, hair colour and eye colour. Body reality is dynamic as our bodies undergo constant physiological changes. We may be more aware of some of these than others, for example the physiological changes that occur during puberty as pubic hair, breasts or facial hair develop. These will have a dramatic effect on body reality and inevitably affect body image, self-image and self-esteem. From birth to older age, there are clear examples of how body reality alters.

Body ideal

Body ideal represents how we believe our body should look and perform. This body ideal is influenced by the beliefs, norms and attitudes that we develop from early childhood as part of our primary socialisation.

During adolescence, the body ideal appears to require constant updating in the light of new trends, the media offering examples of the most recent 'role models', for example popular music bands and their accompanying style of dress. The adolescent age group has, more than any other, to adjust body reality with respect to variations in fashion and social behaviour. Both body piercing and tattooing have recently been on the increase (Langford, 1996), are attractive to young people and may be considered to be a permanent body reality change, but there are implications relating to an alteration in body ideal as fashion changes or a person ages.

Body ideal includes how we think we should smell and age, what we should weigh, and how our body should be proportioned, for example the size of our breasts or penis. Body ideal is also influenced by cultural standards: over the past two decades a focus on exercise and fitness, to produce a slim, toned body, has led to a 'body-conscious' society (Sundeen et al., 1994).

Body presentation

Body presentation is linked with body ideal and represents how we present our body to others in a social context and in intimate situations. Body presentation

Activity 3

Think about how you present your body to others. Write down what you do, for example through the use of make-up, clothes and hairstyle, in order to 'face the world' when you go out to meet others.

Does this change depending on whom you are meeting and what you are doing?

body reality
the body as it actually is in terms of its objective physical characteristics

body ideal
how we believe our body should look and perform, this being influenced by our beliefs and attitudes and by changes in fashion

body presentation
how we present our bodies to others in a social context, including our clothes, make-up and hairstyle

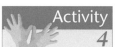

Activity
4

Breast and testicular self-examination should be a routine part of personal health care. Do you examine yourself? List the reasons why you do or do not regularly practise this self-examination.

Ask your close friends the same question. What reasons do they give for regularly self-examining? What reasons are given by those who do not?

includes how we dress, adorn our body, groom and use posture and gesture (Price, 1990, 1998). It also involves how we smell: whether or not we choose to wear deodorant and/or perfume, and what type of perfume we want others to smell on us, can play an important part in how we want to be perceived and the association that society makes with particular smells and perfumes. We have a level of control over how we present our body to others, but we are also influenced by what is expected of us, for example policies regarding how and when uniform should be worn, or guidelines on what is acceptable at work. We are then aware of the limits and boundaries of how we can present our body to others, as can be seen with those working in the community as a community psychiatric or district nurse.

Being unhappy with our body image affects how we behave and inevitably affects those around us, even if this unhappiness is temporary. If we feel good about our body image and others notice this and offer positive comments to support us, this will usually positively affect our self-image so that we feel good about ourselves and discern approval.

■ What Is Altered Body Image?

altered body image

the state of distress and lowered self-esteem that occurs when coping strategies to deal with changes in body reality, ideal or presentation are overwhelmed

Early developments, particularly from childhood to adolescence, pregnancy and ageing are evident through visual physiological changes to body reality and are perceived as part of normal human functioning. **Altered body image** may not be evident through obvious physiological change to the normal body, but, even with a lack of external evidence for the observer, it may still have a devastating effect. Price (1995) defines altered body image as:

> A state of personal distress, defined by the patient, which indicates that the body no longer supports self-esteem, and which is dysfunctional to individuals, limiting their social engagement with others. Altered body image exists when coping strategies (individual and social) to deal with changes in body reality, ideal or presentation, are overwhelmed by injury, disease, disability, or social stigma.

This definition appears to recognise the importance of people in their social and cultural environment, their spiritual awareness and its significance for how they perceive their altered body image.

loss of self model

a model that aims to understand altered body image by considering loss of psychological self, loss of socio-cultural self and loss of physical self

Loss of self model

Blackmore (1989) applies Watson's (1980) description of 'loss of self' by using three concepts to explain altered body image: loss of psychological self, loss of socio-cultural self and loss of physical self.

Loss of psychological self occurs when a person's self-concept and self-esteem is diminished, and loss of socio-cultural self is seen when a person experiences a loss of social identity, social role, family grouping or linkage with his or her cultural background. Loss of physical self refers to a loss of bodily function or functions, a body part or parts or the quality of physiological functioning. 'Loss of self' will affect the person in different ways depending on the disease, illness or trauma and the treatment involved, how the person perceives these and their significance to the person's life. Consider, for example, a man who has experienced ostomy surgery: the mutilation and relocation of a body orifice could have a serious effect on his body image.

CONNECTIONS

Chapter 5 explains ostomy surgery.

Loss of psychological self

Loss of psychological self will include the man feeling as though he has returned to an infantile stage of development, unable to control his excretory functions. This may affect how he views his masculinity and sexuality. He may question his sexual role and functioning, asking questions such as, 'Do I smell?', 'Am I still attractive?', 'Will my partner still find me attractive?', 'Will people be able to see my ostomy bag?', 'Will I still be able to have sex?' and 'Will my partner still want to have sex with me?' A man involved with sporting activities may question how other men perceive him: is he seen as disabled?

Loss of socio-cultural self

Loss of socio-cultural self arises because society has particular attitudes towards excretion. For adults, urination and defaecation usually occur in private and are not usually discussed with others. There is also the stigma that is attached to having a disease of the bowel. Postoperatively, there may be a degree of unpredictability as the body adjusts to the physiological change and the person adapts to using an appliance. During this time, he may chose to isolate himself socially. Family relationships can be affected: apart from the change in role within the partnership or family, temporary or otherwise, to that of patient, the man has to decide how to include his partner and other family members in the knowledge of his illness and its effects on his day-to-day life. Added to this is any cultural and religious attitude towards excretion, which may be a problem when caring for a stoma site, for example in keeping the right hand clean for preparing and eating food (Bell, 1989).

Loss of physical self

Loss of physical self can occur in different ways after surgery. The loss of the normal way of defaecating can cause difficulty, and having to adapt to wearing a bag on your stomach can affect how you view your body. Physical changes may include the effects of other treatments after surgery for stoma formation, such as radiotherapy, which can cause fatigue, sore skin, nausea and vomiting. Chemotherapy can lead to hair loss, skin discolouration and infertility. Sexual problems and a decreased libido are suffered by a high percentage of patients (de Marquiegui and Huish, 1999), and the general quality of body functioning can be affected (Blackmore, 1989).

Examples of altered body image

'open' altered body image

an alteration in body image that can be clearly seen by others

'concealed' altered body image

an alteration in body image that is hidden from others

There are many different types of altered body image, some examples of which (Table 7.1) can be placed in either an 'open' or a 'concealed' category. A woman who has recently developed anorexia nervosa may not be seen as experiencing anorexia nervosa by others, but if her illness progresses and her eating patterns change, this, along with weight loss and other physiological changes, will lead to her illness becoming 'open' and evident to others.

Along with this idea of altered body image being open or concealed goes the consideration of whether or not an injury, illness or disease is permanent or temporary. Individuals may not know this in the early stages of their condition as a prognosis may not have been given, but once a diagnosis and prognosis have been given, there will be an idea of whether or not there is any permanence. This information will influence how the person adapts and manages any alteration to his or her body image.

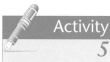

Activity 5

Think of a patient whom you have cared for who was experiencing altered body image. Write down what you observed and found out about this patient.

The role of the nurse

Assessment

It is important to assess how people perceive their bodies and how this influences their self-image and self-esteem. Observing the way someone presents, for example their posture, hair, dress and make-up, can provide important information. Conversations about the patient's cultural background, age and occupation can further help the nurse to make sense of the patient's body image and self-image. Specific questions can be asked, for example how much importance the patient places on appearance and physical functioning. The nurse will then start to understand the significance of health and illness for the patient. If a body image change has occurred because of illness, or is about to occur from surgery, what effect might this have on the patient's future body image, self-image and self-esteem? Watson's (1980) loss of self model can be used as a framework to assess the significance and context of altered body image for the patient.

Table 7.1 Examples of altered body image

Congenital	Hereditary	Degenerative	Trauma
		OPEN	
Muscular dystrophy	Huntington's	Parkinson's disease	Facial burns
Cleft palate/lip	chorea	Multiple sclerosis	Amputation
Spina bifida	Retinitis	Arthritis	
Facial birthmarks	pigmentosa		
	Hair loss		
	Acne		
	Psoriasis, eczema		
		CONCEALED	
Hypospadias	Diabetes mellitus	Conduction deafness	Burns to main body Body scarring (abuse)

Psychological	Surgical	Medical	Miscellaneous
		OPEN	
Anorexia nervosa	Mastectomy	Medication	Tattoos
Schizophrenia	Reconstruction	Chemotherapy	Body piercing
Obsessive disorders	Amputation of limb	Psychotropic	Limb prosthesis
	Miscarriage	Hormone	Pregnancy
	Disfigurative	replacement	Obesity
	surgery, for	therapy	Use of a wheelchair
	example for cancer	Alopecia	Birthmarks
	of the neck	Halitosis	Intravenous
	Breast reduction/		infusion
	enhancement		
		CONCEALED	
Nasogastric tube	Circumcision	Sexually	Crohn's disease
Body dysmorphic	Hysterectomy	transmitted	
disorder	Orchidectomy	diseases	
Body scarring	Lumpectomy	Medication	
(cutting)	Stoma	Peri-anal abscess	
Bulimia nervosa	Termination	Caesarean section	
		Impotence	
		Sterility	
		Premature	
		ejaculation	

Source: Adapted from Salter (1997) and Price (1990).

During the assessment process, the nurse may have contact with the patient's relatives and friends; assessing their perception and expectations of the patient, and how the relative or friend is managing the situation, is important. How well informed are they? What strategies are they able to use to manage their own feelings about the patient's altered body image? Are they able to continue supporting the patient (Price, 1990)? If the altered body image is permanent, how will this affect the relationship on a psychological, socio-cultural and physical level? It is important to recognise the needs of relatives and friends and be proactive with the support and information they require. It is also important to be aware of issues of confidentiality for the patient: communication with relatives, partners and friends should ideally only be undertaken with the patient's permission. Some of the areas considered above could be discussed with the patient, relatives, partner and friends together.

Nursing skills

Any change in body image, particularly when the change is viewed as negative, requires time for adjustment. For some patients, a full adjustment may be too difficult to contemplate or totally accept as they feel vulnerable and not in control of their situation. The nurse should be available to listen to the patient's concerns and fears when the patient feels ready. It may be that the individual is only able to take in a small amount of information at any one time.

CONNECTIONS

Chapter 9 provides further information on bereavement.

As previously discussed, alteration in body image is a loss and can affect the patient in different ways depending on what the altered body image signifies. The manifestation of this loss is to experience a grief reaction, which may include anger and denial.

Once the patient has experienced the altered body image, there should be a period of rehabilitation, perhaps involving access to specialist practitioners such as stoma care or breast care nurses. The adaptation to any change in body image will be influenced by a number of factors: gender, age, the severity of the change in body image, pre- and postoperative preparation including patient or client education, beliefs and values, coping mechanisms and sexual functioning.

CONNECTIONS

Chapter 11 looks at therapeutic communication amd working in groups.

Patients will observe anyone who cares for them to ascertain their reactions towards and acceptance of the change in body image (Salter, 1997). The qualities and skills of the nurse will help patients to adjust and find their own way of coming to terms with this alteration in their body image. Nurses must not, however, underestimate the challenge that this brings to the patient but must value and respect the process of adjustment. In turn, nurses have a responsibility to ensure that they are able to work with the patient in a meaningful way on both a physical and a psychological level, undergoing regular clinical supervision with someone who is able to help them make sense of the caring relationship they have formed.

Casebox 7.1

Sally is a 24-year-old married mother of two young children, who was admitted 3 weeks ago to an acute mental health unit for the treatment of her depression. She has been given antidepressants and has attended counselling sessions with her key worker. Sally is being prepared for discharge home to her supportive family and will receive regular visits from a community psychiatric nurse. Sally has stated to her key worker that she is worried about sleeping with her husband in case he wants to be intimate with her. She has also stated that she does not feel very attractive and thinks that she is 'right off sex'.

What could be the main reasons for Sally feeling this way?

■ Any long stay in hospital can influence how people feel about themselves. Not being able to attend to our 'body presentation' in our normal way may mean that we become dissatisfied with how we look as the gap between our body presentation and body ideal widens.

■ The antidepressants that Sally has been prescribed may also affect her sexual functioning and libido. She may have become more aware of this as the antidepressants have started to work and she begins to focus her attention on being back at home.

■ Sally's body weight and appearance may have changed during the time she has felt depressed. This too could affect how she perceives and feels about her body.

Casebox 7.2

Janice is a 38-year-old woman who has been living with her partner Lisa for 11 years. Janice has been diagnosed with Crohn's disease after suffering from chronic diarrhoea, abdominal pain and weight loss for nearly a year, and after a number of admissions to hospital. She has been taking medication to treat the diarrhoea and analgesics to reduce the pain. Her physician has informed her that she has a partial obstruction of her small bowel and has referred her to a surgeon who believes that surgery may be necessary to remove the obstruction. Janice has also been told that she will require a temporary stoma. She is devastated and has asked whether she can discuss this with Lisa before she agrees to surgery.

List some of the concerns that Lisa may have concerning the formation of a stoma.

■ How the stoma will look? How it will function? How will Janice manage the appliance? How will it affect her everyday life? How will she broach the subject with Lisa, and what effect will this have on their relationship? One of Janice's worries could be whether she may need a permanent stoma in the future. Janice will also be working out how to cope with social situations and any other activities that could involve others becoming aware of her stoma.

■ Human Sexuality

Health professionals are often uncomfortable with the issue of sexuality even though it is part of everyday life. For various reasons, individuals who cope reasonably well with the uncertainties of sexuality in their own lives find this much more difficult when in a professional role. In this section, we will be looking at why sexuality can in general create difficulties, and why the situation can be even more complicated in the context of health care.

The most common responses to the challenge of understanding human sexuality are either to ignore it and hope it goes away, or to make some hard and fast rules in an attempt to make it easier for everyone. Neither of these approaches has been proved to work particularly well, so we will be advocating a different way: to accept the intricacies and paradoxes of human sexuality, to try to understand them and to work with them.

Dos and don'ts

Activity 6

If you had to choose just one sexual behaviour to be entirely forbidden, what would it be? Ask a few other people what they would forbid and then ask yourselves why.

What is so bad about these examples of sexual behaviour? The reasons are usually complicated!

Sex and sexuality are fundamental to what humans are, so if nurses ignore this part of people's lives, they are missing a large chunk of the whole person. It is also potentially harmful to people not to have their sexuality acknowledged. The French philosopher Michel Foucault has written extensively about sexuality, describing the 'triple edict of taboo, non-existence and silence' surrounding sexuality (Foucault, 1978). But what does he mean by this? By using the word 'taboo', he is referring to the largely unwritten rules on sexual behaviour, the beliefs and myths that have developed over time. These appear to be real, but a closer examination reveals that humans have created these systems to guide their behaviour. We will be exploring the derivations of some 'common sense truths' in the history of sexuality, below. First, however, try Activity 6.

'Non-existence' is Foucault's way of expressing one of the ways in which sexuality is dealt with, that is, by totally denying its existence and repressing any mention of sex and sexuality. Many health-care practices appear to be attempting to do this, and it was only relatively recently in Western society that this approach has waned. Foucault's mention of 'silence' is linked to the idea of non-existence but conveys a subtle difference: 'silence' suggests a notion that sex and sexuality exist but are not to be talked about, just accepted as given, suffered in... well, silence. To get a better idea of these concepts, try Activity 7.

The skill of the nurse in dealing with sexuality is to balance the biomedical realities of sexual function, sexual health and the reproductive process with what sexuality means to the individual, this personal meaning relating to what we looked at in Activity 2 above. It has to do with the way in which a person has been brought up, current thinking in society in general, race, culture and religion. The Nursing and Midwifery Council (NMC) makes it plain in the *Code of Professional Conduct* (NMC, 2002) that nurses must respect each individual's point of view. It is also a requirement that the individual's views be actively included in care-planning (point 2.1).

The nurse's role

The ways in which nurses will encounter sexuality can be divided into two. The first group involves situations in which a patient or client's condition is likely to have a direct and obvious effect on sexual functioning and sexuality. Examples are a young woman having a hysterectomy, a man having prostate surgery that may lead to impotence, and a girl with extensive burns to her body and face. More positive examples comprise orthodontic treatment, cosmetic plastic surgery and in vitro fertilisation (IVF). To develop your thinking, spend a little time considering Activity 8. (It is interesting to note that many of the examples of health interventions that 'obviously' relate to sexuality are also linked to body image.)

A second way in which nurses encounter sexuality is in the sense that 'everyone has one'! Many writers believe that sexuality is a fundamental component of the person, that you are not 'you' without it. Nurses routinely have access to peoples' most intimate details but are open to criticism for often ignoring this crucial component of any individual's life. This is not to say that nurses should pry unnecessarily into an individual's private life – it is rarely necessary for them to know any details of a patient or client's sexual functioning and relationships. However, nurses should be sensitive to this crucial aspect of their client's lives and confident and competent in discussing sexual issues whenever they arise. Research consistently demonstrates that nurses need to improve in both these arenas (Gamel, 1993; Meerabeau, 1999).

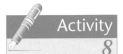

Activity 7

Think about how important sexuality is to you – your gender, your sexual orientation, fancying people, being fancied, mistakes, being a parent, dreading being a parent, your body and how it feels, your wardrobe, your haircut... the list is endless.

Now think about services you have participated in and the service users you have worked with. Is any of this richness expressed in what is written or said about them, the buildings in which the services are provided, the materials promoting the service?

Do the services have specific policies or guidelines to help workers to deal with issues of sexuality?

Activity 8

Divide a piece of paper into two columns, one labelled 'Health interventions with a negative impact on sex and sexuality', the other 'Health interventions with a positive impact on sex and sexuality'. Carrying on from the examples in the text, write as many items as you can under each heading.

Having done this relatively quickly, reconsider the interventions you have chosen. Are they as clearly good or bad as you first thought?

IVF, for example, is a positive intervention to help couples meet their need to have children, but the difficulties that couples receiving such treatment can experience are well known, regularly appearing in TV documentaries and popular novels.

Casebox 7.3

Rob is 33 years old and has a learning disability. Until recently, he lived in his family home, but he has now chosen to move to a housing association flat and live on his own. He regularly visits his local health centre for a minor health problem, and the nurses have got to know him quite well. Rob has begun to talk to them about how he would like to have a girlfriend but is starting to feel down because he is still on his own.

Sant Angelo (2000) suggests some probable features of the lives of people with learning difficulties that may well apply in Rob's case:

■ A high incidence of sexually abusive experiences

■ Multiple experiences of bereavement and loss

■ Difficulties in talking about emotions

■ Limited sex education

■ Limited expectations and low self-esteem

■ A lack of assertiveness about sex and relationships

■ A lack of privacy.

What simple interventions could be made with Rob to empower him to achieve his desired lifestyle?

■ Rob could be encouraged to talk about his feelings. If his needs were simple advice and education, the health centre nurses

might be able to provide this. If Rob's needs went beyond this, he could be offered access to other services, for example self-help groups run by people with learning disabilities, the learning disability community nursing service, a range of independent and voluntary services to help him increase his social network, counselling and other services as appropriate. Most importantly, Rob needs to be listened to with respect and sensitivity so that he can find the best way to achieve his goals.

Sexuality and self-awareness

Self-awareness is an important attribute for nurses generally but is perhaps especially needed in the case of sexuality, given the subject's possible sensitivity. It is perfectly acceptable for nurses to have strong views on issues relating to sexuality, but it is potentially harmful to impose these blindly on patients and clients. Being a nurse does not mean having to subscribe to a particular set of beliefs about sex and sexuality, but it does mean appreciating that there are many viewpoints, yours being simply another. It is an essential skill to know what your standpoint is and how that relates to other peoples'. Whatever our views are, they did not come out of nowhere, so it may help to know where our beliefs originated, giving us a chance to consider them a bit more closely. The next section will thus review some of what is known about historical views of sexuality as many of our present beliefs have a long, but not always distinguished, history. Before reading this section, spend some time on Activity 9 as it should make the material more relevant.

An historical perspective on sexuality

The object of exploring history is to trace the derivation of ideas that are believed to be the 'truth' and to investigate the diversity of sexual codes.

Prehistoric times

What we know here derives mainly from cave paintings, which show men and women in various sexual poses. Magical qualities were apparently attributed to the sex act. Many figurines have been found of women's bodies, the reproductive aspects being obviously out of proportion, so it would seem that fertility was the main concern.

Ancient Egyptian society

Sexual symbolism was a large part of religious life, phallic symbols and a preoccupation with fertility being highly evident. Some prostitution occurred in the temples, and intercourse with a virgin was considered to be very potent. But despite this apparently orgiastic approach, Egyptian laws on adultery are among the earliest known recorded laws governing morality. Women were at this time seen as the property of men.

Ancient Greek society

The Greeks apparently had an altogether more aesthetic and tolerant attitude towards sex and sexuality. They had a far more bisexual approach too: the procreation of children was obviously still of the utmost importance, but, especially among higher echelons of society, a love between men was sometimes considered to be on a higher plane. The earliest known recorded accounts of lesbian sexuality, written by a woman called Sappho, can also be attributed to the Greeks. What seems probable is that the concept of 'homosexual' as a special kind of person, or even as a specific activity, would have been alien to people living in this era.

Roman society

Roman civilisation encompassed a wide range of communities, so it is probably misleading to suggest that there was a single approach to sexual practice. It is,

Activity 9

Where do you think the following ideas originate from? We are not suggesting that they are right or wrong, but you may find yourself agreeing or disagreeing. Asking yourself why will help towards developing self-awareness:

● Gay and lesbian individuals should have freedom of sexual expression

● Anal sex is unnatural

● Children should not be taught about sex

● Women are the passive receivers of male sexual advances.

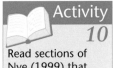

Activity 10

Read sections of Nye (1999) that particularly interest you.

however, known that Galen (a Roman physician c.200 AD) recommended sex as being healthy; he suggested that abstaining from sex could cause anxiety and health problems. Again, women's position in society was inferior to that of men.

Ancient Jewish society

Jewish culture was unique in the sense of having clear delineations of sexual behaviour. Sex was for procreation only, homosexuality, incest and masturbation being forbidden. This culture is very important to Western society as a large portion of it came to us through Christianity; an example will illustrate how 'absolute truths' are largely misleading in discussions of sexuality. One of the most famous stories from Ancient Jewish writing, known to us as the Old Testament, concerns the destruction of the cities of Sodom and Gomorrah. For many generations, it was taught that the cities were destroyed because the citizens practised forbidden sexual acts, including anal intercourse, and as a result of this teaching, anal intercourse came to be known as sodomy. Wilton (2000), however, points out that Bible scholars now believe that the cities were destroyed because of their lack of hospitality to strangers – in a desert society, this was much more a matter of life and death. This alteration of the meaning of the original Old Testament by the Bible interpreters of the past illustrates beautifully how thinking about sexual behaviour is constantly manipulated to achieve political ends.

Middle Ages

It was not really until the Middle Ages that any strong views on sex emerged in Europe, these deriving from the Christian Church. This was partly the result of the growing belief that spiritual activities were superior to physical ones. St Thomas Aquinas (1225–1274), thought to be influential in terms of Western ideas about sexuality, made the distinction between sins against other people and those against nature (that is, God), which were much more serious. Sinful sexual activities (most serious first) were:

- Bestiality
- Homosexuality
- Sexual intercourse in an 'unnatural' position
- Masturbation

These sexual activities were considered sinful because they offended the 'natural' order. This way of looking at sexuality became very influential and lingers to this day.

Seventeenth and eighteenth centuries

Despite the apparently extreme approach to sexuality recommended by writers such as Thomas Aquinas, real life was for most people probably not closely guided by these principles. Sexual behaviour was not strongly regulated in practice until the seventeenth and eighteenth centuries, when various factors combined to make states begin to legislate and enforce that legislation. An enormous number of factors is involved but two are of prime importance (Davenport-Hines, 1990).

Spread of syphilis across Europe

Syphilis was practically epidemic in Europe from the late fifteenth century onwards. This is significant for two main reasons. First, the prevalence of syphilis was blamed on whoever was liked least at the time – other nationalities, prostitutes, immoral men. The disease was also no respecter of social status, kings as well as their subjects contracting it! Second, it became apparent that the only safe form of sex was with one partner, in other words monogamy.

Revolutions across Europe

As unrest and revolution spread across Europe, culminating in the French Revolution of 1789, governments were extremely concerned about social order. It was thought then, as now, that the mainstay of social order was the family, so sexual expression outside family-based monogamy became increasingly targeted. Sexual modes of expression gained labels and were in some cases made unlawful; if they were already unlawful, they were pursued more vigorously by the authorities. Male homosexuality is an example of this, the result being that gay sex was practised in secret and became a potential source of guilt.

From the nineteenth century to today

Looking back, we tend to see the Victorian era as the height of widespread sexual repression, but at the same time the natural sciences and medicine were developing at an enormous rate, and with them a scientific interest in sexuality. This is exemplified by the work of writers such as Havelock Ellis and Freud, who started the lengthy process towards making the study and discussion of sexuality important and above all respectable.

■ Gender

gender

a social group's interpretation of being a man or a woman. It concerns the status and role of the sexes rather than their physical characteristics

Gender is a crucial issue in health care and nursing, going way beyond the physical characteristics of being male or female. The study of gender is the study

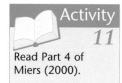

Activity 11

Read Part 4 of
Miers (2000).

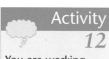

Activity 12

You are working
with a school nurse
in a secondary
school and have
become involved in
the sexual health
component of the
curriculum. This
involves planning
and running a
series of sessions on
sexual behaviour
for a group of 12-
year-old boys and
girls.

Should the boys
and girls be taught
separately? Do they
need to be taught
different things?
Can stereotyped
gender differences
be avoided?

of how being a man or a woman has an impact on how much money you have, how well educated you are, what diseases you are most likely to have, your life expectancy, mental health, diet and weight. The literature on gender needs to be studied in its own right (see Activity 11, for example) to do it justice, but nurses can learn from the major finding of the social science literature on gender – that gender operates through members of a society learning to make assumptions about the roles and capabilities of the sexes. Most societies are heavily biased to the advantage of men, so the widely held assumptions about women, for example, that women are physically and mentally weaker than men, that women gossip and men think deep thoughts and so on, tend to discriminate against them.

Nurses can contribute towards reducing health inequalities based on gender by challenging the unsupported (and often false) assumptions about the differences between men and women. Nurses can also help by acknowledging that men and women often have different approaches to health, this acknowledgement being called gender sensitivity (Miers, 2000).

Sexual Orientation

There is now an enormous amount of material available on what is known about sexual orientation, this being found in academic literature, books, films, television programmes, newspapers, magazines and so on. Despite this, however, gay and lesbian individuals can still experience discrimination in society in general and in the health services in particular (Wilton, 2000). In recognition of this, the Royal College of Nursing (RCN, 1994) issued a statement guiding nurses in how to combat discriminatory practice and make positive health contributions to lesbians and gay men. The main difficulties seem to come from a combination of factors, but you may find it useful to ask yourself these questions:

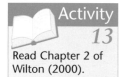

Activity 13

Read Chapter 2 of
Wilton (2000).

1. Do I know much about gay, lesbian, transvestite, transsexual and other alternative lifestyles?
2. Do I really know how I feel about people who have sexualities different from mine?

Your answers will indicate the way to competent and effective nursing practice with people who have alternative sexualities. Make it your business to find out more about the richness and diversity of our sexual lives and discover whether you have some unsupported prejudices that influence your behaviour without your really being aware of it.

This is quite deep and difficult, so an example of nursing practice may make the point clearer: read Casebox 7.4 below before you continue.

Desire

Casebox 7.4 demonstrates that being aware of sexuality in your practice does not require superhuman interpersonal skills or encyclopaedic knowledge. It mainly concerns listening, observing and showing some sensitivity to different viewpoints.

One way of viewing alternative sexualities is to think of all sexuality in terms of desire. Some men like tall women with brown hair who want a family. Some women like men who are reliable and have a steady job. As far as we know, there are no specific labels for these desires, and the people who practise them are left to do so without interference. But, a man who likes men with brown hair who want a family, and a woman who likes reliable women with steady jobs, may well experience interference. We all have preferences in terms of what kinds of person and activity arouse us sexually. Use Activity 14 to think about your own desires.

It is difficult to avoid the conclusion that society chooses what is acceptable sexual behaviour, albeit often unclearly and often based on outdated and unacceptable prejudices. Some of the restrictions, for example laws against rape and sex with children, obviously benefit us, but others are more difficult to justify outside artificial and misguided belief systems.

■ Sexuality and Skilled Nursing Care

Even a cursory exploration quickly reveals the complexity, richness and changeability of human sexuality, further examination demonstrating that if nursing is to take an holistic approach it can no longer routinely ignore this aspect of human life. But the depth and diversity of human sexuality can at times make it seem unmanageable. The **PLISSIT model** (Fogel and Lauver, 1990) attempts to make issues of sexuality more manageable for nurses. It categorises a nurse's potential interventions into four levels, each becoming increasingly intimate and needing more specialist knowledge. The idea behind the model is that all nurses can include sexuality in their practice but that they should operate at the level at which they feel safe and well informed. The four levels are:

● *Permission:* It is suggested that the sexual history should be a routine part of the assessment, thus raising sexuality as a legitimate concern and giving patients permission to ask questions about it in relation to their own care. Although this is implied to be most basic level, its success is dependent on a non-judgemental and accepting approach on the part of nurses

● *Limited information:* Misconceptions and myths are clarified at this level. Many of the difficulties people experience when dealing with their sexuality can be solved very quickly by good-quality, evidence-based information. To

Activity

14

Describe your ideal partner(s). If you can, write this down, although imagining will work too. What do they look like, what do they wear, what are they interested in, how do they treat you? How would the relationship run: a quick fling, living together, a big white wedding, eloping to an exotic destination? Would there be children?

Now think about this ideal scenario you have created. Does it have a specific label that conjures up your desire in complete detail? Are there debates in Parliament over what age you should be before you are allowed to indulge your desires? Would these lead to you being shunned by your family?

PLISSIT model

a model comprising four levels of nursing intervention to take sexuality and body image into account

A lesbian woman (we will call her **Dawn**) was in a medical ward for some straightforward treatment. Many of the staff were cold and remote towards her because of her sexuality. Dawn did not say much and was quite bad-tempered in her interactions with the health-care staff. One of the nurses, Lucy, noticed this and found it upsetting, although she could not think of a specific intervention that would help. Then, Lucy saw Dawn's partner Julie walking across the hospital car park. Lucy turned to Dawn, smiled and said, 'Hey, Dawn, that's great, your partner Julie is coming to visit you!' Dawn's demeanour immediately softened and she started to chat about their home life together. From then on Dawn would talk freely to Lucy and was more co-operative. The nursing care that Dawn received was therefore more effective, and her treatment was successful.

Why do you think Lucy's simple intervention made such a difference?

Have you had, or heard of, similar experiences?

be told that many people have similar difficulties, and to be given a few simple solutions, can be very liberating and take very little time. All the nurse needs is a sound (but not necessarily encyclopaedic) knowledge base and a straightforward, adult communication style

- *Specific suggestions:* These can relieve anxiety, promote creativity and help individuals to solve their own problems in partnership rather than being the passive recipients of advice
- *Intensive therapy:* The person is referred to a specialist sex therapist, who may also be a nurse. If nurses are to make competent interventions, it is important that they be clear about the limitations of their knowledge and skill. In some cases, the solutions may not be simple, so expert intervention is needed.

Modernisation of services and sexuality in nursing

The PLISSIT model is a very useful tool and goes a long way towards emphasising the importance of sexuality in nursing practice. The model can potentially relieve anxiety among nurses who are so concerned about not being 'experts' that they altogether ignore issues of sexuality. It is, however, important to build on the helpful principles established in the PLISSIT model and take them further by putting them into the context of current and future health-care trends. To do this, we will take a brief look at government policy for health and social care and UKCC policies for the preparation of nurses.

The education and preparation of nurses is now based on the principles underlying *Fitness for Practice* (UKCC, 1999). This report tackled many of the difficulties facing nursing, among them a series of competing demands, one of which is particularly relevant for our current investigation into body image and sexuality. The report talks about health care in the future demanding that nurses have 'high technical competence and "scientific rationality"', but about there being at the same time a 'continuing need for "human" qualities and the time to express them' (UKCC, 1999). Body image and sexuality are clearly very human qualities, which have in the past been overlooked by an overreliance on the disease-orientated medical model of care.

At a national, more structural level, government policy for the health-care services is also relevant to our discussion. It is clearly the intention for future health services to be driven by the people who use them. The version of the NHS Plan directed towards nurses emphasises holistic care, listening to patients, respecting their dignity and including them in their own health care (DoH, 2001). The Plan as a whole aims to reduce health inequality, prevent discrimination and help individuals to know more about, and take responsibility for, their own health. All of these aims are partly met by nurses taking account of body image and sexuality, which can have an impact far beyond more obvious biomedical concerns.

As we have seen, sexuality can relate to people in different groups having different amounts of power: adults and children, men and women, heterosexual and homosexual. These differences in power sometimes lead to abuse, perhaps linked to a powerful person or group not being willing to accept views other than their own. The UKCC's (2001) competencies for registration as a nurse make clear the stance of professional nursing by promoting respect for individuals and communities. The document goes on to discuss nurses practising without prejudice in an antidiscriminatory manner.

So nurses *do* need to be sensitive to each individual's notion of body image and sexuality in their face-to-face interactions, as demonstrated in the PLISSIT model, but the broader picture needs to be taken into account if our care is to be truly holistic.

■ Chapter Summary

To conclude the chapter, we need to bring body image and sexuality back together again: looking at them separately makes the material easier to absorb, but they are inextricably linked in our daily lives. If we consider our bodies and health, either to celebrate our good fortune or to bemoan an unkind fate, some part of that consideration relates to sexuality. This could encompass our gender, our orientation, whether we think others will find us attractive or the physical ways by which we express our sexual selves. This process accelerates considerably when perceptions of our bodies change, as is nearly always the case when we access the health services. So, to practise holistic care, nurses need to be aware of body image and sexuality, and how they are linked. These links take many forms, but we propose here a four-factor analysis taking into account the complexity of human life and providing a framework within which nurses can work.

1. *Intimacy:* Nursing can be extraordinarily intimate at times, so it is not safe to be unaware of the range of potential impacts on a person.

antidiscriminatory practice

practice that aims to acknowledge the sources of oppression in people's lives and actively works to reduce them

2. *Antidiscriminatory practice*: without discrimination body image and sexuality would cease to be a difficulty in individuals' lives. It is only because humans choose to make judgements about each other, based on particular characteristics, that we become concerned about how we look or how we express ourselves sexually. Antidiscriminatory practice regularly appears in the competencies required for nurses (UKCC, 2001) and is an especially important way of working in terms of body image and sexuality. Practising in an antidiscriminatory way means both acknowledging the sources of oppression in people's lives and actively working towards reducing them (Thompson, 1998). So although you may be very accepting of a person who is gay, you also have to work to make sure that your colleagues are equally as accepting.

empowerment

working with individuals to enable them to find their own solutions and progress independently

3. *Empowerment*: this can be an elusive concept (see Thompson, 1998, for a readable overview), but put simply it means focusing your work on enabling the individuals around you to find their own solutions and progress independently. Health-care professionals have traditionally held tremendous power over individuals, often with a great unwillingness to share it, but there is no place for this approach in the modern health services – individuals need to regard themselves as having a large say in their own destiny. The issues surrounding body image and sexuality are often related to personal power, so nurses can make a positive contribution by understanding how much power they themselves hold because of often being perceived as 'experts'. Patients undoubtedly need us to have expertise but they can do without experts. In addition, by practising in an empowering way, nurses can actively demonstrate how power can be successfully shared.

partnership

the situation that occurs when separate individuals or groups contribute as equals to devising a useful solution to a problem

4. *Partnership*: empowerment does not imply that nurses should not actively help individuals, but instead means that the care given should occur within a particular type of relationship – a partnership. Working in partnership with clients prevents them relying too much on professionals and services, in other words becoming dependent.

This framework applies very strongly in nursing practice related to body image and sexuality. Dealing with these issues may well leave people feeling vulnerable and distressed, for example when they are facing a mastectomy, the use of a stoma or disfigurement. Running the nurse–patient relationship as a partnership in such high-emotion circumstances has several benefits for both parties. Partnership means that a nurse can retain the vital qualities of warmth and genuineness, but because these are not 'leading' the process, dependence is avoided. This makes practice safer professionally for the nurse as well as better for the patient or client, who needs to be able to deal with the world in his or her own right. Health-care staff will not always be around, so it is much better for the clients to learn to use their existing support networks (family, friends and so on) or be helped to find new ones (such as specialist support groups and voluntary services).

It is misleading to suggest that dealing with body image and sexuality issues is always easy, but a little knowledge and a lot of openness, acceptance and willingness to talk will form a strong foundation for competent practice.

● Test Yourself!

1. Using your own words, describe what is meant by the term 'body image'.

2. Give five examples of surgical procedures not evident to others (concealed) that could affect body image.

3. What are the three fundamental interrelated concepts used by Price (1990) to define body image?

4. Name some factors that may affect the sexual experiences of people with learning disabilities.

5. Which society is thought to have the earliest recorded laws on morality?

6. What are the four principles suggested as a framework for practice related to body image and sexuality issues?

Further Reading

Carlowe, J. (1997) Face values. *Nursing Times* **93**(42): 34–5.

Grogan, S. (1999) *Body Image. Understanding Body Dissatisfaction in Men, Women and Children.* Routledge, London.

Harrison, T. (ed.) (1998) *Children and Sexuality: Perspectives in Health Care.* Baillière Tindall, London.

References

Bell, N. (1989) Sexuality and the ostomist. *Nursing Times* **85**(5): 28–30.

Blackmore, C. (1989) Altered images. *Nursing Times* **85**(12): 36–9.

Chilton, S. (1984) Identity crisis. *Nursing Mirror* **158** (13 June): ii–iii.

Davenport-Hines, R. (1990) *Sex, Death and Punishment: Attitudes to Sex and Sexuality in Britain since the Renaissance.* Fontana, London.

De Marquiegui, A. and Huish, M. (1999) A woman's sexual life after an operation. *British Medical Journal* **318**: 178–81.

DoH (Department of Health) (2001) *The NHS Plan – an Action Guide for Nurses, Midwives and Health Visitors.* DoH, London.

Fogel, C. and Lauver, D. (1990) *Sexual Health Promotion.* W.B. Saunders, Philadelphia.

Foucault, M. (1978) *The History of Sexuality,* Vol. 1. *An Introduction.* Penguin, Harmondsworth.

Gamel, C. (1993) Nurses' provision of teaching and counselling on sexuality: a review of the literature. *Journal of Advanced Nursing* **18**(8): 1219–27.

Goffman, E. (1961) *Asylums: Essays on the Social Situation of Mental Patients and Other Inmates.* Anchor, New York.

Kitzinger, S. (1985) *Woman's Experience of Sex.* Penguin, London.

Langford, R. (1996) The hole truth. *Nursing Times* **92**(40): 46–7.

McCrea, C.W., Summerfield, A.B. and Rosen, B. (1982) Body image: a selective review of existing measurement techniques. *British Journal of Medical Psychology* **55**(3): 225–33.

Meerabeau, L. (1999) The management of embarrassment and sexuality in health care. *Journal of Advanced Nursing* **29**(6): 1507–13.

Miers, M. (2000) *Gender Issues and Nursing Practice.* Macmillan – now Palgrave Macmillan, Basingstoke.

Nye, R.A. (ed.) (1999) *Sexuality.* Oxford University Press, Oxford.

Nursing and Midwifery Council (NMC) (2002) *Code of Professional Conduct.* NMC, London.

Price, B. (1990) *Body Image: Nursing Concepts and Care.* Prentice Hall, London.

Price, B. (1995) Assessing altered body image. *Journal of Psychiatric and Mental Health Nursing* **2**(3): 169–75.

Price, B. (1998) Cancer: altered body image. *Nursing Standard* **12**(21): 49–55.

RCN (Royal College of Nursing) (1994) *The Nursing Care of Lesbians and Gay Men: An RCN Statement.* RCN, London.

RCN (Royal College of Nursing) (2000) *Sexuality and Sexual Health in Nursing Practice.* RCN, London.

Salter, M. (1997) *Altered Body Image. The Nurse's Role.* Baillière Tindall, London.

Sanderson, E. (1985) Nursing patience. *Lampada* **4**: 36–7.

Sant Angelo, D. (2000) Learning disability community nursing: addressing emotional and sexual needs. In Astor, R. and Jeffereys, K. (eds) *Positive Initiatives for People with Learning Difficulties: Promoting Healthy Lifestyles.* Macmillan – now Palgrave Macmillan, Basingstoke, pp. 52–68.

Savage, J. (1987) *Nurses, Gender and Sexuality*. Heinemann, London.

Sundeen, J., Stuart, G.W., Rankin, E.A.D. and Cohen, S.A. (1994) *Nurse–Client Interaction*. C.V. Mosby, St. Louis.

Thompson, N. (1998) *Promoting Equality: Challenging Discrimination and Oppression in the Human Services*. Macmillan – now Palgrave Macmillan, Basingstoke.

UKCC (United Kingdom Central Council for Nursing, Midwifery and Health Visiting) (1999) *Fitness for Practice: The UKCC Commission for Nursing and Midwifery Education*. UKCC, London.

UKCC (United Kingdom Central Council for Nursing, Midwifery and Health Visiting) (2001) *Requirements for Pre-registration Nursing Programmes*. UKCC, London.

Watson, J. (1980) Altered body image and the self. In Brown, M.S. (ed.) *Nursing and the Concept of Loss*. John Wiley & Sons, New York.

Wilton, T. (2000) *Sexualities in Health and Social Care: A Textbook*. Open University Press, Buckingham.

8

Movement and Mobility

Contents

- The Musculoskeletal System
- Exercise and Well-being
- Impaired Mobility
- Physical Health
- The Pressure Issue

- Psychosocial Health and Implications for Nursing Practice
- Disability and Adaptation
- Chapter Summary
- Test Yourself!
- References

Learning outcomes

Movement is vital in many activities, for example in seeking food and avoiding danger. As disease or ageing impairs mobility, the nurse has an important role in promoting the remaining mobility and independence, and enhancing the client's well-being. On completing this chapter, you will be able to:

- Describe the musculoskeletal system, skin, lever systems and movement

- Appreciate the importance of physical activity and movement throughout the life span, as well as the importance of exercise on health and physical fitness

- Understand some of the diseases and conditions affecting the musculoskeletal system and mobility

- Appreciate the impact of impaired mobility on social, psychological and physical health

- Understand the development of pressure sores and the nursing care involved in their prevention

- Appreciate the role of the nurse when caring for the client with impaired mobility.

There are also a number of activities throughout the chapter to enhance learning.

Although other sources can provide the necessary information, the activities in this chapter refer to the following texts:

Brooker, C. (1998) *Human Structure and Function*, 2nd edn. C.V. Mosby, London.

Hinchliff, S.M., Montague, S.E. and Watson, R. (1996) *Physiology for Nursing Practice*, 2nd edn. Baillière Tindall, London.

Mobility is generally defined as the ability to move about freely (Ismeurt et al., 1991). For a person to stay fit and healthy, and homeostasis to be maintained, movement is vital. We need, for example, to be able to move to seek out, prepare and eat food. We move hurriedly to escape from danger, and twist and turn when sitting or standing just to make ourselves comfortable. There are, however, some people who, through age, disease or injury, lose their ability to move freely, becoming to some degree dependent upon others. A particularly important aspect of the nurse's role when caring for such clients is to promote independence and provide a feeling of well-being.

The Musculoskeletal System

Muscles

The human body is composed of a number of moving parts, perfectly designed for each of the movements that our bodies carry out each day, for example eating, speaking, walking and running. The muscles adjust themselves and become finely tuned to these regular movements and actions; if, for example, certain muscles are used more frequently and for longer, they increase in size and become stronger. They can also work for long periods of time without tiring; that is, their stamina increases. In contrast, muscles that are used infrequently become weaker and reduced in size.

There are three types of muscle, each of which has a different function and is made up of a different kind of tissue:

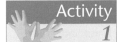

Activity 1

Open and clench your fingers as often as you can. How many times can you do this before you get tired?

These muscles are normally used only for gripping things and do not have much stamina. Thus they will tire quite quickly.

- Smooth muscle (non-striated involuntary muscle)
- Cardiac muscle
- Skeletal muscle (striated voluntary muscle).

Smooth muscle

The muscle layers of the body's internal organs, such as the stomach and intestines, are made up of smooth muscle. This smooth muscle, albeit a lot slower to act than skeletal muscle, expends a lot less energy when contracting. Smooth

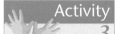
Activity 2

In the back of each hand, the tendons that run from the forearm muscles to the middle and ring fingers are connected. Place your hand palm down on a table, curl your middle finger up but stretch out the others. Your ring finger is completely immovable.

Activity 3

When our hands are inactive, tension from the muscles and tendons adopting their natural resting positions causes the fingers to be slightly bent.

Clasp your hands, interlocking the fingers while keeping the forefingers straight and parallel. Now let your muscles relax. What happens to your forefingers?

muscle is responsible for automatic (autonomic) actions such as peristalsis. It is not possible to control the actions of this muscle voluntarily so it is also known as involuntary muscle.

Cardiac muscle

The walls of the heart are composed of cardiac muscle, which is also involuntary.

Skeletal muscle

The body contains approximately 640 skeletal muscles, most of which are attached to the bones of the skeleton by tendons. Skeletal muscles are arranged in the body in parallel bundles, the cells forming a striped pattern; they are thus known as striped or striated muscles. Skeletal muscles are also known as voluntary muscles as we are able to control their action. They move a part of the body by contracting and pulling on the bone to which they are attached. In order for the body to push, pull and make all its other movements, skeletal muscles are usually arranged in pairs, one on each side of a bone, enabling the bone to be pulled in either direction.

Skeletal muscles also tend to work in groups, adjusting and shifting for each of the movements that the body makes. As you move or bend your leg, for example, the muscles in your calf, thigh and buttocks adjust to deal with the leg's new position. This involves some muscles contracting as they take up the strain and others relaxing as the strain is moved away.

Bones and joints

The framework of the body, or its 'inner scaffolding', consists of bones and joints. These are extremely flexible, adapting to the many demands placed upon them throughout life. Exercise, for example, helps to make the bones stronger and more resilient, and encourages the joints to stay supple and healthy.

Bones

cartilage

a non-vascular supporting connective tissue found in the joints, thorax, larynx, trachea, ear and nose

Bone is a complex organ and is continuously remodelled throughout life. As we pass from childhood into adulthood, the composition of our bones changes. A baby's skeleton has more than 300 bones, but many are formed from softer, flexible **cartilage**. During childhood, this cartilage becomes replaced by true bone, so by the time adults have reached their mid-twenties, the skeleton has a final number of 206 fully matured, hardened bones.

There are two types of bone in the adult skeleton:

- *Compact bone:* which makes up 80 per cent of the skeleton and is found in the shaft of long bones such as the femur
- *Trabecular bone:* which comprises the remaining 20 per cent of the skeleton and is found in the vertebrae, the pelvis and the ends of the long bones.

Bones have a number of functions including:

- Supporting body tissue and providing the skeletal framework
- Protecting the body's organs
- Enabling the body to move
- Acting as a store for mineral salts.

Approximately one-third of each of the body's bones is made up of water, making them not hard and rigid but slightly soft and flexible. Bones have their own blood and nerve supply; they require nutrients and also detect sensation. In other words, bones are alive. When food is scarce, essential minerals are transported from the bones to places where they are needed more urgently.

A typical bone consists of a hard, dense, outer shell called compact bone. This is composed of hundreds of tiny cylindrical units known as Haversian systems, which provide much of the bone's strength. The tube-shaped Haversian units lie in the directions of the greatest stresses on the bone. In the femur, for example, they lie lengthways in the bone shaft, so the bone resists buckling. Weight for weight, bone is stronger than wood, concrete or steel. If the human skeleton were made of steel of equal strength to bone, it would weigh five times as much.

Osteoblast cells found within the Haversian systems produce a substance called bone matrix. This consists of a mixture of microscopic crystals containing minerals, which make the bone tissue in the walls of these tubes hard, and bundles of fibres made from collagen, which give the tissue some elasticity and resilience. As a result, bones, being slightly flexible, tend to bend rather than snap under a small amount of stress.

Within the compact bone lies a spongy substance known as spongy, trabecular or cancellous bone, and in the centre of the bone is a soft jelly-like substance called bone marrow. In children, red marrow occurs in all the bones of the skeleton and makes nearly all the body's new blood cells. From about 5 years of age, red marrow in the limb bones is replaced by yellow marrow, which consists mainly of fibrous connective tissue and fat, and produces far fewer blood cells than does red marrow. At around 25 years old, the production of blood cells takes place in only a few bones, mainly the spine, sternum, collar bones, hip bones and skull.

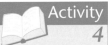

Activity 4

Read and make notes from Hinchcliff et al., 1996, pp. 261–76, or Brooker, 1998, pp. 381–8.

Activity 5

To appreciate the strength of the Haversian systems, gather about 60 straws, a lump of plasticine and a book.

Cut two rounds out of the plasticine about 3 in in diameter. Using one of these rounds, make a tower with the straws, putting the straws in all directions. Make a second tower, but place the straws upright around the edge of the plasticine in a ring. Now press the book on each. You should find that the circular arrangement is much stronger.

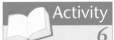

Activity 6

Read and make notes from Hinchcliff et al., 1996, pp. 284–94, or Brooker, 1998, pp. 369–78.

Joints

Bones are linked together by movable joints, without which it would be impossible to move – we could not nod or shake our heads, run or reach out and grasp things. Human joints are not dissimilar to mechanical joints. For a mechanical joint to function effectively, there needs to be a special smooth, hard-wearing substance where the two parts come into contact. In the body, this substance is cartilage. **Synovial fluid**, found within human joints (Figure 8.1), acts as an oil, lubricating the surfaces of this cartilage and allowing movement to occur smoothly. The body's joints work as a unit, constantly maintaining and occasionally repairing themselves to give the body a lifetime of service.

There are a number of different types of synovial joint, including:

- *Ball and socket joints*, found in the hips and shoulders
- *Hinge joints*, found in the elbows, knees, toes, fingers and ankles
- *Pivot joints*, found in the elbows and vertebral column
- *Gliding joints*, found in the shoulder girdle, hands, feet and vertebral column
- *Saddle joints*, found in the hands at the base of the thumbs
- *Ellipsoid joints* found in the wrist, hands and feet.

Synovial joints permit a number of ranges and types of movement:

synovial fluid

a viscous fluid that acts as a lubricant for joints and tendons

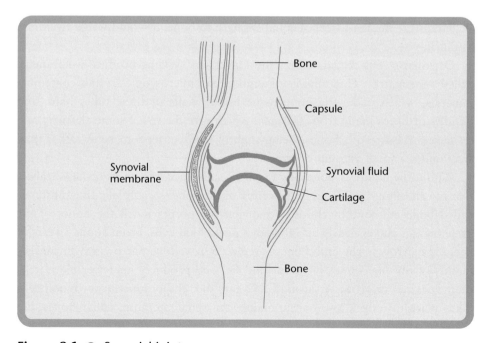

Figure 8.1 ● Synovial joint

- *Flexion:* which causes the angle between the bones to decrease, for example as the palm of the hand is moved towards the shoulder
- *Extension:* which causes the angle between the bones to increase, for example when the palm of the hand is moved away from the shoulder
- *Abduction:* which moves the bone away from the midline of the body, for example when moving the arm out to the side
- *Adduction:* which moves the bone towards the body's midline, for example moving the arm back to the side of the body
- *Rotation:* the movement of a bone around its own axis; the radius, for example, is caused to rotate when the palm of the hand is turned up and then down.

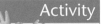

Lever systems and movement

Movement in human beings occurs as a result of lever systems. A lever can be visualised as a rigid bar that rotates around a pivot or **fulcrum**. Basically, a lever moves a load using effort. There are three main types of lever system (Figure 8.2a–c), and the body has examples of each, the bone acting as the lever, the

fulcrum
the pivot point of a system

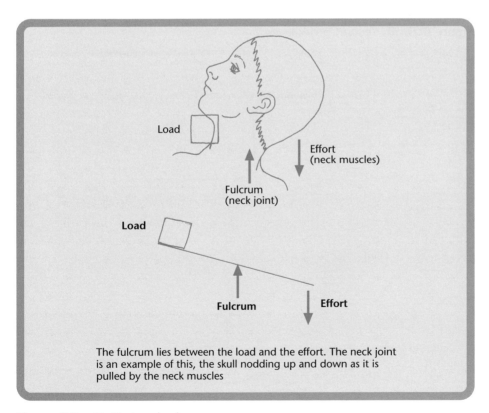

The fulcrum lies between the load and the effort. The neck joint is an example of this, the skull nodding up and down as it is pulled by the neck muscles

Figure 8.2a ● First-order lever

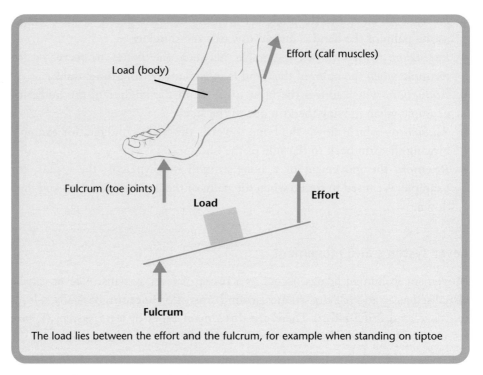

Figure 8.2b ● Second-order lever

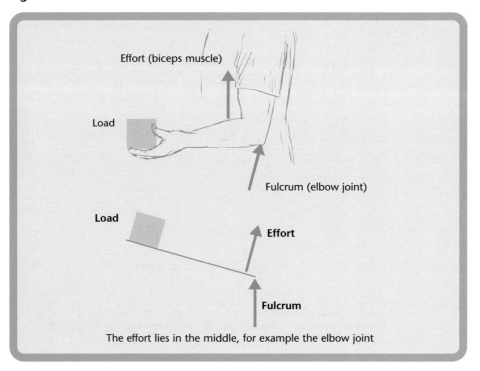

Figure 8.2c ● Third-order lever

muscle supplying the effort, and the body parts, supported by the bone, comprising the load. An example of a first-order lever is the neck joint; in this type of lever, the fulcrum is positioned between the load and the effort. A second-order lever is one in which the load is placed between the fulcrum and the effort, for example when standing on tiptoe. In third-order levers, the effort lies between the fulcrum and the load; this can be seen at the elbow joint.

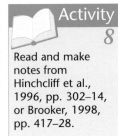

Activity 8

Read and make notes from Hinchcliff et al., 1996, pp. 302–14, or Brooker, 1998, pp. 417–28.

Exercise and Well-being

Physical activity and movement are basic human needs, important throughout the whole of the life span. As babies and toddlers, we move our limbs around, crawl, walk, jump and run. Between the ages of 2 and 5, children develop many skills, for example those necessary to wash, dress and eat, these requiring not only mobility, but also dexterity. Most adolescents have boundless energy and are constantly on the move, frequently involved in a number of physically demanding leisure activities such as football and swimming. As individuals pass through adolescence, work, hobbies and pastimes engage them in movement.

The increasing number of elderly people need to be able to move if they are to maintain their independence. If this group exercises regularly, osteoporosis (see below), a problem of increasing magnitude in the elderly, can be prevented or slowed down. Exercise interrupts bone loss and even encourages new bone mass. Furthermore, if the bones are strengthened, they are less likely to fracture. Evidence suggests that a lack of exercise and physical activity can lead to a decrease in fitness and an increase in dependency. Findings from a recent report suggest that individuals over 55 years of age who failed to carry out tasks of daily living were unable to do so as a result of inadequate strength (Allied Dunbar National Fitness Survey, 1992). A study involving manual workers found that only 4 per cent of those aged between 55 and 60 years old were able comfortably to sustain a walking jog (Bethell, 1992). Although reduced fitness may not result in significant debilitation in this age group, such a reduction in fitness in older age groups may lead to a lack of independence.

There are a number of factors that may prevent people exercising, including a lack of time, a lack of interest or self-discipline and a lack of understanding of the benefits of exercise. Individuals may also be unaware of how to gain access to suitable exercise programmes. Furthermore, older people may under-estimate their physical capabilities, seeing exercise as an activity for the young. The development of an appropriate activity programme can, however, mean the difference between dependence and independence, isolation and integration (Dinan, 1994).

■ Impaired Mobility

During a life span, there are a number of diseases and conditions that can affect the musculoskeletal system and therefore mobility. Some of these disorders are briefly described below.

Muscular dystrophy

muscular dystrophy
___
a group of diseases characterised by the progressive atrophy of symmetrical groups of muscles

Muscular dystrophy is a condition affecting the skeletal muscles; it is an umbrella name for a group of neuromuscular conditions. Symptoms may vary and can appear at birth or later on in life, but they always involve a progressive wasting and weakening of the muscles. The cause of this breakdown and death of muscle fibre is still unknown despite continuing research. The damaged fibres attempt to regenerate but fail, and slowly, over several years, the muscle tissue is destroyed, to be replaced by fibrous tissue and fat. The result is a gradually increasing weakness and loss of muscle bulk that causes difficulty in walking and in the use of the arms and that may, over a period of many years, be increasingly disabling.

Osteoporosis

osteoporosis
___
a condition in which there is thinning of the compact bone by resorption, enlargement of the Haversian systems and a loss of trabeculae from cancellous bone. Bones become fragile and porous, and may fracture spontaneously

bone resorption
___
the digestion of bone tissue by osteoclasts, a type of macrophage found in bone

Osteoporosis can develop over many years, usually becoming apparent in the over-60 age group. It is particularly prevalent in postmenopausal women although it can occur in childhood or young adults. It affects 1 in 3 women and 1 in 12 men.

Osteoporosis involves thinning of the cortical bone by resorption, enlargement of the Haversian systems and a loss of trabeculae from the cancellous bone. Bones are fragile and porous, and may fracture spontaneously. Problems encountered include deformity and disability, causing pain, debility and in some cases death. Osteoporosis may also occur as a result of deficient oestrogen secretion during the menopause or because of the predominance of **bone resorption** over secretion during old age.

Osteoarthritis

osteoarthritis
___
a condition in which the joints undergo degenerative changes

Osteoarthritis is a degenerative joint disease. Although the condition is common in the 50–70-year-old group, it can occur in individuals as young as 20. Osteoarthritis occurs in both men and women, and although the cause of this disease is unknown, it is thought that heredity, trauma, congenital factors and pre-existing diseases play a part.

When a joint is affected by osteoarthritis, the normally smooth cartilage becomes rough and cracked, eventually being destroyed. This is thought to occur as a result of digestion of the cartilage by enzymes. During this process, spurs of new bone can be seen at the joint margins. These may then break off and appear in the joint cavity. Osteoarthritis can cause tremendous pain in the movable joints, particularly the large weightbearing joints such as the hips, and joints in the hand. The joint may also become enlarged and, following a period of rest, stiff.

Rheumatoid arthritis

Rheumatoid arthritis is a chronic inflammatory disease affecting the connective tissue. It is three times more common in women than men, normally occurring at an age – between 40 and 50 years – when career and family responsibilities are greatest. The cause of rheumatoid arthritis is not known, but it may be related to an immune mechanism, involve metabolic factors or result from a virus.

Similar to osteoarthritis, rheumatoid arthritis affects the joints. The synovial membrane and joint capsule become inflamed and swollen, which results in the formation of granulation tissue. This leads to fibrous scar tissue, adhesions and possibly **calcification**. Symptoms commonly include pain, stiffness, fatigue and systemic manifestations such as anaemia. The ability to remain active is compromised.

Falls

The changes occurring in the joints and muscles as people grow older include:

- A decrease in lean muscle mass
- An increase in body fat
- A decrease in muscle strength
- **Demineralisation** of the bones.

Osteoarthritis, rheumatoid arthritis and osteoporosis are conditions that are fairly prevalent in the elderly, and as a result of these diseases joints may stiffen and muscle tone may decrease. The individual often develops an awkward gait, and mobility becomes impaired. Rising from a sitting position or getting in and out of a car becomes, for example, increasingly difficult. Impaired gait and loss of mobility, combined with other physical changes that occur in the elderly, including impaired vision, a confused mental state and a decreased ability to maintain equilibrium, predispose the individual to falling. Contextual factors such as poor lighting, an unfamiliar environment, loose slippers, cluttered equipment and furniture also increase this risk.

People who suffer from impaired mobility will have an associated loss of

---

Activity 9

Read and make notes from Hinchcliff et al., 1996, pp. 314–19, 278–83 and 294–301.

rheumatoid arthritis
a chronic inflammatory disease affecting the connective tissue

calcification
the deposition of mineral salts in a tissue

demineralisation
the loss of calcium and phosphorus from bone

Casebox 8.1

Jane Foster is 65 years old. As a result of an old fracture to her femur, she has a slight deformity of her leg, which interferes with walking. She also has poor vision. Jane is a private person and has no living relatives. The only social contact she has is occasional with a neighbour. Jane is a regular smoker and also likes to drink. Her mother suffered from osteoporosis, and Jane is concerned that she may develop this disease.

Describe the clinical picture of osteoporosis and identify three factors that can lead to its development. What advice would you give Jane in order to prevent osteoporosis?

■ Osteoporosis is initially a silent disease. It can develop over many years and normally becomes apparent in the over-60

age group, being particularly common in postmenopausal women. Bones may fracture spontaneously, leading to deformity and disability.

■ Age, the menopause, heredity, diabetes mellitus, hyperthyroidism, Cushing's syndrome (from the oversecretion of glucocorticoids) and acromegaly (from excess growth hormone) are all contributory factors.

■ Lifestyle characteristics known to lessen bone loss and fracture risk include: the maintenance of fitness (everyday activities such as dressing, washing and eating help); regular exercise such as running, jogging, swimming and walking to stimulate bone strength; the prevention of falls (reducing environmental hazards, for

example loose carpets, wires, footstools, bath hazards, poor lighting and slippery floors); and taking care while wearing bifocal spectacles when walking down stairs.

■ Jane should eat a nutritionally sound diet (calcium and vitamin D being essential). As people with a high alcohol intake have an increased risk of osteoporosis, Jane should be advised to cut down.

■ Smoking, too, is to be avoided as it doubles the risk of osteoporosis, also causing an early menopause and reducing body weight, which lowers bone density.

CONNECTIONS

Chapter 4 outlines the functions and sources of calcium and vitamin D.

Casebox 8.2

David Jones is 72 years old and has a moderate-to-severe learning disability. He cannot speak and his behaviour has been described as autistic. He is also partially sighted. After many years in hospital, he now lives in a small residential home. David has recently developed

'obsessional and ritualistic' behaviour and is continually moving around the room touching, picking up and moving objects.

What factors may lead to David having a fall? How might the risk of a fall be prevented?

■ David's partial vision and continual movement may contribute to a fall.

■ The risk of falling can be reduced by tackling environmental hazards, for example not moving the furniture, and by ensuring that David is wearing his glasses.

independence affecting their social, physical and psychological health, with implications for nursing practice. We will now explore this in more detail.

■ Physical Health

The client with impaired mobility may suffer from a number of problems affecting several of the body's systems, as outlined below.

Circulatory system

When a person moves, for example during walking, the muscles contract and press upon the veins, causing them to empty. This maintains venous circulation and prevents venous stasis. If, however, an individual is immobile, the legs fail to assume or maintain vasoconstriction, resulting in pooling of the venous blood. In this situation, a deep vein thrombosis can form in the leg veins. The danger is that this clot, or a portion of it, may become detached and be swept into the pulmonary circulation, causing a pulmonary embolism.

stasis

halting of the normal flow of a fluid

CONNECTIONS

Chapter 6 also explains deep vein thrombosis and pulmonary embolism, their precipitating factors and how to reduce risks.

Nurse's role

It is essential that the nurse observes for the signs and symptoms of a deep vein thrombosis or a pulmonary embolism. In the case of a deep vein thrombosis, signs include a painful, swollen calf. With a pulmonary embolism, there is chest pain and a cough. The nurse's role also involves assisting the client with active and passive exercises and isometric exercises of the extremities.

passive exercises

exercises in which the patient's limb is put through a range of movement by another individual

isometric

muscle contraction with minimal muscle shortening so that there is no movement

Respiratory system

The effect of impaired mobility on the respiratory system is reduced ventilation of the lungs. This lowered ventilation, combined with reduced movement, leads to a decreased stimulation of coughing. Secretions consequently build up in the bronchi and bronchioles, leading to chest infection.

auscultation

examination by listening to sounds in the body using a stethoscope

CONNECTIONS

Chapter 6 explains the nurse's role in supporting breathing and coughing.

Nurse's role

It is essential that the nurse observes the client for an inability to cough and raise secretions. It is also important to carry out auscultation of the chest for signs of moisture, and to reposition the patient frequently. In order to prevent pneumonia, deep breathing exercises need to be undertaken at regular intervals (at least every 2 hours), and the client must be encouraged to cough.

Gastrointestinal system

CONNECTIONS

Chapter 5 explains how such constipation can occur.

Altered diet and fluid intake, combined with a lack of activity, can result in constipation in those clients with impaired mobility.

Nurse's role

CONNECTIONS

Chapter 5 identifies reasons for the development of constipation.

It is important that the nurse obtains a clear picture from the client of his usual bowel habits and whether or not he takes anything regularly for constipation. The nurse also needs to observe the client's food and fluid intake. A fluid intake of 2–3 litres a day should also be encouraged, along with a diet high in fibre. The client also needs to be encouraged to be as active as possible. Stool softening agents and suppositories are sometimes needed.

Urinary system

Urinary stasis can be caused by impaired mobility, resulting in the development of a urinary infection or urinary calculi (stones). These occur when crystalline substances such as uric acid, calcium phosphate and oxalate, which are normally excreted in the urine, crystallise out of solution.

Nurse's role

CONNECTIONS

Chapter 5 lists the types of urinary stone and some of their causes.

It is important that any history of urinary problems is identified. In male patients, this may involve hesitancy and frequency because of an enlarged prostate gland. It is essential that the nurse records the fluid intake and output, and that drinking is encouraged. The signs and symptoms of bladder infection and renal stones must be sought.

Musculoskeletal system

Clients with reduced mobility suffer from muscle weakness and atrophy. Bone growth and bone destruction are also affected, leading to osteoporosis.

The nurse's role in mobilising joints

An essential role of the nurse is to help prevent problems of the musculoskeletal system. Passive exercises of the affected limbs, along with active and isometric exercises of the unaffected limbs, should be regularly carried out.

Each of the joints has its own specific range of movement, usually maintained by the numerous activities that we undertake during our daily lives. These movements stretch the muscles, ligaments and tendons that surround and support each joint, so clients with impaired mobility may experience a loss of function of their joints, resulting in shortening of the muscles, ligaments and tendons. When this occurs, **contractures** can quickly develop, which can then give rise to further problems. If a foot is allowed to contract in a position of foot drop, for example, the foot will probably not be able to support the foot and leg, and walking will be virtually impossible. A vital role for the nurse when dealing with a client with impaired mobility is to ensure that joints are kept as mobile as possible. In order to do this, each joint must be put through a range of passive and/or active movements several times a day to prevent stiffness and contractures.

> **contractures**
> permanent shortening of muscles and other tissues as a result of disuse, injury or disease

The joints that require exercising include the shoulders, elbows, wrists, neck, fingers, hips, knees, ankles and toes. Exercises not only help to keep the joints mobile, but also promote venous return and lymphatic flow, and prevent excess demineralisation of the bone. Clients who are able to move can put their limbs through each of the movements themselves. Each of the body's joints has a normal range of movement:

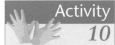

Activity 10

In front of a long mirror, observe the full range of movement of each of your joints.

- *Neck:* the neck muscles rotate or flex the neck depending on whether the muscles of one or both sides are contracting
- *Shoulders:* the shoulder joints are able to rotate as well as flex forward and extend backward. Abduction of these joints occurs when the shoulders move away from the body and adduction when the shoulders move towards the body
- *Elbows:* the elbow joints allow the lower arm to flex towards and to extend away from the upper arm
- *Hips:* the body's hips rotate in a circular motion. They are also able to flex towards the body, and extend and hyperextend away from the body. Adduction occurs when the leg moves towards the body, and abduction when the leg moves way from the body
- *Knees:* both knee joints are able to flex and extend.

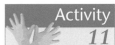

Activity 11

Find out whether your practice setting has access to physiotherapy services. If possible, arrange to spend some time with the physiotherapist, observing how clients with impaired mobility are treated.

When the nurse carries out passive exercises for the client, it is important that the client does not experience any discomfort. Both the limbs and the joints involved must be supported during the exercises. If the client has a weakness or paralysis of one side of the body, it is important that she is taught how to exercise the affected side herself.

Another way in which the nurse can promote activity is to encourage clients to become involved in their own care, for example moving independently in bed or a chair, sitting up to wash and eat, and brushing their own teeth; this will increase strength and endurance.

> **CONNECTIONS**
> *Chapter 4 explains the importance of an upright body posture on swallowing and digestion.*

■ The Pressure Issue

A particularly important aspect of care of the client with impaired mobility is that of pressure areas.

Pressure sores, also referred to as decubitus ulcers (ulcers developed through lying down) or bed sores, can be defined (Collier, 1997) as:

> skin ulcerations that occur because of unrelieved pressure in combination with the effects of other variables.

Pressure sores are costly in terms of both an extended stay in hospital and extra medication. The direct cost to the NHS for pressure sores has been identified as being between £150m and £600m per annum (Morison and Moffat, 1994), but this figure does not take into account the increased suffering incurred by the client. In most cases, pressure sores are avoidable, so this incidence can be seen as an indicator of the quality of health care. It is therefore extremely important that everything is done to prevent their development.

In order to understand pressure sores, it is necessary to have an understanding of the anatomy and physiology of the skin. To reinforce this information, the structure of the skin will be summarised below. Pressure sore development is then examined, along with the associated risk factors.

pressure sores

tissue destruction as a result of tissue overlying a bony prominence being subjected to prolonged pressure from an external object

Skin

CONNECTIONS

Chapter 10 also reviews the functions and structure of the skin.

The skin (Figure 8.3) is the body's heaviest organ, that of an average adult weighing about 4–7 kg, approximately one-twelfth of the body's total weight. The skin has a large surface area, which spans approximately 2 m². As well as its role as a sensory organ, it has a number of physiological functions including the control of body temperature, the excretion of water and salt, the manufacture of vitamin D, the screening of harmful ultra-violet rays from the sun and the protection of the inner organs.

The skin is composed of two layers of tissue:

1. The outer *epidermis*.
2. The inner *dermis*.

Epidermis

The skin is continually subjected to mechanical injury. The cells of the basal cell layer within the epidermis are continuously renewed, and it is from these cells that the rest of the epidermis is formed. In 1 minute, 30,000–40,000 skin cells

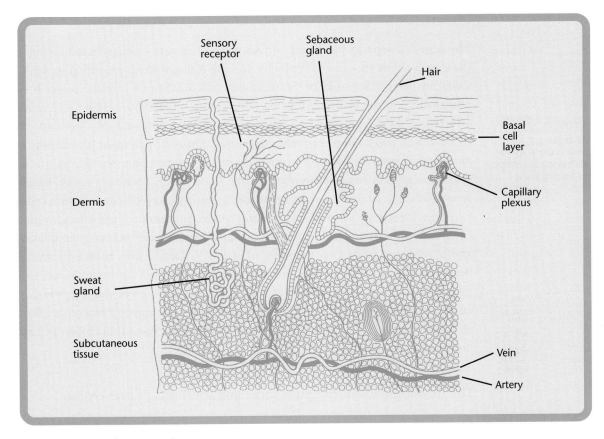

Figure 8.3 ● Skin in section

fall from the body, and each year up to 4 kg of skin wears away and flakes off our body's surface. Gradually, over a period of about 2 weeks, cells are pushed towards the surface of the skin from the basal layer, during which time their structure and activity change. While still in the basal layer, they begin forming a protein called keratin, this formation of protein being continued as they move towards the surface. Eventually, as the cells reach the stratum corneum (the outer layer of the epidermis), they are like flattened bags of protein and the intracellular organelles have disappeared.

The stratum corneum is the major barrier to the loss of water from the body. It has two actions that restrain the movement of water and limit the loss of water from the skin's surface. First, the matrix in which the cells of the stratum corneum are embedded is rich in lipid. This substance is almost impenetrable to water, which makes it extremely difficult for water molecules to move out of the epidermal cell. Second, protein inside the epidermal cells attracts and holds on to water molecules. As a consequence, the surface of the skin is normally dry, with very little water lost.

Dermis

The dermis comprises a network of two types of protein – collagen and elastin – the elastin giving the skin its flexibility and the collagen fibres providing strength. Collagen plays a key role in the formation and healing of pressure sores. It is fundamental in the protection of the body's microcirculation, helping to protect **interstitial fluid** from pressure. The dermis is also composed of a network of blood vessels and a number of other structures. These include sweat glands, which are found all over the skin and secrete a dilute salt solution on to the skin's surface; sebaceous glands, found everywhere in the body except non-hairy areas, which secrete sebum containing a mixture of lipids; sensory receptors; and defence cells.

There are variations in skin in relation to age, environment and ethnic origin. Patches of skin that receive greater wear and tear respond by becoming thicker and tougher, as is seen on the soles of feet of someone who habitually walks barefoot. The skin also varies between different parts of the body. Non-hairy (glabrous) skin, as on the palms of the hands and the soles of the feet, has, for example, an extremely thick epidermis and numerous sensory receptors. Skin with hair follicles (hairy skin), as is found on the scalp, has a thin epidermis and many sebaceous glands.

interstitial fluid

the portion of extracellular fluid that fills the spaces between the cells of tissue

The development of pressure sores and methods of prevention

CONNECTIONS

Chapter 1 includes the case history of a lady who is at risk of pressure sores.

Pressure sores usually develop as a result of external pressure causing occlusion of the blood vessels and endothelial damage to the arterioles and the microcirculation.

Certain bones, for example the shoulders, elbows, hips, sacrum and heels, lie close to the skin at pressure points. When a person lies or sits, the skin becomes compressed between the bone and the surface of the bed or chair and is stretched. This external pressure is transmitted from the surface of the skin to the bones underneath, compressing the tissue in between. The pressure increases 3–5 times as it travels through the skin, as illustrated by McClemont's cone of pressure (Figure 8.4) (McClemont, 1984). At a bony prominence such as the sacral bone, for example, the pressure rises from 50 to 200 mmHg.

This affects the blood supply to the area, and if the occlusion of the blood vessels is maintained, anoxia and a build-up of potentially harmful waste ensue. Suddenly releasing the pressure will result in an increase in blood flow, reaching a level much greater than usual. The resulting red flush is known as reactive hyperaemia. This flush lasts for approximately one-half to three-quarters of the occlusion time. If the vessels of the skin are left intact, there will be no permanent damage, but if they are damaged, tissue changes will occur, cell membranes rupture and toxic intracellular materials be released. The risk of pressure sore development is greater if the pressure is prolonged.

Pressure sores are caused by unrelieved pressure in combination with other

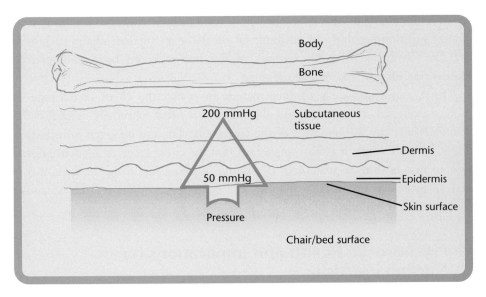

Figure 8.4 ● Cone of pressure (adapted from McClemont, 1984)

factors, including impaired mobility, poor nutritional status, diabetes, incontinence, reduced fluid intake and oedema. Age is also important as the skin changes as a person gets older, contributing to the likelihood of skin breakdown. There is a decrease in vascularity and elasticity, and the skin becomes drier. The subcutaneous fat layer of the skin thins, and there is also a reduction in the number of temperature and touch receptors. Therefore, as a person grows older, the skin becomes more easily damaged and takes longer to heal.

During the nursing assessment of a client with a pressure sore, each of the above factors must be taken into consideration. Furthermore, a full description of the altered skin is essential. A standard classification system should be used to describe the sore, identification of the stage of sore development helping to determine the most effective intervention. A photograph of the sore, with an indication of its size, is extremely valuable. Such a photograph not only identifies the extent of the problem, but can also be used to evaluate the treatment regimen.

A particularly important feature of treatment is that a consistent approach should be adopted by all those health-care professionals involved in the client's care. Initial care interventions involve identifying those clients at risk of pressure sore development and acting to prevent pressure sores. Once a pressure sore has begun to develop, intervention will occur in accordance with its stage of development. This care will, however, centre upon relieving pressure. Basic nursing interventions involve positional change or the relief of pressure, and the use of an appropriate mattress when the patient is in bed. Such mattresses include circulating air mattresses, water beds and egg-crate mattresses. If the client is seated or in a wheelchair, special cushions need to be used. Those clients who

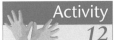

Activity
12

Find out whether your unit uses a pressure sore risk calculator. Obtain a copy and try to identify the original source, for example the Norton scale.

CONNECTIONS

Chapter 10 provides further information on wound care and identifies a useful pressure ulcer website.

CONNECTIONS

Chapter 5 discusses bladder and bowel management.

spend long periods of time in a wheelchair need to be encouraged and taught to change position regularly by pushing up on the arms of their chairs to relieve pressure. Isometric flexion exercises of the buttocks can be encouraged to increase circulation and relieve pressure.

Other important areas of care include involving the client in a range of motion exercises, ambulation and skin care. It is often extremely helpful if the client's family can become part of the treatment plan and be given information about pressure sores. It is also important that the client receives adequate nutrition so that healing is promoted. If albumin is being lost from the sore, a diet high in protein is essential. A bladder and bowel programme will be necessary for incontinent patients.

■ Psychosocial Health and Implications for Nursing Practice

Clients' attitude, acceptance and motivation greatly influence how they cope with their disability. They should be allowed to make decisions involving care at their own pace and be allowed to work within their own limitations. It is vital that those with impaired mobility receive information and support from the nurse. In this way, clients can begin to regain control over their lives and implement coping strategies. The development of a trusting relationship between the nurse and the client enables the client to explore his or her emotional reactions to the illness. This may include feelings of isolation and rejection, and also a sense of loss, for example a loss of self-esteem, a loss of status within the family or a loss of independence.

The duration of an individual's illness, intermittent hospitalisation, increased financial strain and emotional and social burdens all place the family under terrific pressure. It is therefore important that the client is not viewed in isolation but that the needs of the whole family are considered because the support offered by the family has a great influence on how a person responds to illness and also has a bearing on compliance with treatment and rehabilitation. The nurse should thus identify failures of understanding of the illness in both the client and the close family and friends. If, for example, the family does not appreciate the role of exercise in reducing pain and stiffness, the client may find it hard to incorporate this into the daily routine. Similarly, if a spouse has a poor perception of the disability and pain, she may not acknowledge any problems and offer support (Symmons et al., 1996).

When dealing with clients with impaired mobility, the nurse needs to help them to appreciate that their roles may have changed. If clients are unable to return to work, the despondency that this may cause will have repercussions for the whole family. The loss of a job may cause boredom and a lack of self-esteem

(LeGallez, 1993). The nurse needs to encourage and support clients in this situation, perhaps referring them to the disability employment officer for advice on
retraining, or actively involving them in a support group. The patient will also
require information on benefit entitlement, which can be obtained from the
Department of Health and Social Security.

It is clear that the nurse has a number of responsibilities when providing care
for the client with impaired mobility. These include:

- Providing an opportunity for both client and family to articulate their feelings and emotions about the disorder; care provision can then be based on a
  joint appreciation of the condition
- Providing information on the condition for all family members and the client,
  the aim being a shared understanding and awareness of the symptoms and
  the goals of treatment
- Referral to outside help, for example social workers
- Joint goal-setting and sharing of responsibility, enabling the client to recognise and accept the help and emotional reassurance provided by the family,
  while also helping family members to respect the individual.

Disability and Adaptation

An individual's social roles provide a link between that person and society as
social roles are determined by society and occupied by individuals. If these roles
are disrupted, for example during the working years or the transitional adolescent years, the effects can be extremely disturbing. The manner in which an individual acts within society has much symbolic value. Dressing ourselves has, for
example, connotations of autonomy, adulthood and independence, but even this
simple act may prove impossible for someone with impaired mobility. Thus, the
social and psychological effects of impaired mobility can be devastating.

The causes of impaired mobility vary greatly and may alter throughout the
course of an illness. Immobility, whatever the cause, can, however, pose a threat
to an individual's normal pattern of interdependence with others, which may be
particularly traumatic for children and adolescents striving to become independent. In these instances, even mild alterations to relationships can be
extremely traumatic. There may be a feeling of being a burden on others, which
might be so strongly felt that help will not be sought when it is needed. Alternatively, individuals may not go out with friends because they think they are an
encumbrance. Clients may also worry about the effect that their condition may
have on their schooling and future job prospects: How will they fare in the job
market? Will employers be biased against them? Will they be limited in their
choice of career?

> **CONNECTIONS**
>
> *Chapter 7 explores
> these issues in
> greater detail.*

The emphasis by today's society on physical achievement and appearance may have disastrous effects on individuals who suffer impaired mobility. In juvenile chronic arthritis, for example, girls who have mildly effused knees may be grossly embarrassed and feel unable to wear short dresses. Teenagers with mobility problems may have only a slight limp but may feel too embarrassed to go out with their friends. Individuals confined to wheelchairs will be unable to participate fully in the usual physical adolescent activities, and a lack of suitable transport may exacerbate this problem.

Thus, people who experience an alteration in mobility often lack confidence in their abilities, which can result in a withdrawal from social activities and a feeling of physical and emotional isolation. Individuals may develop an extremely negative self-image as a result of changes brought about by the disease itself, the visibility of the treatment regimen and their perceptions of how they are viewed by others. If depression, non-compliance and withdrawal from social situations are to be understood, it is essential that these issues are recognised.

The growing number of elderly disabled living alone increases the risk of social isolation, which, along with loneliness, can lead to a deterioration in both physical and mental health. Research has identified that those elderly who are living alone are more likely to suffer from dietary insufficiencies (Walker and Beauchene, 1991). They also suffer losses in relation to their independence, social network and financial status (Drake, 1999). Low self-esteem may develop as a result of feeling unable to support others. Loneliness in the elderly can ultimately result in depression, with a risk of self-neglect or suicide (Palinska et al., 1990).

Stereotyping is an important issue confronting the disabled. It means that disabled people may be expected to behave in certain ways, for example to be the passive recipients of care. When they comply with this, their behaviour reinforces people's attitudes that they are inferior and incapable of making their own decisions. If, however, they do not conform to this role, they are viewed in a negative fashion (French, 1994). It is important that a positive attitude is developed towards disabled people and that the nurse fully understands the meaning of disability.

Aids to normal living when mobility is compromised

Equipment can help to minimise the disabling effects of impaired mobility and also make caring for a disabled person easier. A range of equipment is available for the disabled (Maczka, 1990), including:

- Beds and accessories, for example mattresses, coverings to protect the bed, alarms for clients suffering enuresis, and self-lifting aids
- Chairs, for example ones that adjust and are mobile, high seats, sandbags, footstools and cushions

- Reading and writing aids such as tape-recorders and radios, page turners, and aids for clients with hearing difficulties
- Eating and drinking aids, for example adapted cutlery and plates, drinking aids, non-slip materials and bibs
- Hoists and lifting equipment such as electric hoists, lifts and stair climbers, and hoists to gain access to cars
- Walking aids, for example frames, crutches and walking sticks
- Household equipment such as kitchen utensils, cooking appliances and equipment for washing and cleaning
- Clothing, for example special clothes adapted for wheelchair users, hosiery and extra waterproof clothing
- Made-to-measure footwear.

CONNECTIONS
Chapter 4 looks at ways of helping people who need support with food and fluids.

CONNECTIONS
Chapter 3 contains a section on moving and handling.

Local hospitals, residential homes and day centres may hold some of the above equipment, so it may possible to try it out. If equipment is unavailable, many firms will arrange for a demonstration in the client's home. Disabled Living Centres are also available for individuals to find information about apparatus. Although items are not on sale in these centres, advice on the sources of supply and cost can be obtained.

The Department of Health and Social Security provides several benefits for the disabled person, but those who are disabled frequently fail to claim benefits that they are owed. Contributory factors may include a lack of information and knowledge, and an inability to fill in an application form. Consequently, several thousands of pounds of benefits remain unclaimed each year (Drake, 1999). Benefits currently available for the disabled include:

CONNECTIONS
Chapter 7 investigates body image in greater depth.

Casebox 8.3

Susan Burton was diagnosed as having juvenile chronic arthritis 10 years ago at the age of 4. During her childhood, she experienced very few problems and participated in most physical and social activities. Recently, however, Susan has become withdrawn. She no longer enjoys swimming or other sports, and she very rarely goes out with her friends.

What factors may have contributed to Susan's behaviour?

What can be done to help her?

- Altered body image, for example as a result of swollen joints, and impaired gait may have contributed to Susan's behaviour.

- Provide support, and encourage Susan to explore her emotions. Involve her family and close friends in discussions. Also encourage Susan to go out with her friends and resume her social and physical activities.

- Attendance Allowance
- Industrial Injuries Disablement Benefit
- Disability Living Allowance
- Disabled Person's Tax Credit
- Pneumoconiosis, Byssinosis and Miscellaneous Disease Benefit Scheme
- Workmen's Compensation (Supplementation) Scheme
- Severe Disablement Allowance
- Invalid Care Allowance
- Incapacity Benefit
- Statutory Sick Pay
- Vaccine Damage – lump sum payments.

More detailed information on benefits can be obtained from the Department of Health and Social Security.

Chapter Summary

This chapter began by examining those structures involved in movement and mobility: the musculoskeletal system, the skin and lever systems. Physical activity and movement throughout the life span, as well as the effects of exercise on health and physical fitness, were also explored. This was followed by a brief description of the diseases and conditions that affect mobility, and the impact of impaired mobility on social, physical and psychological health. Finally, the role of the nurse when caring for these clients was discussed.

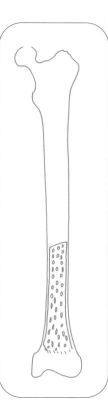

● Test Yourself!

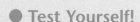

1. Label the long bone illustrated.

2. What are the three major components of bone?

3. Where is compact bone found?

4. What are the functional units of these bones?

5. What are the functions of skeletal muscle?

6. What is muscle tone?

7. When the muscles are at rest, what percentage of the cardiac output do they utilise?

8. What are the functions of joints?

9. Where would you find a third-order lever system in the body?

10. Where would you find a gliding joint?

11. What is the range of movement of a ball and socket joint?

12. How does exercise affect health and physical fitness?

13. What are the effects of immobility on each of the body's systems?

14. What is a pressure sore, and what nursing care is involved in pressure sore prevention?

References

Allied Dunbar National Fitness Survey (1992) *A Report on Activity Patterns and Fitness Levels.* Belmont Press, Northampton.

Bethell, H.J. (1992) In praise of exercise. *Care of the Elderly* **4**(3): 150.

Collier, M. (1997) Pressure area care: knowledge for practice. *Nursing Times* **93** (Supplement): 1–4.

Dinan, S. (1994) Fighting fit and over 50. *Practice Nurse* **9**: 441–9.

Drake, R. (1999) *Understanding Disability Policies.* Macmillan – now Palgrave Macmillan, London.

French, S. (1994) The disabled role. In French, S. (ed.) *On Equal Terms: Working with Disabled People.* Butterworth-Heinemann, Oxford.

Ismeurt, R.L., Arnold, E.N. and Carson, V.P. (eds) (1991) *Concepts Fundamental to Nursing.* Springhouse, Pennsylvania.

LeGallez, P. (1993) Rheumatoid arthritis: effects on the family. *Nursing Standard* **7**(39): 30–4.

Maczka, K. (1990) *Assessing Physically Disabled People at Home.* Chapman & Hall, London.

McClemont, E. (1984) Pressure sores. *Nursing* **2**(21) (supplement).

Morison, M. and Moffat, C. (1994) *A Colourful Guide to the Assessment and Management of Leg Ulcers,* 2nd edn. Times Mirror International, London.

Palinska, L.A. (1990) The biocultural context of social networks and depression among the elderly. *Social Science and Medicine* **30**(4): 441–7.

Symmons, D., Jones, M., Osborn, J., Sills, J., Southwood, T.R. and Woo, P. (1996) Paediatric rheumatology in the UK: data from the British Paediatric Rheumatology Group register. *British Journal of Rheumatology* **23**(11): 1975–80.

Walker, D. and Beauchene, R.E. (1991) The relationship of loneliness, social isolation, and physical health to dietary inadequacies of independently living elderly. *Journal of the American Dietetics Association* **3**: 300–4.

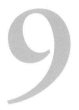

Dying, Death and Spirituality

Contents

Learning outcomes

This chapter is concerned with dying, death and loss. It will introduce you to the concept of death and begin to examine some of the principal aspects of palliative care. At the end of the chapter, you should be able to:

- Reflect on the nature of death in today's society

- Discuss the concept of death

- Explore how and when people die

- Identify the key principles of palliative care

- Discuss the principles of pain and symptom control

- Reflect on the nature of communication with patients who are dying and their relatives

- Identify the measures required in caring for a body after death

■ Consider your role in bereavement

■ Reflect on the spiritual nature of human beings and its importance in health care.

For most of us, death seems a long way off. We hopefully enjoy our lives and are more interested in living life to the full than worrying about dying. Wilson (1975) suggests man cannot live to the full until he has confronted death, but although this may be very true, it might also be argued that with today's healthy lifestyles and an expectation of life until well into our 80s, there is no reason to concern ourselves with death. Whatever the truth of these arguments, you have as a nurse chosen to enter a profession in which you will inevitably be confronted by death. You therefore need to be able to care not only for people who are dying, but also for their relatives through this process and beyond as they are confronted by grief and bereavement and perhaps having to learn to live alone. In addition, there is a need to care for yourself and your colleagues. We are after all dealing with one of the most powerful and emotional periods of life – the transition from the living, known world to the unknown world of death.

A word of caution here: some of the discussions and exercises in this chapter may be distressing if you have recently been bereaved or have someone close to you who is dying. Feel free to miss out this chapter and revisit it when you feel the time is right for you.

■ Awareness of Death

Surely our attitudes to death and to life would be less riddled with fears and anxiety, if we recognised death and talked and taught about it as part of normal human experience. (Collick, 1986)

Perhaps you have not given death very much thought, or perhaps you have experienced death in your life and it has loomed large in your thoughts. Whichever is true, you are encouraged here to think about how death is viewed by society today.

It is suggested that we live in a death-denying society. In other words, even in the face of the obvious we find it difficult to accept that we will one day die. We rarely discuss the subject, and for many death takes place hidden away in institutions such as hospitals, hospices and nursing homes. It might be argued that this blind spot occurs partly because very often we have no need to think about death. For most of us, longevity has become the norm and we can be optimistic about achieving our three score years and ten. Modern science and better health care could, it is suggested, leave us with a life span of up 120 years. So if this is the case, why should we concern ourselves with a far-off event? Nevertheless, the knowledge that we will one day die always lurks in the background. Death may face us at any time of life, sometimes suddenly and unexpectedly, sometimes creeping slowly upon us.

> This existence of ours is as transient as autumn clouds.
> To watch the birth and death of beings is like looking at the movements of a dance.
> A lifetime is like a flash of lightening in the sky,
> Rushing by, like a torrent down a steep mountain.

> (The Buddha, in Rimpoche, 1992)

Although most people recognise the inevitability of death, it is to a large extent kept in the shadows. Death rattles away at the edge of our awareness (Yalom, 1980), and in modern Western society we have fewer and fewer reminders that we will one day be faced by the reality of death. The emergence of a life-limiting disease can, however, awaken hidden fears that have lain only in the shadow of our awareness. Society's death-denying approach, in which dying is hidden away in institutions, death is rarely talked about, and funeral rituals and mourning have become minimised, has little power over keeping death at bay (Aries, 1981). As Morgan (1995) comments, 'death refuses to die' – death can strike at any moment and we may be very unprepared for it:

> When you are strong and healthy,
> You never think of sickness coming,
> But it descends with sudden force
> Like a stroke of lightning.

> When involved in worldly things,
> You never think of death's approach;
> Quick it comes like thunder
> Crashing round your head.

> (Milarepa, in Rimpoche, 1992)

Rimpoche (1992) suggests that, deep down, we know we cannot avoid facing death forever and that the more we can accept the impermanence of life, the greater freedom we can find in living. It is up to you to decide how far you will explore your own personal living and dying, but you might wish to consider this advice by La Rochefoucauld (in Walter, 1990): 'Death and the sun are not to be looked at steadily', but 'As with the sun, so with death: without staring at it, the wise person lives in its light'. Whatever your personal explorations involve, you have chosen a profession in which you will inevitably be faced with people who are dying and people who are bereaved. Although many people in society never have to face death until middle age or beyond, you will inevitably have to confront it. As Collick (1986) suggests, 'death is a crisis for the dying and for the living for which both are usually wholly unprepared'. A large part of understanding death and dying is achieved by learning through experience rather than being taught, and you might like to start this process by reflecting on some of the losses in your life.

Activity

1

Think of some of the losses in your life. Don't think just of deaths but of all sorts of loss, such as the loss of security the first time you went to school, or when a brother or sister first left home. What effect did these losses have on you? What did you do to cope?

■ Where and How People Die

There is evidence to suggest that most people would prefer to die in their own home (Townsend et al., 1990), yet most people still die in an institutional setting. Table 9.1 shows that a significant number of people, whether or not their condition is cancer related, die in NHS hospitals. It is also evident that a considerable number of people with non-cancer-related conditions die in nursing and residential homes. Despite this, many people do spend much of their last year of life in their own home but are admitted when their condition worsens and their families feel that they are no longer able to cope (Barclay, 2001). This clearly has implications for how care is provided and where resources are needed. People, of course, do die at all ages and from a variety of causes, including suddenly from illness and accidents. In addition, although much of the literature on caring for the dying focuses on people dying from cancer, the main causes of death in England and Wales continue to be diseases of the circulatory systems such as heart attacks and stroke.

Table 9.1 Place of death for cancer and non-cancer patients

	Cancer (%)	Non-cancer (%)
NHS hospitals	48.3	55.0
Voluntary hospices	13.3	0.2
Psychiatric hospitals	0.3	1.0
Own home	25.8	19.9
Nursing home	7.3	10.9
Residential home	3.6	9.6
Other home/places	1.6	3.4

Source: Office of National Statistics (1997), England and Wales.

Activity

2

Look at Table 9.2. What are the main causes of death for people under the age of 65?

Work out the average age for men and for women for all causes of death. What does the table tell you about life expectancy for men and for women?

Table 9.2 Mean age at death from selected causes, by sex

Cause	Mean age at death	
	Male	Female
All	71.9	78.2
Stomach cancer	71.9	76.6
Colon cancer	71.5	75.7
Lung cancer	71.1	71.5
Skin cancer	62.0	66.4
Female breast cancer	–	68.9
Cervix cancer	–	62.5
Prostate cancer	77.6	–
Leukaemia	67.0	69.9
Diabetes	72.9	77.8
Ischaemic heart disease	73.2	80.1
Stroke	76.9	82.0
Bronchitis, emphysema and asthma	73.1	74.6
Liver disease	56.9	60.9
Injury and poisoning	46.5	63.9
Car accidents	38.8	49.1
Suicide/self-inflicted	43.9	50.1

Source: Office of National Statistics (1997), England and Wales.

It is also useful to reflect on the age at which people die. Mortality tends to be high during the first year of life, decreasing during childhood and then gradually rising with age from 15 years onwards (Victor, 2000). However, unless you are a midwife or a children's nurse, the majority of people you care for will be 65 years or older and dying from a wide range of conditions, of which the cancers comprise just one specific collection of conditions. Table 9.2 shows the mean age of death from selected causes.

Having considered how and where people die, it is useful to consider what we mean by dying and how we define someone as being dead.

■ When Am I Dead?

If nurses are to care for people who are dying in a way that is positive, it is important to recognise that we are alive until we are dead, and that we should have the opportunity, should we choose, to live to our full potential. Life exists on a continuum from conception to death. During this time our health varies and is affected by many factors in our internal body environment and by external influences. Despite efforts to deny death and to preserve life, death continues to be the inevitable earthly end and the last stage of life.

CONNECTIONS

Compare this with the criteria for cardiac arrest found in Chapter 6.

This end-point of life that we call being dead is not as easily defined as one imagines. The common understanding of death is the absence of vital signs, that is, a cessation of breathing, a lack of a palpable heart beat and fixed dilated pupils. In most cases of expected death, these remain the usual criteria, but the situation has been complicated by modern technology, which allows people to be kept alive on life-support machines. Establishing the exact moment of death in such circumstances requires different criteria, such as brain death tests, to cope with this technologically supported extension to life (Veatch, 1995). Furthermore, although most Western societies try to make a clear distinction between being alive and being dead, some societies have a much wider differentiation. Such societies consider the person to be alive for a considerable period after most Western cultures would regard them as dead, other cultures grieving for people as if they were dead in a way that most Western societies would hold to be inappropriate because the person would still be considered to be alive (Rosenblatt, 1997). But have you ever heard anyone in our own society say, 'For me she died a long time ago; now there is just an empty shell'? Perhaps in some circumstances we too have different definitions of death.

Whichever way we look at death, dying has no easily definable point. When does light become dark, and when does day become night? These are arbitrary and manmade divisions. We are all dying until we reach that ill-defined point we call death. Or put in a more positive way, life continues until a decision is made that we have reached that end-point we call death.

◼ When Am I Dying?

Understanding the point at which someone is defined as dying is itself a grey area. Davis et al. (1996) emphasise that a diagnosis alone is not enough. Someone, whether it is the patient, a carer or the medical staff, needs to reach a position at which they accept the condition as being terminal. Nevertheless, dying and being in a terminal condition is not necessarily the same thing. A prognosis suggesting that there is no obvious curative treatment does not mean the person does not have much active living to do, and even the terminal phase will differ from person to person. The whole process of dying may take various directions and shapes. Death may be sudden or lingering, expected or unexpected; it may progress slowly and then take a sudden downturn, or the process may move up and down before finally declining to death (Glaser and Strauss, 1968). For some, there may be little opportunity to reflect on the process, but many others have the opportunity for living fully right up until the moment of death. Although dying is a time of crisis, it can also be a time of opportunity for change and positive growth (Yalom, 1980).

The point of this discussion is that if we are to care for people who are dying, we first need to acknowledge that there are many grey areas: just as the person who is dying is facing uncertainty, nurses too have sometimes to face ambiguity and uncertainty. It is, however, important to focus on the fact that people are living until they are dead and that they deserve the highest quality of life that is attainable. One positive way at looking at this is to view care of the dying from a health-promotion perspective.

Health Promotion and Dying

CONNECTIONS

Chapter 2 provides more details on Our Healthier Nation.

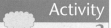

Activity
3

Imagine you are asked to look after a 67-year-old woman who is in the terminal stages of an illness. What would be your main concerns over how to care for her?

The concepts of health and death rarely fit comfortably together, yet if life exists until death 'health for all' must include all people from birth up to the end of life. The White Paper *Our Healthier Nation* (DoH, 1999) is targeted at helping people achieve healthier, more fulfilling lives. Although it makes no reference to care of the dying, it might be hoped that some aspects of the White Paper would be interpreted and acted upon within the scope of those who are defined as dying. Good health is described by the White Paper as requiring a confident and positive outlook and being able to cope with the ups and downs of life. Health is not just about how long people live but about quality of life, ensuring that they are not robbed of dignity and independence; it is equally important to all people whatever their clinical health status.

Seedhouse (1997) emphasises the importance of allowing people to achieve their maximum potential for health whatever their starting point. This health-promoting perspective thus allows a more positive view of the dying process. It is also a view that gives patients a choice. How they choose to do their dying may be very different from how we might choose to do ours, but their decision should always be respected. This perspective on death and dying fits well the philosophy of caring for the dying usually referred to as **palliative care**.

palliative care

care provided to people whose condition is no longer amenable to curative treatment

Definitions of palliative care

'Palliative care' is the term used to refer to the care of patients whose condition is not amenable to curative treatment. Such conditions invariably lead to the person's death, but the length of time involved is extremely variable. The World Health Organization's (1990) definition of palliative care is:

> The active total care of patients whose disease is not responsive to curative treatment. Control of pain and other symptoms, and of psychological, social and spiritual problems is paramount. The goal of palliative care is achievement of the best quality of life for patients and their families.

and that it:

- affirms life and regards dying as a normal process
- neither hastens nor postpones death
- provides relief from pain and other distressing symptoms
- integrates the psychological and spiritual aspects of care
- offers a support system to help patients live as actively as possible until death
- offers a support system to help the family cope during the patient's illness and in bereavement.

The term 'terminal illness' tends to hold highly negative connotations and can lead to patients receiving appropriate care far too late in their condition, whereas palliative care can and should start at the time of diagnosis, in some cases several years before the person reaches the terminal stages of the illness.

The growth of modern palliative care grew out of the work of Dame Cicely Saunders who opened St Christopher's Hospice in Sydenham in 1967. A former nurse, she moved into the world of medical social work before finally training as a doctor. Through her work, she became very conscious of the poor care and distress of patients who were dying. Her vision was for people to die free of pain and that they should be enabled to live until they died, supported by skilled carers and with their physical, psychological, spiritual and social needs addressed. Dame Cicely Saunders caught the imagination of the country and the world, and by the year 2001 over 93 countries throughout the world had initiated hospice and palliative care interventions (Hospice Information Service, 2001).

Palliative care has now become a speciality in its own right, initially emerging through the work of the hospice movement. Specialist palliative care is now, however, provided in a variety of settings, including hospices. These may be independent voluntary or fall within the NHS. Many hospices also have a day unit providing a range of facilities from symptom control to counselling and complementary therapies.

Palliative care may also be offered in the home, supported by the primary care team, and may involve a Macmillan nurse. Macmillan nurses are invariably clinical nurse specialists funded by the organisation Macmillan Cancer Relief, and although they predominantly work in the community, some may be employed as part of the hospital palliative care team. In addition, Marie Curie nurses offer hands-on care to patients at home, usually spending their whole shift caring for one individual. These nurses are usually part charity and part NHS funded, and range from care assistants who have specialised in this area to highly trained palliative care nurses.

Hospital palliative care teams offer support and symptom control to patients

terminal illness

refers to a prognosis suggesting that there is no obvious curative treatment. 'Terminal care' is the term reserved for the care provided to patients in the last days, weeks or sometimes months of their life

hospice

voluntary or NHS-funded establishments where palliative care is provided. Hospices attempt to provide the best possible quality of life for the final stages of an illness. This includes family support and bereavement services

in general hospital wards. This is often where palliative care begins, early intervention usually meaning better managed palliative care.

Whatever the setting palliative care involves a number of specialised professionals including:

- Clinical nurse specialists in palliative care (often Macmillan nurses)
- Consultants in palliative medicine
- Social workers
- Clinical psychologists
- Other supporting professionals, such as physiotherapists, occupational therapists and in some cases complementary therapists.

One of the criticisms of palliative care has been its predominant focus on people with cancer, but although much has been learnt from the experience gained while caring for those with cancer, there is now a desire to make such expertise available in the care of people with other chronic diseases. There is also a considerable need to extend this expertise into nursing homes, where more and more people will end their lives (Komaromy et al., 2000). To this end, a **palliative care approach** is advocated in addition to specialist palliative care.

The aim is for the palliative care approach to become an integral part of all clinical practice whatever the illness or its stage (NHS Executive, 1996). So, for example, this would include not only patients with cancer, but also those with dementia, chronic heart disease, stoke and respiratory disorders, and those at the end of life in nursing homes. It is this notion of a palliative care approach that can be practised by all health-care professionals and supported by specialist palliative care teams. Like the definition of palliative care above, it is underpinned by key principles advocated by the NHS Executive (1996). These are:

- A focus on quality of life, including good symptom control
- A whole-person approach, taking into account the person's past life experience and current situation
- Care that encompasses both the person with the life-threatening disease and those who matter to that individual
- A respect for patient autonomy and choice, for example over place of care, treatment options and access to specialist palliative care
- An emphasis on open and sensitive communication, extending this to patients, informal carers and professional colleagues.

This palliative care approach is very significant to the nurse because it acknowledges the importance of all nurses providing palliative care rather than this just being something left to specialists in the field.

---

palliative care approach

a philosophy of care suggesting that all people with life-threatening illness should receive quality care and that this should be provided by all health-care professionals rather than just by specialist palliative care services

---

Activity

4

Think of each of the NHS Executive's key principles and make some notes about what they mean for nursing practice in caring for the dying.

The above discussion emphasises that palliative care is a team activity. It is not just about different team members doing their job but about working together jointly in the best interests of the patient and the family. Here, however, we will focus on the role of the nurse within the team.

The nurse's role

The nurse's role in palliative care is about caring for the living, so it is primarily about providing high-quality nursing care. We will focus here on some of the important elements required to provide quality care to people facing death as a result of their illness, but first try to think of the sort of person you would like to care for you or a member of your family; what sort of person would they be, and what sort of skills would you want them to have?

It is always difficult to pin down the specific skills required to be a good nurse, but Saunders (1978) offers some help in this when she talks of 'being with' people when they are suffering. It is as if we walk alongside them offering support as and when it is needed. Saunders identifies the characteristics required for this role:

- Respect the identity and integrity of other human beings
- Be sensitive and non-judgemental
- Know when to listen and when to speak
- Have the knowledge and skills to intervene in a way that promotes the best quality of life as perceived by the patient.

Not too difficult a list to read or understand perhaps, but each item requires considerable skill and expertise. It is perhaps a skill that can be learnt only through experience, coupled with hard work on ourselves, through reflection, and a developing self-awareness.

Davies and O'Berle (1990) also provide a useful framework that encapsulates those elements expressed by Saunders. The dimensions they describe in Figure 9.1 emerged from work interviewing patients and their families, and although the research reflects care delivered by specialist palliative care nurses, these dimensions are relevant to any nurse who subscribes to the palliative care approach.

Valuing is very much a core element and relates to respecting the person and being **non-judgemental**. These terms are discussed in Chapter 11 and are part of the core conditions that Rogers felt were necessary for a therapeutic relationship. This relational aspect of caring becomes increasingly important in the care of the dying. It is through this that we connect (*connecting*) with patients and their relatives. It is hard to describe what this actually means but it bears similarities to empathy. It is about listening, having a caring attitude that says 'You

CONNECTIONS

Chapter 13 contains a range of strategies to enable you to develop this skill.

CONNECTIONS

Chapter 12 will help you to enhance your self-awareness.

non-judgemental

accepting the values of others

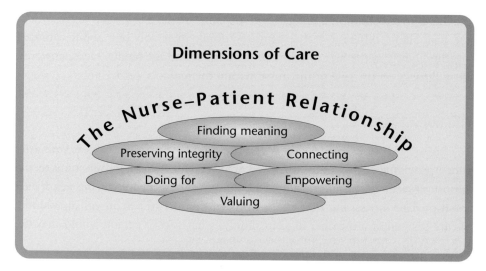

Figure 9.1 ● Dimensions of care (adapted from Davies and O'Berle, 1990)

CONNECTIONS

Chapter 11 outlines a range of strategies and suggestions to help you develop the skill of empowerment.

are important.' It means giving quality time to the person, even if this is only a couple of minutes.

One of the great anxieties facing people who are dying is losing control, which easily happens when vulnerable people are faced with powerful professionals and sometimes find themselves in a strange institutional environment. It is therefore important not to disempower people but to allow the person to care for themselves and make decisions for themselves as much as is possible (*empowering*). This can be very difficult, particularly when you are faced with what might appear to you an irrational decision, such as refusing some form of treatment. It is at such times that the need to be non-judgemental, coupled with being supportive, becomes increasingly important.

Facing death may be a daunting prospect and a time when people question why and what has life been about. They seek to sort out their life and the meaning it has for them (*finding meaning*) and for others around them. This is part of the spiritual aspect of our lives and will be dealt with more thoroughly later in the chapter.

People who are dying often need a lot of physical care and emotional support; families too may feel inadequate and frightened. At such times, nurses may need to provide much of the care (*doing for*), including pain and symptom control. This may be carried out by an individual nurse but is supported by a team approach. There is an inherent danger here of taking over from the patient and relatives so it is important in 'doing for' that this is, whenever possible, carried out in negotiation with the person and family to avoid disempowering them.

The final element of care is *preserving integrity*. Caring for the dying can be a challenging experience and it is important for nurses not to lose sight of their own self, their ability to maintain a positive view of themselves and their capacity to feel valued by themselves and by others. This may mean reflecting on the care given and exploring the meaning of life and death. In maintaining integrity, it is important that the nurse has good support within and outside her professional arena. Becoming emotionally involved with and upset for someone who is dying is not a loss of integrity: it is quite normal sometimes to feel emotional turmoil, just as it is quite normal sometimes not to feel any emotional attachment. Loss of integrity comes about when these emotions incapacitate the nurse and there is a loss of self-esteem and self-worth, perhaps associated with guilt and inadequacy. At such times it is important to seek help and support.

CONNECTIONS

Chapter 13 is relevant to work on your ability to think about these issues.

CONNECTIONS

Chapter 12 will help your self-awareness in such situations.

■ The Concept of Pain and Symptom Control

Pain and symptom control is an important and specialist area when caring for the dying; a detailed and technical discussion will therefore be left to other texts to explore. Nevertheless, it is important to have an introduction to some of the concepts related to pain and pain management and the diversity of potentially unpleasant symptoms that need careful management in those who are dying.

Although not all patients with a life-limiting disease will experience pain, it remains one of the most feared symptoms (Clark, 1993). According to Faull et al. (1998), pain occurs in 75 per cent of patients with advanced cancer and 65 per cent of those dying from all other causes. Pain is not, however, a straightforward sensory experience but an inclusive one that is moderated by emotional, social and spiritual elements as well as physical influences. This is known as the 'concept of total pain'. We can usually tolerate quite intense pain if we know that it will go away and that it is not ultimately associated with our impending death. For individuals with a life-limiting disease, the pain is not only often chronic, but also a constant reminder that it is part of a disease process that will result in their death.

CONNECTIONS

Pain assessment is described in Chapters 1 and 6.

Pain is a highly personal and individual experience and as such requires detailed assessment and management that goes far beyond simply prescribing **analgesics**. As such good pain management requires a considerable input from the nurse in terms of assessing the non-physical aspects of pain. But the physical aspects are important too, and prescribing the right analgesic at the right time and via the right route is very important. The World Health Organization (1996) advocates the use of a three-step analgesic ladder (Figure 9.2) when managing pain. This concept is basically simple but is for most patients effective in minimising their pain. **Non-opioid analgesics** for mild pain may include paracetamol; **opioids** for mild-to-moderate pain may include drugs such as dihydrocodeine; and opioids for severe pain may include morphine. You may wish to look these drugs up in your drugs handbook.

analgesics
pain-relieving drugs. An absence of pain is termed 'analgesia'

non-opioid analgesics
analgesics such as paracetamol and non-steroidal anti-inflammatory drugs, for example aspirin

opioids
drugs such as morphine derived from the opium poppy; these are controlled drugs

adjuvant

a drug that is not in
itself an analgesic but
can help with the
analgesic effect

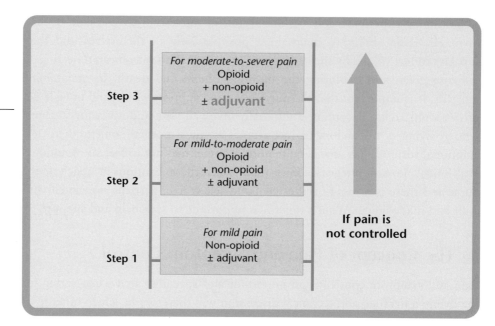

Figure 9.2 ● Three-step analgesic ladder (adapted from World Health Organization, 1996)

This method of pain control has been accepted worldwide as a valuable model. You are not expected to have a full grasp of its prescribing implications but instead to recognise that effective analgesia is available to patients. If the patient is to remain relatively pain-free, pain management should be started early and analgesics given regularly, if possible by mouth. With early intervention, most patients start at step 1, but it is perfectly acceptable to start at step 2. What is essential is to get the patient as pain-free as possible as quickly as possible if that is what the patient wants.

Other symptoms

CONNECTIONS

*Chapter 5 identifies
factors affecting
constipation and
how to manage
them.*

Other distressing symptoms experienced by the patient are many and varied; some of these are shown in Table 9.3. According to Finlay (1995), the five most common symptoms are pain, weakness, constipation, nausea and vomiting, and dyspnoea. As with pain, a careful and comprehensive assessment of all symptoms is very important. What might be a minor irritation for a healthy individual can be a huge burden to a person approaching the end of their life, draining their energy, self-esteem and enjoyment of life, and leading to insomnia, fatigue and depression. Each additional symptom adds to the patient's total discomfort, yet with good nursing care many of the symptoms are treatable and/or avoidable. It is thus essential to assess thoroughly and regularly, and

Table 9.3 Common distressing symptoms

Gastrointestinal symptoms	Respiratory symptoms	Cardiovascular symptoms
Dry mouth	Choking	Dehydration
Nausea and vomiting	Cough	Oedema
Constipation	Dyspnoea	Haemorrhage
Diarrhoea		
Anorexia		
Neurological and psychological symptoms	Urinary tract symptoms	Skin symptoms
Loss of concentration	Frequency	Pressure sore
Insomnia	Incontinence	Fungating lesions
Weakness and fatigue	Dysuria	Pruritis
Anxiety and fear	Bladder spasm	Disfigurement
Depression/sadness		
Confusion		

This is not a definitive list of symptoms but outlines some of those commonly encountered.

Source: Adapted from Cooke (2000).

never dismiss any symptom of which the patient complains. Although some of the symptoms involved require specialist intervention, many can be managed by good-quality nursing care, including caring therapeutic communication.

■ Communication

What is special about communication when caring for the dying? Maybe nothing. Students often tell me that death holds no fear for them, that they are happy to talk about death. In the safety of the lecture room perhaps, but when confronted by a frightened patient and anxious relatives, meaningful communication can become more difficult. What do you say to someone who is facing death? How do you respond to the relatives and friends? Perhaps part of the difficulty lies in our deep-rooted fears of death, referred to earlier in the chapter. Because these fears lie essentially in our subconscious, we may not even be aware of their existence. There are, however, other more overt fears that may get in the way of open communication. Buckman (1998) identifies the following fears commonly encountered in health-care professionals:

● There is a fear of the pain *we feel* because of patients' and relatives' distress. Sometimes we almost hurt for them

- We fear being blamed by patients for their condition and ultimate death, as if it were our fault. This blaming does sometimes happen as patients and relatives struggle to understand why nothing can be done to cure them. Nursing and medical staff also struggle with how to manage a condition that is not amenable to treatment
- We fear not knowing what to say because we have never been taught what to say. Indeed, talking about dying is not like other clinical procedures: although you can have guidelines, there is no script for the right thing to say. But if we always wait for the right thing to say, we may end up with nothing being said, a common scenario. With the right intent and a little courage, we will gain experience and become more confident in effective therapeutic communication
- In a similar way, our desire always to have the right answer can make it difficult for us to say, 'I don't know.' Yet we may have many unanswered questions, and trying to flannel with patients and relatives will only lead to mistrust. An honest 'I don't know' can lead to a much more open communication and a developing trust between the patient and the health professional
- Talking to patients and relatives can sometimes result in their giving an emotional reaction. This can lead to fears of how to manage this reaction and how to manage other staff members who may feel that you have 'upset' the patient. Discussing life and death issues is, however, upsetting, and we need to be prepared for a whole variety of possible reactions and learn how best to manage them
- Many people have fears about their own death. Some of these lie in the person's awareness and some may be subconsciously held. Health-care professionals are, however, regularly confronted by death, so it is more difficult for them push such fears aside and out of their thoughts
- Some nurses wonder how much they should express their feelings and fear that to do so would be unprofessional. Although it is important to remain in control of the situation, it is rare for patients or relatives to see emotion as unprofessional, and indeed a lack of any emotion can be seen as insensitive
- Finally, there is a fear of the hierarchy. What am I allowed to say? How should I respond when asked questions? Will the hierarchy blame me, especially if they have differing views about talking to patients?

These fears can lead to nurses using blocking or distancing tactics to avoid talking to the patients. They may avoid the patients altogether, use small talk, give false reassurances, ignore or not pick up on cues, use jargon, deal only with the positive or pass the buck (Faull et al., 1998). This may result in patients and relatives being left stranded in an uncertain world; the barriers erected may encourage them to withdraw into themselves and become even more anxious and depressed.

Learning to cope with these fears comes easier to some than others. We all have a unique background that affects how we manage such situations, and it is important that you are gentle with yourself and develop your abilities gradually. Just reading this chapter will certainly not be the answer, and perhaps a good place to start is reflecting on your own thoughts and experiences of death. Some guidelines can, however, help in providing at least a little scaffolding to support you through your learning:

- Listen to patients and their relatives. Don't feel you have to have the answers; just listen and care
- Remember that not everyone wants to talk about their illness or about dying, so don't force it on people, but do be sure it is not just you that is avoiding the issue
- Don't deny people their feelings by telling them not to worry or not to be silly. Acknowledge their feelings by saying something like 'It must be worrying' or 'It seems you are very frightened'
- Offer openings such as 'Is there anything you would like to talk about?'
- Don't distance yourself. Sit with the person and, when appropriate, use touch as a way of connecting with them
- Be prepared for a variety of emotions, including anger. This is rarely personal but may be an expression of the person's fear, uncertainty and loneliness
- Don't be offended if they choose someone else to talk to. We can't always be the right person, but this does not mean that you are not a good nurse or not good at communication.

> **CONNECTIONS**
>
> *Chapter 11 discusses some of the core skills in good communication, including an introduction to breaking bad news. You might wish to review this now in the light of the discussion on communication in death and loss.*

■ Last Offices

'Last offices' is the term used to describe the last elements of care carried out after a person has died. For many nurses, this is their first contact with death, and handled sensitively it can be a positive experience. Much of the procedure is not founded on research, but is based on myth and ritual. Nevertheless, ritual can itself be an important part of caring and should not be dismissed lightly. Much of the laying out of the dead provides an avenue for the nursing staff to offer their last opportunities for care and may for some act as a final closure. Procedures for last offices will vary and also depend on whether the person has died in hospital, at home, in a nursing home or in a hospice. There are, however, some broad, very practical aspects to the procedure, and the following principles outlined by Cooke (2000) need to be followed. Examine your local policy on last offices and reflect on each of these aspects of care:

last offices
final procedures carried out after a patient has died

- Appropriate care should be given to the bereaved relatives. If possible, give them the opportunity to be with the deceased before the body is removed from the ward. Prepare the area by removing as much clutter and as many clinical items as you can. Ensure that there are chairs next to the bed for the relatives to sit on

- You will need to be guided by local procedures for preparing the body, but in essence individuals can be left in their nightwear; leaving a hand exposed allows the relatives to touch and hold the person. Covering the face with a sheet can make death frightening and unnecessarily mysterious for the relatives (Henley, 1986). Relatives should not be discouraged from talking to, hugging and kissing the person; this, after all, may be the last time they are close together

- It is not a necessary routine to wash the patient, but a judgement should be made on whether, for example, a man should be shaved. If nurses choose to wash the patient as a way of saying goodbye, this will often be acceptable as long as it does not infringe any religious or cultural norms for the patient

- Be careful not to do anything that would have been out of the ordinary for the person when alive: do not, for example, put lipstick on a woman who would normally never have worn it

- Offer to stay with the relatives, but be equally prepared to leave them alone in privacy. Relatives will need to be given advice and help with what to do next. They may wish to talk to the doctor or nurse to ask about the circumstances of the death. It is important for them not to be left with many unanswered questions, and it is helpful for them to have a contact person should questions arise at a later date

- Ensure that there is appropriate support for the staff. Death will not always be an upsetting experience, which is perfectly acceptable. On some occasions and for some staff, it may, however, be an upsetting experience, so be alert to your own feelings and the feelings of the staff around you. Be supportive and if necessary take 'time out' to reflect on what has happened. It is always useful to identify someone in your life whom you can talk to at such a time, even if this is only at the other end of the telephone

- Provide appropriate support for other patients as they are invariably aware when someone has died. Do not try to hide the facts from them – they have a right to know – particularly in long-stay wards or nursing homes, and they may need an opportunity to talk

- Provide dignity and privacy for deceased patients, treating them with the respect you would have given when they were alive

- Protect staff, other patients and relatives from infection and hazards. You should consult local procedures for infection control measures, but essentially those who have died are no more or less infectious then when they were alive. Universal precautions should still, however, be used. Body bags may need to be used for infectious patients

Activity 5

Ask a children's nurse and a community nurse how they manage last offices. Identify the differences and try to work out a rationale for these.

Look at the *Royal Marsden Hospital Manual of Clinical Nursing Procedures* (see further reading) for details of last offices and requirements for different faiths.

Look at the Age Concern website www.ageconcern.org.uk and search for the information contained in 'What happens when someone dies'.

- Ensure a respect for the religious and cultural beliefs of the patient and family. If possible, find out from the family before the patient dies what specific procedures are required afterwards. Then ensure that these are adhered to
- Comply with the relevant legal requirements. Always check whether the coroner needs to be informed of the death; if so, drains, catheters, tubes and so on should normally be left in situ
- Ensure the care and safe custody of patient's property
- Provide prompt and effective communication with other wards and departments. Remember that many people are involved – relatives, porters, mortuary staff, doctors, chaplains, infection control nurses and patient administration staff.

Bereavement

Death can release a whole variety of emotions. Some people may hardly be affected: perhaps the relationship was not very strong, or the death may have been a relief as it marked the end of suffering. For others, death can be very difficult to come to terms with. C.S. Lewis (1961), tormented by the death of his wife, opens his book with the comment:

No one ever told me that grief was so like fear. I am not afraid but the sensation is like being afraid. The same fluttering in the stomach, the same restlessness, the same yawning. I kept on swallowing.

What these emotions and feelings relate to and what purpose they serve have been the subject of great debate for many years. Do we have to work through grief in a series of stages, and do we eventually have to let go of the lost person before we can get on with life? The debate remains in a state of flux so only a brief outline of some of the models proposed will be described here.

Many recent models of **bereavement** stem from the work of Freud and his contemporaries. Freud (1917) saw **grief** as a process to be worked through, something he called 'griefwork'. He hypothesised that, to recover from grief, the person needed to let go of all the energy invested in their loved one before they could invest that energy in another (Freud, 1917). Although most of the bereavement models have since changed and developed, this concept is still central to many of them. One of the models emerging from this tradition is that of Worden (1983), who describes a 'tasks of grief' model in which the bereaved work through a series of tasks. These tasks are:

bereavement
the state of having lost someone significant

grief
a natural human expression and reaction to a loss

- To accept the reality of the loss
- To experience the pain of grief

- To adjust to an environment no longer containing the loved one
- To relocate the deceased and move on.

Parkes (1996) describes grief as a psychosocial transition in which the bereaved individual has to readjust to a new world without the deceased person. Every aspect of life becomes changed and they have to adapt to this new and altered world. Parkes also identifies a number of stages involved in the grieving process: shock and alarm; searching; anger and guilt; and finally gaining a new identity. Central to this theory is letting go of the old world and adapting to the new.

A widely published model is that of Kubler-Ross (1969), who also describes a staged model consisting of denial, anger, bargaining and acceptance. Her initial work was in fact based on people who were dying. She talked to many terminally ill patients and observed the way in which they were attempting to adapt to their illness and impending death. The work of Kubler-Ross opened up a whole new way of caring for those who were dying. The stages she observed and described were similar to those which people appeared to pass through when bereaved.

Although the theories described here all add something to the understanding of grief, they are also open to criticism in that people rarely follow such a neat pattern of bereavement and are just as likely to want to maintain a connection with the deceased as to let them go completely (Klass et al., 1996; Walter, 1999). In a study of bereaved parents, Rubin (1993) found that they still maintained a firm attachment to their child up to 13 years after the death, and there is reason to believe that such an attachment may continue for as long as the parent lives.

More recent studies have placed a greater emphasis on people's individual experience of grief, which is in turn considerably influenced by culture and social norms. It is not unusual in our current society for people to expect the bereaved to get over their grief very quickly, yet for many it is a long and sometimes painful struggle. So much depends upon the relationship with the deceased, the person's usual coping strategies and the support available. In addition, factors such as the mode of death, for example a prolonged illness, suicide or an accident, can have a profound impact on how the bereaved person copes. The death of a child may be especially difficult to cope with and requires careful and sensitive management.

An alternative approach to the bereavement process has been proposed by Stroebe and Schut (1999). They have suggested a dual-process model in which bereaved people oscillate between working at their grief and expressing their feelings on the one hand, and allowing themselves to deal with everyday tasks and take on new roles on the other (Figure 9.3). This model allows a much more individualised approach to bereavement, taking into account gender and to some extent cultural differences. This model acknowledges that people sometimes need to be fully immersed in the emotional aspects of their loss, whereas on other occa-

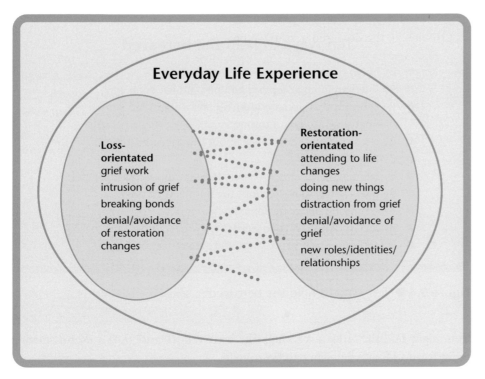

Figure 9.3 ● Dual-process model of bereavement (adapted from Stroebe and Schut, 1999)

sions they need time to adjust to life without the deceased, to manage day-to-day life and to be distracted from their grief. People oscillate between these two, sometimes confronting their grief and at other times avoiding it.

Nurses are for the most part involved with people during the acute stage of grief when someone significant has recently died. It is, however, worth remembering that many people who enter the health-care system, whether in hospital or at home, will have experienced losses during their life. In particular, older people are frequently faced with the death of family and friends, and those who move into nursing home care face many additional losses. Bereavement responses will also be manifest in people who are confronted by a social loss, such as the loss of a job or a relationship, and the associated loss of self-esteem and self-worth. Illness too brings with it many losses, including the physical loss of body parts or body function.

Whatever the cause of the loss, it is important to focus on individuals rather than a theoretical perspective. Listen to their story rather than trying to fit them into any model or stage. Accept them and their way of grieving. Helping people through grief and bereavement relies heavily on your ability to communicate effectively through listening, touch, the use of silence and sensitive responding.

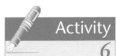

Activity
6

List the types of loss experienced by someone who has to leave their own home and move into a nursing home. What sorts of positive and negative thoughts and feelings might they experience?

Think of all the types of loss that people might experience through ill-health – psychological, physical and social losses.

Ten ways to help the bereaved

- By being there
- By listening in an accepting and non-judgemental way
- By showing that you are listening and understand something of what they are going through
- By encouraging them to talk about the deceased
- By tolerating silence
- By being familiar with your own feelings about loss and grief
- By offering reassurance about the normality of grief
- By not taking anger personally
- By recognising that your feelings may reflect how they feel
- By accepting that you cannot make them feel better

Figure 9.4 ● Ten ways to help the bereaved (adapted from Goodall et al. 1994)

You might find the '10 ways to help the bereaved' (Figure 9.4) a useful starting point for deciding what you can do to help.

Perhaps you could add to the above list 'By recognising the spiritual nature of bereavement' because when someone is bereaved, questions often emerge about the whole nature of life and death. Relatives may need someone who will listen and not judge them but enable them to explore these fundamental questions. The nature of spirituality will be the focus of the next section.

■ Spirituality

CONNECTIONS

Chapter 2 offers an explanation of spiritual health.

Spirituality is not something that belongs only to the dying and to those suffering, but is potentially an aspect of our everyday lives throughout our life. The notion of 'spiritual health' was in fact introduced in Chapter 2. It is, therefore, an important element in all aspects of nursing, and it is discussed here partly out of convenience and partly because it is in times of crisis that many people become more acutely aware of the spiritual nature of life. Rimpoche (1992) comments:

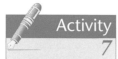

Activity

7

Think about the word 'spirituality', making notes about what you feel the term means to you.

> Spiritual care is not a luxury for the few; it is *the* essential right of every human being, as essential as political liberty, medical assistance, and equality of opportunity. A real democratic ideal would include knowledgeable spiritual care for everyone as one of its essential truths.

So what is spirituality and spiritual care? It is clearly not easy to define, and the danger of defining it is that in doing so you lose its very essence. Walter (1997) argues that when you begin to examine the various definitions, you are left with the question of how some aspects are any different from 'psychological care', 'social care' and religion. However true this might be, spirituality is perhaps more than the sum of its parts: the diverse elements when enmeshed become something new and something very individual. Stoll (1989) captures this sentiment by expressing the relational aspect of spirituality and the religious dimension when she writes:

> Spirituality is my being; my inner person. It is who I am – unique and alive. It is me expressed through my body, my thinking, my feelings, my judgements and my creativity. My spirituality motivates me to choose meaningful relationships and pursuits. Through my spirituality I give and receive love; I respond to and appreciate God, other people, a sunset, a symphony and spring. I am driven forward, sometimes because of pain. Spirituality allows me to reflect on myself. I am a person because of my spirituality – motivated and enabled to value, to worship and to communicate with the holy, the transcendent.

Kellehear (2000) argues that, although spirituality is difficult to define, some level of definition is not only possible, but also important. Definitions provide a platform for debate and practice, and are useful providing we recognise they are dynamic and changing, and that they are open to dissent and challenge.

It is suggested that human beings seek to understand and transcend suffering, desiring to understand and make sense of their situation; this is no more so than when people are faced with death (Kellehear, 2000). Kellehear describes a multi-dimensional model that incorporates the situational, religious, and moral and biographical aspects of spirituality (Figure 9.5). Although not everyone will access all three areas or all of the elements within the areas, they do assume the types of need that co-exist in spirituality. What the areas have in common is that each reflects an attempt at transcendence, in other words an attempt to find meaning from a given life crisis.

I will not attempt to explain all these aspects of spirituality in the model but will try to give a flavour of what Kelleher is suggesting.

Religious

Religion is for many an important aspect of spiritual life. Through this vehicle many seek to find answers and guidance through prayer, meditation and ritual. It is an almost impossible task to describe the particular practices of the many religions, and even within the same religion people will have different interpretations and depths of devotion. Indeed, there is a danger of trivialising people's beliefs if we simply focus on the ritual aspect of their belief system. This makes it even more important to take care in the assessment process.

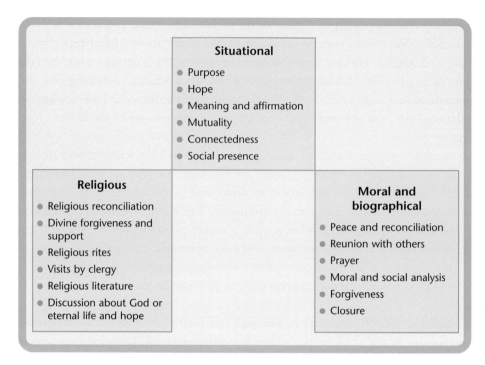

Figure 9.5 ● Dimensions of spirituality (adapted from Kellehear, 2000)

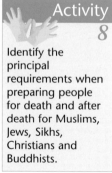

Activity
8

Identify the principal requirements when preparing people for death and after death for Muslims, Jews, Sikhs, Christians and Buddhists.

Rather than simply 'ticking the box', it is important to ask what patients' religion means to them and what they need while they are in our care – do they wish their spiritual leader to visit them, what dietary needs do they have, and so forth? If it is not possible to ask the patient, consult the relatives. If the patient is terminally ill, find out what the potential requirements might be in the terminal stages of the illness and after death. Sikhs, for example, may desire to have prayers said to them during the last stages of their life. Muslims may require that only Muslims touch or prepare the body after death.

In summary, be respectful of religious needs; seek advice and guidance early; keep contact numbers for local spiritual leaders and trusted local interpreters; listen to the needs of patients and relatives; and provide support to allow people to practise and meet their religious needs.

Situational

The situational aspect relates closely to trying to understand and make sense of the situations in which people find themselves. It emerges from the immediate situation, with its attendant medical problems, treatment and environment, be this hospital, hospice or their own home. People seek to discover hope and purpose in the place and situation they are in, to seek hope where there sometimes appears to be none. There can be nothing worse than to tell someone that there is nothing more we can do for them. But if we are to 'die living', there is always hope, hope to see a grandchild born, to paint a final picture, to see the sun rise, to be held by those you love, to be angry and express your emotions, to cry and seek solace, to fight and struggle. There is a need for help in this potentially frightening journey and people may seek the closeness, presence and affirmation of others as they seek to find meaning from their situation.

Moral and biographical

This also involves finding meaning in life but more from a biographical perspective – 'What has my life been about?' It is so easy just living life from day to day that we forget to ask more fundamental questions, but people faced with a life crisis frequently reflect on their life and try to make sense of it. It is also a time to seek forgiveness from loved ones, to say the things often left unsaid and to make amends. This may be done through prayer, which may have no specific religious significance. The nurse can help by using the skills already discussed, giving time, however little, listening, caring, touching, giving a smile, listening to the anger, and providing privacy for visits. For those who are dying, there is a need to bring about some degree of closure on life, to make this a time to sort out and put into perspective their life history.

This section has reflected on the complex nature of spirituality and has suggested that it is concerned with more than religion, being instead something within all of us – even though some may be more aware of this than others. At a time of crisis, however, spirituality may become more central to our thinking. Narayanasamy (2001) suggests that, to develop these skills, nurses need to develop their own self-awareness of spirituality, becoming aware of their own attitudes, values and prejudices and recognising what skills they have and which they are deficient in. Some of the skills needed are listening, trust-building and giving hope, as well as a knowledge of spirituality.

■ Chapter Summary

Death is the inevitable end to life for all of us. As a nurse, you are in a position to help many people with this transition and to help and care for the bereaved who are left. This chapter is only a brief introduction to this fascinating aspect of nursing; it does not pretend to be comprehensive, and in places you have perhaps been left with more questions than answers. You are encouraged to read widely around the subject and to do so critically, but just as important is your ability to learn from experience through active reflection. You may find it useful

Activity 9

Consider the following questions in relation to the branch and client group you will be working with.

● How would you tell your client of the death of a significant person?

● How would you start to talk to someone in your client group about their illness and prognosis? (In the case of a neonate, this will be with the parents. With a child, this may, depending on age, involve the child and his or her parents or guardians.)

● How will last offices and disposal of the dead person be managed?

Be content with not knowing all the answers at this stage, but think about the difficulties these questions pose and carry them around in your head so that you can read, observe and practise as a continuous journey to knowing.

to explore a range of sources of information on death and loss, including novels, poetry and the arts; some suggestions are offered in the further reading below.

This chapter has tried to emphasise the individual nature of caring for people who are dying or bereaved. It has not been possible to include every scenario, but whether you are dealing with a dying neonate or a child, an adult or older person, someone with mental health problems or a learning disability, each requires their individual circumstances to be taken into account.

● Test Yourself!

1. List the common cardinal signs of death.

2. What are the dimensions of palliative care described by Davies and O'Berle (1990)?

3. What does the term 'total pain' mean?

4. What does the term 'analgesic ladder' mean?

5. What, according to Finlay (1995), are the five most common symptoms seen in the dying patient?

6. What does the term 'last offices' mean?

7. What are the elements of loss-orientated grief and restoration-orientated grief, as described by Strobe and Schut (1999)?

8. Identify at least four ways in which you can help bereaved relatives.

9. What are the three elements of spirituality, as defined by Kellehear (2000)?

10. Make notes on your feelings about caring for the dying. What would you like to do to develop your skills and abilities in this area of nursing care?

Further Reading

Dickinson, D., Johnson, M. and Katz, J.S. (eds) (2000) *Death, Dying and Bereavement*. Sage, London. This book provides a useful collection of papers and articles, including cultural and ethical issues.

Hill, S. (1977) *In the Springtime of the Year*. Penguin, London. This is a useful novel as it explores how two people experience different reactions to grief, neither fully understanding the other.

Lewis, C.S. (1961) *A Grief Observed*. Faber & Faber, London. The story of the philosopher and writer, well known for his Narnia books. Lewis writes movingly of his feelings following the death of his wife. You might also like to watch the film *Shadowlands*, which is meant to recount the journey experienced by Lewis and his wife as she becomes ill and ultimately dies.

Further Reading continued	Mallett, J. (ed.) (2000) *Royal Marsden Hospital Manual of Clinical Nursing Procedures,* 5th edn. Blackwell, Oxford. A very helpful evidence-based manual on clinical procedures.	Nyatanga, B. (2001) *Why Is it So Difficult To Die?* Mark Allen, Dinton Quay, Wilts. A useful and recent book for health-care professionals exploring many aspects of death and loss.

References

Aries, P. (1981) *The Hour of Our Death.* Knopf, New York.

Barclay, S. (2001) Palliative care for non-cancer patients: a UK perspective from primary care. In Addington-Hall, J.M. and Higginson, I.J. (eds) *Palliative Care for Non-cancer Patients.* Oxford University Press, Oxford.

Buckman, R. (1998) Communication in palliative care: a practical guide. In Doyle, D., Hanks, G. and Macdonald, N. (eds) *Oxford Textbook of Palliative Medicine.* Oxford University Press, Oxford.

Clark, D. (1993) *The Future for Palliative Care: Issues of Policy and Practice.* Open University Press, Buckingham.

Collick, E. (1986) *Through Grief: The Bereavement Journey.* Darton, Longman & Todd, London.

Cooke, H. (2000) *When Someone Dies: A Practical Guide to Holistic Care at the End of Life.* Butterworth-Heinemann, Oxford.

Davies, B. and O'Berle, K. (1990) Dimensions of the supportive role of the nurse in palliative care. *Oncology Nurses Forum* **17**: 87–94.

Davis, B.D., Cowley, S.A. and Ryland, R.K. (1996) The effects of terminal illness on patients and their carers. *Journal of Advanced Nursing* **23**: 512–20.

DoH (Department of Health) (1999) *Our Healthier Nation.* DoH, London.

Faull, C., Carter, Y. and Woof, R. (eds) (1998) *Handbook of Palliative Care.* Blackwell, Oxford.

Finlay, I. (1995) The management of other frequently encountered symptoms. In Penson, J. and Fisher, R. (eds) *Palliative Care for People with Cancer.* Edward Arnold, London.

Freud, S. (1917) *Mourning and Melancholia.* Standard edition, Vol. XIV, 1957. Hogarth Press, London.

Glaser, B.G. and Strauss, A.L. (1968) *Time for Dying.* Aldine Press, Chicago.

Goodall, A., Darge, T. and Bell, G. (1994) *The Bereavement Training Manual.* Winslow, Bicester.

Henley, A. (1986) *Good Practice in Hospital Care for Dying Patients.* King's Fund, London.

Hospice Information Service (2001) *Palliative Care Facts and Figures.* www.hospiceinformation.co.uk.

Kellehear, A. (2000) Spirituality and palliative care: a model of needs. *Palliative Medicine* **14**: 149–55.

Klass, D., Silverman, P.R. and Nickman, S.L. (1996) *Continuing Bonds: New Understandings of Grief.* Taylor & Francis, London.

Komaromy, C., Siddell, M. and Katz, J. (2000) The quality of terminal care in residential and nursing homes. *International Journal of Palliative Nursing* **6**: 192–200.

Kubler-Ross, E. (1969) *On Death and Dying.* Macmillan, New York.

Lewis, C.S. (1961) *A Grief Observed.* Faber & Faber, London.

Morgan, J.D. (1995) Living our dying and our grieving: historical and cultural attitudes. In Wass, H. and Neimeyer, R.A. (eds) *Dying: Facing the Facts,* 3rd edn. Taylor & Francis, Washington.

Narayanasamy, A. (2001) *Spiritual Care: A Practical Guide for Nurses and Health Care Practitioners,* 2nd edn. Mark Allen, Dinton Quay, Wilts.

NHS Executive (1996) *A Policy Framework for Commissioning Cancer Services: Palliative Care Services.* NHS Executive, London.

Office of National Statistics (ONS) (1997) *Mortality Statistics: England & Wales 1996, General.* Stationery Office, London.

Parkes, C.M. (1996) *Bereavement: Studies of Grief in Adult Life.* Routledge, London.

Rimpoche, S. (1992) *The Tibetan Book of Living and Dying.* Rider, London.

Rosenblatt, P.C. (1997) Grief in small-scale societies. In Parkes, C.M., Laungani, P. and Young, B. (eds) *Death and Bereavement Across Cultures.* Routledge, London.

Rubin, S.S. (1993) The death of a child. In Stroebe, M., Stroebe, W. and Hansson R.O. (eds) *Handbook of Bereavement: Theory, Research and Intervention.* Cambridge University Press, Cambridge.

Saunders, C. (1978) *The Management of Terminal Illness.* Arnold, London.

Seedhouse, D. (1997) *Health Promotion: Philosophy, Prejudice and Practice.* John Wiley & Sons, London.

Stoll, R. (1989) The essence of spirituality. In Carson, V. (ed.) *Spiritual Dimensions of Nursing Practice.* W.B. Saunders, Philadelphia.

Stroebe, M. and Schut, H. (1999) The dual process model of coping with bereavement: rationale and description. *Death Studies* **23**: 197–224.

Townsend, J., Frank, A.O., Fermont, D., Dyer, S., Karran, O., Walgrove, A. and Piper, M. (1990) Terminal cancer care and patients' preference for place of death: a prospective study. *British Medical Journal* **310**: 415–17.

Veatch, R.M. (1995) The definition of death: problems for public policy. In Wass, H. and Neimeyer, R.A. (eds) *Dying: Facing the Facts,* 3rd edn. Taylor & Francis, London.

Victor, C.R. (2000) Health policy and services for dying people and their carers. In Dickenson, D., Johnson, M. and Katz, J.S. (eds) *Death, Dying and Bereavement,* 2nd edn. Sage, London.

Walter, T. (1990) *Funerals and How To Improve Them.* Hodder and Stoughton, London.

Walter, T. (1997) The ideology and organisation of spiritual care: three approaches. *Palliative Medicine* **11**: 21–30.

Walter, T. (1999) *On Bereavement: The Culture of Grief.* Open University Press, Buckingham.

Wilson, M. (1975) *Health is for People.* Darton, Longman & Todd, London.

Worden, W.J. (1983) *Grief Counselling and Grief Therapy.* Tavistock, London.

World Health Organization (1990) *Cancer Pain Relief and Palliative Care.* Technical Report Series 804. WHO, Geneva.

World Health Organization (1996) *Cancer Pain Relief.* WHO, Geneva.

Yalom, I.D. (1980) *Existential Psychotherapy.* Basic Books, New York.

Chapter

Wound Management

10

Learning outcomes

The purpose of this chapter is to explore the nursing management of wounds. After working through it, you should be able to:

- Identify and discuss some of the issues surrounding accountability in wound management

- Define the term 'wound' and discuss wound classification

- Describe the use of risk assessment tools in your current area of work

- Describe the recognised stages of the healing process, linking this to the structure and function of healthy skin

- Describe the factors affecting wound healing

- Describe and explain each element of the optimum environment for wound healing

- Describe how each stage of the nursing process may facilitate the nursing management of wounds.

> The chapter contains a number of activities that will help to deepen your understanding of this complex topic. Some of these activities require you to access and read the additional texts listed below (or substitute another recommended anatomy and physiology text if necessary).

Additional texts for this chapter are:

Bale, S. and Jones, V. (1997) *Wound Care Nursing: A Patient Centred Approach*. Baillière Tindall, London.

Clancy, J. and McVicar, A. (1995) *Physiology and Anatomy: A Homeostatic Approach*. Edward Arnold, London.

Morison, M. (2000) *The Prevention and Treatment of Pressure Ulcers*. C.V. Mosby, London.

Thibodeau, G.A. (1992) *Structure and Function of the Body*, 9th edn. Mosby Yearbook, St Louis.

■ A Professional Perspective

tissue viability

the sustained health, growth and repair of body tissues

The maintenance of **tissue viability** and the management of wounds is an area of practice that falls clearly within the domain of the professionally qualified nurse. It is an activity that is considered to be important in terms of both patient comfort and care, and the financial strain placed upon service providers (Cullum and Dealey, 1996).

It has been suggested that the key elements in establishing sound practice include the provision of evidence-based education and the development of good communication networks (Allison, 1995; Edwards, 1995). You may have noticed some of the many journal articles concerned with tissue viability and wound management, and you may also be familiar with multidisciplinary associations such as the Wound Care Society, the Tissue Viability Society, the European Wound Management Association and the European Tissue Repair Society. It soon becomes apparent that tissue viability and wound management is a high-profile area of nursing activity. Many NHS Trusts employ clinical nurse specialists for tissue viability with the distinct remit of managing and co-ordinating care, teaching and research in wound management.

It is, however, important to remember that this area of nursing practice is one that most, if not all, practitioners will encounter, both pre- and postregistration.

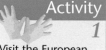

Activity 1

Visit the European Pressure Ulcer Advisory Panel website at www.leahcim. demon.co.uk/ epuap) to review its contents and identify any additional relevant websites. Download any potentially useful information.

Accountability in Wound Management

CONNECTIONS

Chapter 16 explores the four types of accountability.

Inherent in the concept of professionalism is the notion of service and with this the 'duty of care' that is entered into during practice, for which the professional practitioner is held accountable (UKCC, 1989; Carpenter, 1993). Whenever a professional nurse assesses, plans, implements or evaluates a care intervention, a duty of care arises. The nurse can be held to account for the knowledge base upon which such an intervention is founded and must be able to demonstrate practice within the limits of such knowledge (UKCC, 1994).

The duty of care defines the minimum standard of practice that a patient can expect. In professional nursing practice, this is informed by the *Code of Professional Conduct* (NMC, 2002) as well as national standards such as *The Patient's Charter* (DoH, 1991), professional guidelines (Nelson, 1997) and local policies, guidelines, protocols and procedures. If the duty of care is breached, it is possible that a case of negligence may be brought against either the service provider (organisation) or the individual practitioner accountable for the nursing care involved.

Accountability and responsibility often become confused; indeed, they are similar concepts. However, a distinction can be made in that in order to be held accountable for something, you must have authority over it. This means that you must be in the position to make a decision about a particular course of action. If you are not in such a position, it is your responsibility to say so.

A number of 'accountability relationships' (Chart 10.1) exist within which professional practitioners are required to discharge their duty of care to the client. There are times when these different relationships can conflict with one another, for example when moral imperatives conflict with managerial ones.

Activity 2

You are in your second clinical placement and it is a busy shift. A health-care support worker has reported to the staff nurse that Mr Lyons has a superficial break in the skin over his sacrum. The staff nurse is setting up a blood transfusion for another patient and asks you to see Mr Lyons and 'put a dressing on his sacrum'. She assures you that you can do this 'because you are in training'.

Looking at the accountability frameworks, what can you be held accountable for here and why? What do you think is your prime responsibility? You may find it useful to discuss this with your colleagues and tutors.

superficial break

the place at which the continuity of the uppermost layer of the epidermis is interrupted

Chart 10.1 ● Frameworks for accountability

- Legal – common, civil, commercial and criminal law
- Managerial – operational policies and procedures
- Organisational – care delivery systems, contracts
- Professional – codes of conduct, mandates from the leading professional bodies, guidelines, recommendations
- Governmental – national standards, citizens' rights
- Moral – personal beliefs and value systems

Source: Adapted from Marks-Maran (1993).

Table 10.1 Clinical governance framework

Key elements of the clinical governance framework	Relationship to wound management
Evidence-based practice	Ensuring that treatment interventions are based on sound research
Clinical effectiveness	Ensuring that we do the 'right things, for the right people, with the right knowledge and skills and at the right time'
Risk management	Ensuring that we assess all possible risks and plan care to minimise these
	Ensuring that we learn from adverse events to prevent future problems
Monitoring clinical practice	Ensuring that we undertake a systematic audit of wound mangement practice, using published gudelines as benchmarking tools
Continuing education and professional development	Ensuring that we keep our knowledge and skills up to date with current developments
Professional self-regulation	Ensuring that we are always able to account for our practice
Dissemination of good practice	Ensuring that we share and learn from examples of good practice with all our colleagues in the multidisciplinary team

Clinical Governance and Wound Management

CONNECTIONS

Chapter 16 also deals with clinical governance.

The recent government policy intiative, clinical governance, helps to provide a framework for professional effectiveness and accountability in all aspects of health-care provision (DoH, 2000). Clinical governance involves integrating a number of existing systems and processes to ensure that the care given is of the highest possible quality. This process is underpinned by legislation through the 1999 Health Act, which charges NHS organisations with a 'duty of quality' to stand alongside the 'duty of care'. We can consider wound mangement in terms of the clinical governance framework, as illustrated in Table 10.1.

What is a Wound?

Having identified tissue viability and wound management as a regular nursing activity, and highlighted the importance of accountability in wound management, the next step is to examine what is meant by the term 'wound' and identify the different types that may be encountered.

Any kind of breach in the integrity of the skin or underlying tissues is commonly described as a wound. Wounds can also be classified according to how they were caused, how deep they are, whether they are 'open' or 'closed', or the method by which they are expected to heal. Examples of how these classifications can be interlinked are illustrated in Table 10.2.

wound

any break in the integrity of the skin and underlying tissues

Table 10.2 Examples of wound classification

Description of wound	Cause	Expected mode of healing (see 'Modes of healing' later in this chapter)	Open or closed
Surgical excision	Removal of skin and underlying tissues during surgery	Secondary intention	Open
Surgical incision	A precise cut made during surgery using either a scalpel blade or diathermy	Primary intention	Closed
Burn	Thermal, electrical or chemical	Secondary intention	Open
Laceration ('cut')	Trauma	Primary/secondary intention	Either
Abrasion ('graze')	Trauma	Secondary intention	Open
Puncture ('stab wound')	Trauma	Secondary intention	Open
Venous ulcer	Pathology (intrinsic), for example chronic venous insufficiency	Secondary intention	Open
Arterial ulcer	Pathology (intrinsic), for example atherosclerosis	Secondary intention	Open
Diabetic ulcer	Pathology (intrinsic), for example diabetes	Secondary intention	Open
Pressure (decubitus) ulcer	Pathology (extrinsic), for example pressure, shear or friction	Secondary intention	Open
Fungating	Pathology (intrinsic), for example carcinoma	Neither	Open

diathermy

the application of high-frequency electric currents via a fine, hand-held rod, producing intense, localised heat that may be used to divide tissue and/or seal (cauterise) blood vessels

atherosclerosis

the thickening and calcification of the arteries and narrowing of their lumens that occurs as a result of the deposition of fatty substances (plaques) along the arterial walls

Activity 3

Find out which risk assessment tools are in use where you work. Ask your clinical assessor/supervisor the following:

How are the risk assessment tools used? How often is each assessment carried out? Who carries it out? How are the results documented and acted upon? How is the client involved in this?

CONNECTIONS

Chapter 4 looks at factors relevant for assessing nutritional status.

CONNECTIONS

Chapter 3 explores risk assessment in relation to moving and handling.

Activity 4

To explore the anatomy and physiology of healthy skin, refer to your recommended texts (for example Thibodeau, 1992, pp. 63–78 or Clancy and McVicar, 1995, pp. 505–23).

Find out the names and characteristics of the two layers of the skin.

Assessing the Risk

The likelihood of certain wounds developing as a result of pathological processes can be assessed. Such wounds are commonly associated with either:

- Intrinsic (internal) factors such as vascular disease or diabetes
- Extrinsic (external) factors such as pressure damage or infection

or a mixture of both. They can be assessed by examining the risk factors commonly associated with the type of wound.

Assessment may be carried out in a variety of ways, using the nursing process. A number of risk assessment tools have been developed to assist nurses and other health-care professionals in exercising their judgement regarding care planning and resource allocation. These include:

- Pressure sore risk assessment tools, for example those of Waterlow (1988) and Norton et al. (1975)
- Diabetic foot ulcer risk assessment tool (Plummer and Albert, 1995)
- Nutrition risk assessment tools
- Manual handling risk assessment tools.

Healthy Skin and the Healing Process

The ability to support the maintenance of tissue viability and manage wounds effectively is underpinned by a sound understanding of the structure and function of normal, healthy skin as well as a working knowledge of the normal healing process.

Healthy skin

The skin (Figure 10.1) is the largest and one of the most important organs in the body, forming the primary organ of the integumentary system, which comprises the:

- Skin
- Hair
- Nails
- Sweat glands
- Sebaceous glands
- Sensory nerve receptors.

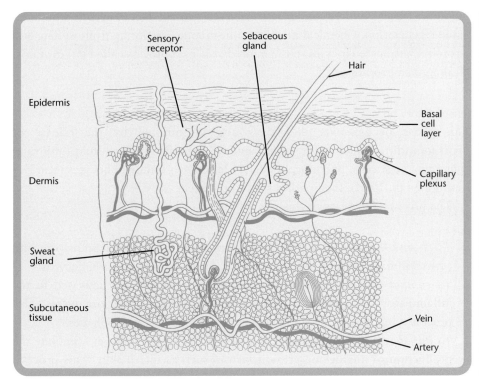

CONNECTIONS

Chapter 8 explains the structure and function of the skin in more detail.

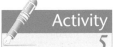

Activity
5

The skin plays a key role in the homeostatic management of the internal environment. Compile a list of the functions of the skin. Discuss the relationships between skin structure and function, sun damage and the ageing process.

Figure 10.1 ● Cross-section of the skin

The healing process

Normal wound healing is often characterised as a complex, but well-integrated, multiphase process. The phases of this process are usually described separately to facilitate understanding, but it is important to remember that there may be evidence of the different phases of healing within the same wound and that each phase overlaps with the next, often running concurrently. The healing process can be reversed or become static in certain circumstances.

The phases of wound healing

Four main phases have been identified.

Haemostasis

Haemostasis involves wound contraction, which decreases the surface area of the wound, thus reducing bleeding and exposure to contaminants. This process is part of the physiological response to blood **extravasation**. Platelets activate

extravasation

leakage of fluid from a blood vessel

kinins

polypeptides present in the blood following tissue injury

chemotaxis

a response involving movement towards or away from a chemical stimulus

prostaglandins

hormone-like substances that affect vasomotor and smooth muscle tone, capillary permeability, platelet aggregation, endocrine and exocrine functions and the nervous system

angiogenesis

the production or growth of new blood vessels

collagen synthesis

the production of supportive, protein-based, fibrous connective tissue

granulation tissue

red, moist, fragile connective tissue that is characteristic of the proliferative phase of the healing process

the kinin system and release platelet-derived growth factor, which stimulates tissue regeneration. Chemical mediators (histamine, adenosine triphosphate and serotonin) attract leukocytes to the injured area by a process called chemotaxis. Healing then progresses.

Inflammatory phase

This phase occurs over 4–5 days and is initiated by the release of prostaglandins, which cause vasodilatation. An inflammatory fluid (infiltrate) containing mast cells, polymorphonuclear leukocytes and lymphocytes (Van Der Kerkhof et al., 1994), then bathes the injured area.

The primary functions of this phase are:

- *To cleanse the area of debris:* monocytes enter the area and transform into activated macrophages. These cells clear the debris through phagocytosis
- *To combat potential infective organisms:* neutrophils are activated in the inflammatory response and clear the site of contaminating organisms. This process is augmented by the phagocytic action of the macrophages
- *To initiate angiogenesis and collagen synthesis:* macrophages stimulate the production of angiogenic growth factors such as interleukin. This process, augmented by the activity of mast cells, initiates endothelial division and angiogenesis as well as the regrowth of sympathetic nerve fibres. Fibroblasts migrate to the wound site, initiating the early stages of the next phase.

Proliferative phase

This phase of the wound healing process occurs over a variable time span and is characterised by the formation of granulation tissue. The fibroblasts produce a framework of collagen fibres that support and sustain the products of angiogenesis. This framework is anchored by fibronectin and bathed in proteoglycans. The successful progress of this phase is dependent upon the oxygen and nutrient supply.

Fibroblast activity is sensitive to oxygen supply, which in turn depends upon the vascularity of the wound and surrounding tissues. The growth of capillary buds from undamaged microvessels, forming a network of loops within the wound, is crucial to the level of oxygen available during the proliferative phase.

Proteins are the source of the 20 amino acids present in the body. These amino acids are described as the building blocks of organic tissue and as such are essential for collagen synthesis, angiogenesis and cell reconstruction (Wells, 1994). If the blood protein level (measured in terms of serum albumin) is low, wound healing will be impaired.

Essential fatty acids, provided from the dietary fat intake, play an important

CONNECTIONS

Chapter 4 explains why we need protein in our diet and investigates sources, types and requirements.

role in cell structure and function. Dietary fat is also the largest source of energy, required for wound healing, as well as providing a source of fat-soluble vitamins.

Carbohydrate, in the form of glucose, is the primary energy substrate required for cellular metabolism. If glucose from carbohydrate is unavailable, amino acids will be oxidised to meet the energy requirements of the wound healing process, thus depleting the pool of amino acids available for reconstruction and tissue repair.

Vitamin C is involved in the metabolism of many amino acids and is required for the formation of cross-linking collagen fibres, facilitating the **hydroxylation** of proline and lysine to hydroxyproline and hydroxylysine – essential components of collagen (Lewis and Harding, 1993). Iron (as well as providing the primary component of haemoglobin, which facilitates the transport of oxygen in the bloodstream) is a co-factor in this process. Vitamin C also enhances wound healing by scavenging potentially harmful **free radicals** from the surfaces of cells. It has been suggested that the antioxidant vitamin E interacts in this process (Davis et al., 1991).

The B vitamins are involved in enzymatic activity (as co-factors) and are also active in collagen cross-linkage, as is vitamin A, which also acts upon cell surface glycoproteins, effecting epithelial cell proliferation and migration. Zinc is another co-factor in the enzymatic activity associated with collagen and protein synthesis and cell growth. The enzyme lysyl oxidase, instrumental in scar formation, contains copper, a trace element. Many enzymes not only contain, but also rely on, manganese as a co-factor for collagen synthesis, and calcium is a mediator for the enzymes involved in collagen remodelling (collagenases).

Two other major processes occur concurrently within the proliferative phase of wound healing – epithelialisation and contraction. The granulation tissue filling the wound bed is gradually resurfaced by epithelial cells, which migrate in from the wound margins or regenerate as 'islands' on the wound surface. As epithelial cells regenerate and migrate over the wound surface, their eventual contact with one another inhibits further migration, and the epithelialisation process is complete. The process of contraction, initiated during the inflammatory phase, is controlled largely by the activity of myofibroblasts. These specialised fibroblasts contain actin and myosin fibrils (the essential contractile components of muscle tissue), and their activity reduces the surface area of the wound.

Granulation, contraction and epithelialisation mark the completion of the proliferative phase.

Maturation phase

This final phase in the wound healing process is concerned with the remodelling and strengthening of the collagen fibres within the wound. The collagen

---

CONNECTIONS

Chapter 4 reviews the role of fat, carbohydrates and vitamins B and C, identifying dietary sources, different types and requirements.

hydroxylation
the formation or addition of a hydroxyl (OH) group

free radicals
unstable, highly reactive compounds containing an unpaired electron or proton

produced during earlier stages is relatively soft, type III collagen, which has been afforded structural strength through cross-linking of the fibres. During maturation, this is replaced with stronger type I collagen, which is organised into bundles lying at right angles to the wound margins. This ongoing process, facilitated by the activity of fibroblasts and characterised by a gradual reduction in vascularity of the wound site, shrinkage and paling of the scar tissue, can continue over a number of years.

Modes of healing

It is common to refer to the healing process as occurring by one of two modes: primary intention or secondary intention.

Healing by primary intention

healing by primary intention

healing occurring in wounds where the skin edges can be apposed so that there is no scar or granulation tissue

Healing by primary intention occurs in wounds where there has been no tissue loss and the skin edges can be brought together, ensuring an absence of dead space in the wound. The four phases of wound healing occur, but there is little granulation tissue produced and minimal wound contraction, epithelial cells migrating along the suture line. Remodelling of the collagen fibres in scar tissue takes place, as previously described, 6–12 months being needed to regain 70–90 per cent of the tensile strength of normal tissue.

Healing by secondary intention

healing by secondary intention

healing in which the edges of the wound are separated, requiring granulation tissue to fill the gap

Healing by secondary intention refers to wounds where there has been tissue loss and the skin edges remain apart. Again, the wound will progress through all four phases of healing, but it will be necessary for the wound bed to fill with granulation tissue, to become resurfaced with epithelium and to contract before and during scar formation.

pus

characteristic fluid composed of exudate, dead tissue debris, macrophages and bacteria

Reference is sometimes made to an additional mode of healing – healing by third intention. In this case, a wound that may be infected or contaminated is left open to facilitate the drainage of **pus** and the formation of granulation tissue. When the complicating factor has been excluded, the wound can be manually closed (for example sutured, clipped or taped), and healing by primary intention can take place.

Factors affecting wound healing

Wounds do not occur in isolation, and care must be taken to complete a holistic assessment. Initial and subsequent assessments should aim to identify any existing or potential problems that will adversely affect wound healing. The numerous factors to be considered during an assessment are illustrated in

Figure 10.2. By reviewing each element in Figure 10.2 and, where possible, discussing these with patients and/or their carers, the nurse will be able to develop an effective care strategy for wound management.

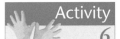
Activity
6

Complications

There are occasions when the wound healing process is interrupted and healing does not progress as anticipated. Commonly observed complications in the wound healing process include the following.

Consider Figure 10.2. Try to explain how each factor affects wound healing and note how they are interrelated.

Now read Chapters 4 and 5 of Bale and Jones (1997). Try to identify how the factors affecting wound healing are reflected in the nursing care of infants, children and adolescents, and how this may differ from the nursing care of adults.

Infection

The normal bacterial colonisation of a wound will not affect the healing process, but an overwhelming number of bacteria, resulting in a clinical infection, will interfere with the healing process by 'locking' the wound into a persistent inflammatory phase. This is characterised by localised heat, pain, cellulitis and an increase in exudate (often purulent in nature).

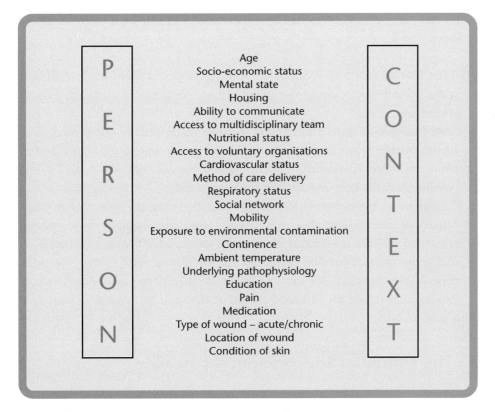

Figure 10.2 ● Factors affecting wound healing

Dehiscence

dehiscence

the separation of a
surgical incision or
wound

'Dehiscence' is the term used to refer to the 'splitting' open of a closed surgical wound. If the collagen fibres that have been laid down are not strong enough to withstand the internal and external tensions applied to the wound, the newly formed layers of the wound will separate. The dehiscence of a wound is often associated with infection and/or the presence of a haematoma.

Haematoma

haematoma

a collection of blood
trapped within the skin
or an organ

Haematoma is the name given to a localised 'pocket' of blood and plasma, which can become a breeding ground for bacteria.

Haemorrhage

Primary haemorrhage (severe blood loss during surgery) and intermediary haemorrhage (severe blood loss immediately following surgery) can affect wound strength by interfering with the function of the fibroblasts. Secondary haemorrhage (blood loss up to 10 days postoperatively) commonly results in haematoma formation and subsequent infection.

Abnormal healing

Abnormal healing is characterised by abnormalities in scar tissue formation and includes:

hypertrophic scarring

scarring caused by the
excessive formation of
new tissue

keloid scarring

the overgrowth of
collagenous scar tissue
infiltrating the
surrounding skin

- *Hypertrophic scarring*, common in young patients. A large amount of scar tissue is laid down along the incision line, resulting in a raised, fibrous wound site
- *Keloid scarring*, more common in patients with heavily pigmented skin. Again, a large amount of scar tissue is laid down, but in this case the scar tissue infiltrates the skin surrounding the wound site, resulting in big, bulbous growths over and around the wound site
- *Contractures:* hypercontraction of the wound during the maturation phase can result in excessive shortening of the associated muscle tissue, which, combined with the presence of fibrous scar tissue, inhibits muscular extension
- *Malignant disease:* because of the intense cellular activity within a wound, there is the potential for chronic wounds to undergo malignant change. Failure to heal over an extended period of time can be associated with such a process.

Activity

7

Can you think of certain measures that could be taken to prevent any of the complications of healing? Discuss your ideas with your colleagues.

■ The Optimum Environment for Healing

It can be seen from the preceding sections that the healing process is not only complex, but also vulnerable to interference from internal and external factors.

Our natural instinct when dealing with vulnerability is to protect; indeed, the efforts that have been made to protect wounds and promote healing have been recorded throughout history (Bale and Jones, 1997).

One glance through a hospital formulary, a look around a modern treatment room or an inspection of the contents of a community nurse's car boot will give an indication of the numerous products currently available to facilitate wound management. Such an array can create a certain amount of confusion when deciding which product will be best suited to which wound. In order to avoid this situation, it is worth remembering that although the characteristics of an 'ideal dressing' have been described (Morgan, 1994), few, if any, of the dressings available conform to every criterion. The choice of dressing material used is *only one* element in creating the optimum environment for wound healing, and the other factors affecting wound healing must also be taken into account.

Thus, the optimum environment at the wound–dressing interface will be:

- *Moist:* research conducted over 30 years ago indicated that re-epithelialisation was enhanced when a moist environment was maintained, both within the wound bed and at the wound–dressing interface. This means that the body must be well hydrated and should not have suffered an extensive loss of skin
- *Protected from bacterial contamination:* the wound requires a physical barrier, and thought must be given to potential sources of infection
- *Protected from particulate or toxic contamination:* again, a physical barrier is required, and the environment must be assessed for potential risks
- *Thermally insulated:* the wound healing process is affected by any variation in the temperature of the wound bed (Morgan, 1994). Not only should any dressing used maintain a stable temperature, but also practices such as frequent, unnecessary exposure of the wound, the use of unwarmed cleansing solutions and changes in the ambient environmental temperature must be assessed
- *Free from excess exudate:* although a moist environment is considered to be conducive to wound healing, excess **wound exudate** (containing microorganisms and wound debris) will interfere with the healing process, causing wound bed oedema. It will also leak on to the surrounding skin, resulting in the maceration of healthy tissue, as well as providing a potential entry portal for infective organisms
- *Well perfused:* gaseous exchange takes place at the wound–dressing interface. A good blood supply will ensure that the oxygen demands of the wound are met, as well as transporting nutrients to, and removing waste products from, the wound site

wound exudate

a translucent, yellow-tinged fluid, rich in proteins and antibodies, which is produced during the inflammatory phase of the healing process

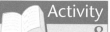

Activity 8

Find a copy of Morgan (1994) or your pharmacy department's formulary of wound management products. Note that the dressings listed are divided into groups, for example hydrocolloids.

Identify the particular characteristics of as many groups as you can and compare them with the elements described in the text. See if you can identify an example (by trade name) for each group.

- *Protected from mechanical damage:* neophyte epithelial cells are extremely delicate and can be easily removed during dressing changes (especially if the dressing material adheres to the wound surface or the surface is rubbed during wound cleansing). Experiments have shown that these cells can also be damaged by the use of certain wound cleansing solutions, for example hypochlorite (Leaper, 1996). Thus, the environment must be assessed for potential hazards that could cause further trauma
- *Undisturbed:* frequent dressing changes, however 'wound environmentally friendly' the dressings are, will interfere with the healing process.

As well as promoting the optimum environment for wound healing, the 'ideal dressing' should be cost-effective, perform in such a way as to maximise the achievement of treatment objectives and be readily available in both hospital and community settings.

Care-planning in Wound Management

CONNECTIONS

Chapter 1 illustrates the five stages of the nursing process.

As you will have discovered from working through Chapter 1, one of the most effective methods available for designing a programme of care interventions is the nursing process. The five stages of the nursing process form the framework for a systematic and holistic review of nursing care, based around a problem-solving approach. One of the benefits of adopting a systematic approach such as this is that you will be able to demonstrate clearly through documentation not only the decision-making processes involved in designing care interventions, but also – and most importantly – the effectiveness of those interventions.

A good way of exploring care-planning in detail is to use a client profile. The profile described in Casebox 10.1 will form the basis for a detailed analysis of care-planning in wound management.

Assessment and nursing diagnosis

CONNECTIONS

Chapter 1 expands on the skills of assessment.

Morison (1991) suggests that a holistic assessment should form the foundation of any wound management programme. This is an essential nursing activity, the role of the nurse being to collate and manage the information gathered during the assessment in order to generate nursing diagnoses and inform subsequent decision-making. You will recall that the skills required to gather information include:

- Listening
- Observing
- Using verbal and non-verbal communication
- Questioning

Casebox 10.1

Mrs Rosen is a 74-year-old widow and a bilateral amputee with a past medical history of severe arterial disease and non-insulin-dependent diabetes mellitus. She lives in a residential home and maintains regular contact with her two children and their families. Mrs Rosen is able to get around independently, using her wheelchair. She is a sociable, chatty lady who enjoys the company of others. Mrs Rosen normally smokes 40–60 cigarettes a day.

Mrs Rosen has been admitted to hospital for the management of the pressure ulcers that have developed over her ischial tuberosities. On admission to hospital, she appears relaxed and eager to find out about her new surroundings. She is wearing a urine drainage bag on her leg, and this is attached to a urinary catheter. As the ambulance crew transfer Mrs Rosen into bed, she winces several times but quickly regains her composure. There is a damp patch where she has been sitting on the ambulance trolley.

Mrs Rosen sets about organising her belongings; she has a large assortment of sweets, biscuits and fizzy drinks as well as her toiletries, cigarettes and lighter. She moves around the bed with ease, reaching over to pull the locker and table nearer. Having made herself comfortable, she calls the nurse over, apparently eager to do anything she can to assist in the admission process.

- Physical examination
- Measurement.

In order to design a comprehensive wound management programme for Mrs Rosen, it will be necessary to review each of the following assessment criteria, identifying any actual or potential problems and stating the related nursing diagnoses. The wound management assessment criteria (adapted from Hallett, 1995) are:

- General physical condition
- Mental state
- Mobility
- Nutritional status
- Continence
- Concurrent disease
- Cardiovascular status
- Pain
- Skin
- Risk assessment.

You will probably have identified the problems described below.

ischial tuberosities

the bony protuberances present on the ischium (the curved bone that forms the base of each half of the pelvis), commonly known as 'the sitting bones'

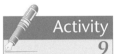

Activity 9

Using the information presented in Casebox 10.1, write an assessment of Mrs Rosen and identify any actual or potential problems using the assessment framework in the text.

General physical condition

Although Mrs Rosen has a degree of disability associated with bilateral amputation of her legs, she demonstrates a high level of independence. She does not appear to have any difficulty breathing, either at rest or on exertion. Neither does she appear to show any signs of malaise. There is insufficient information, at this stage, to identify any problems.

Mental function

Mrs Rosen is alert and appears orientated. She appears to be keen to participate and initiates conversation with the nursing staff. She is aware of her immediate needs and takes steps to meet them independently. No actual or potential problems have been identified.

Mobility

Mrs Rosen's mobility is limited. She is confined to a wheelchair when out of bed but can move herself around the bed using her upper body. She cannot transfer from one surface to another independently.

Actual problems

- Mrs Rosen will be subject to unrelieved pressure while sitting in her wheelchair
- She will be subject to additional pressure while in bed
- Mrs Rosen is unable to transfer independently.

Potential problems

- Mrs Rosen might experience fatigue because of the effort she puts into moving around the bed, and this may lead to unrelieved pressure while in bed
- She may lose her balance while moving around in bed, and this may result in injury
- Mrs Rosen may have a reduced ability to manoeuvre her wheelchair because of the unfamiliar surroundings
- There is a risk of injury (to either Mrs Rosen or the staff) while facilitating movement and manual handling.

Nutritional status

Mrs Rosen is a non-insulin-dependent diabetic who appears to have a very sweet tooth! The presence of the wounds means that she requires additional protein and vitamins in her diet to effect wound healing.

Actual problems

- Mrs Rosen has an undesirably high sugar intake
- Mrs Rosen has enhanced protein, vitamin and mineral requirements.

Potential problems

- Mrs Rosen may develop poor diabetic control
- She may display delayed wound healing.

Continence

Mrs Rosen appears to suffer from urinary incontinence, indicated by the presence of an indwelling urinary catheter. It would also, however, appear that the catheter is leaking.

Actual problems

- Mrs Rosen has urinary incontinence, managed by the use of an indwelling urinary catheter
- The catheter seems to be leaking
- Mrs Rosen is unable to get to the toilet independently.

Potential problems

- Mrs Rosen is at risk of developing a urinary tract infection
- There may be trauma associated with the presence of the catheter
- Mrs Rosen may suffer skin excoriation from leakage of urine
- Her wound may be contaminated by leaking urine
- Mrs Rosen may suffer from constipation as a result of immobility
- She may experience faecal incontinence because of immobility, which will result in both wound contamination and psychological distress.

Concurrent disease

Mrs Rosen suffers from non-insulin-dependent diabetes mellitus. No actual problems have been identified.

Potential problems

- Mrs Rosen may develop a poor control of her diabetes because of her dietary sugar intake
- Diabetes is associated with impaired wound healing.

Cardiovascular status

Mrs Rosen has severe arterial disease, which has led to the amputation of both her legs. She is also a heavy smoker, with no apparent intention of giving up. This will further compromise her cardiovascular system.

Actual problems

- Arterial disease implies an impaired blood flow to wound sites and impaired healing. Mrs Rosen is a smoker; smoking exacerbates the effects of cardiovascular disease as well as being a causative factor for it. It is also a health and safety hazard while Mrs Rosen is in hospital.

Potential problems

- Mrs Rosen may suffer withdrawal symptoms if she reduces or eliminates her nicotine intake
- Further deterioration of her cardiovascular system will lead to multisystem failure.

Pain

Although Mrs Rosen did not verbally complain of any pain, her facial expression during manual handling indicates that she might have experienced some.

Actual problems

- Mrs Rosen is not voicing her experience of pain
- Pain will cause a stress reaction that will interfere with the healing process.

Potential problems

- Mrs Rosen, although she appears cheerful and talkative, may be frightened
- Mrs Rosen may be reluctant to cause a fuss
- It may be difficult to assess the level and nature of Mrs Rosen's pain and the effectiveness of any interventions
- Increasing pain may further limit Mrs Rosen's mobility.

Skin

Mrs Rosen has pressure sores over her ischial tuberosities. It is unclear how many wounds are present or what their status is. There is insufficient information to describe any problems at this stage.

Risk assessment

Mrs Rosen has been admitted with pressure injuries and is therefore at risk of developing additional wounds. There is, however, insufficient information to complete a full risk assessment at this stage.

You may be surprised at how much information can be gathered from the careful reading of a client profile, but certain areas need clarification so that problems can be better identified and accurate nursing diagnoses made. You will now need to use the other skills of enquiry, taking into account the factors affecting wound healing described in Figure 10.2 above, to enhance the data you have already gathered.

Now tackle Activity 10. Your answer may include the following.

General physical condition

You will want to know more about Mrs Rosen's respiratory status. Does she have a cough or a wheeze? Are there any signs of **cyanosis**? Has Mrs Rosen recently suffered from any chest infections? Does she have a history of respiratory disease? What is her general state of well-being?

You will need to use the skills of observation, questioning, listening and physical examination. Your sources of information are likely to be Mrs Rosen's:

- Verbal responses
- Non-verbal responses
- Vital signs: measurements of blood pressure, respiratory rate and depth, pulse rate and rhythm, and body temperature.

You may also gather additional information from her:

- Previous medical and nursing notes
- Relatives and carers.

Mental function

Although Mrs Rosen appears to be adjusting well to the situation, you will need to observe and listen carefully to detect any signs of distress or disorientation. Be aware of the reactions of visitors: are they at all concerned about Mrs Rosen's behaviour?

Mobility

It is necessary to assess the extent of Mrs Rosen's mobility and identify what types of aid to mobility and manual handling may be required. A thorough assessment of mobility can only be effected by a direct observation of Mrs Rosen

Activity 10

Imagine that you are Mrs Rosen's named nurse and are conducting her initial assessment as part of the admission process. Think carefully about how you can augment the information already gathered from the patient profile.

Review your assessment and identify any additional information required, specifying how you would obtain this.

cyanosis

the blue tinge that appears in the skin and/or mucous membranes when the blood oxygen supply is diminished

FOUNDATIONS OF NURSING PRACTICE

over a period of time (minimum 24 hours) and will need to be repeated regularly. This will also involve questioning.

Your sources of information will include:

- Mrs Rosen
- Members of the nursing and multidisciplinary team
- Staff at the residential care home
- Mrs Rosen's community nurse.

Continence

You will need to establish why a urinary catheter is in situ and how long Mrs Rosen has had a catheter. You will also need to establish whether the catheter is leaking and try to ascertain the cause. In addition, it will be necessary to find out whether there is infection present and whether the catheter is causing Mrs Rosen any discomfort. In order to promote continence and prevent constipation, you will need to establish Mrs Rosen's normal bowel habit. This assessment, like the others, will be ongoing and will rely on your skills of observation, questioning, listening, measuring and recording.

Your main sources of information here are Mrs Rosen's:

Chapter 5 deals with urinary assessment.

- Verbal responses
- Physical signs and symptoms: cloudy and/or offensive urine, which on urinalysis may show proteinuria or haematuria; pain, discomfort or retention of urine.

Additional information can be gained by liaising with the staff at the residential care home, thus building up a complete picture of Mrs Rosen in her normal environment.

Nutritional status

CONNECTIONS

Chapter 4 looks at some factors to consider when assessing nutritional status.

It will be useful to establish how much sugary food Mrs Rosen consumes and how often. Try to find out how much she understands about diet and diabetes. You could ask Mrs Rosen if she can remember what she has eaten over the past 24 hours and what her favourite foods are. You will also need to establish whether Mrs Rosen is underweight, overweight or obese. It is also vital to know whether there is a degree of protein energy malnutrition. You will use the skills of questioning, listening, observation, measuring and recording.

Sources of information will include:

- Mrs Rosen
- Her family

- Carers in the community
- The results of medical investigations such as blood tests.

Concurrent disease

In order to enhance your information relating to Mrs Rosen's diabetes, it will be necessary to establish a pattern of blood glucose level over a period of time, starting with a baseline level on admission. You will also need to know whether Mrs Rosen is excreting glucose in her urine. It is important to establish whether she is taking any medication to control her diabetes and whether this has been taken regularly, as prescribed.

Cardiovascular status

The extent of any arterial disease present and Mrs Rosen's understanding of her condition and prognosis should be clarified. You will need to establish the possibility of negotiating a reduction in the number of cigarettes she smokes. Is she willing to give them up for a trial period? How does she feel about this? Your ability to question, listen and observe will be vital in gaining accurate information from:

> **CONNECTIONS**
> *Chapter 6 explains cardiovascular assessment.*

- Mrs Rosen
- Medical colleagues
- Medical notes
- Carers in the community.

Pain

You will need to establish whether Mrs Rosen is experiencing pain and, if so, its nature, intensity, location, duration and precipitating factors (for example movement or wound dressing changes). You will also need to ascertain Mrs Rosen's feelings about pain control and prevention.

> **CONNECTIONS**
> *Chapter 1 illustrates pain assessment.*

Skin

Assess the quality of the skin in terms of hydration, thickness, elasticity and integrity. Establish exactly how and where the integrity of the skin has been breached, assessing each wound individually and recording:

- *Wound site:* anatomical location
- *Wound dimensions:* diameter or length/width and depth
- *Pressure sore grading:* a numerical value given to pressure sores relating to their severity (Reid, 1994)
- *Wound bed status:* the percentage of wound bed occupied by necrotic tissue (eschar), slough, granulation tissue and epithelial tissue. You may also aim

necrotic
dead, devitalised

eschar
dead tissue, characterised by its dry, crusty, black appearance, which adheres to the wound bed

slough
shed dead tissue resulting from injury or inflammation

to establish which stage of wound healing is apparent (although this is not always possible)

- *Exudate:* is the level high, medium or low? Is it increasing or decreasing? Is the exudate purulent or bloodstained?
- *Infection:* are there any signs or symptoms to indicate a wound infection?
- *Surrounding skin:* is it intact? Well perfused? **Macerated?** Inflamed? Eczematous?
- *Expected mode of healing.*

maceration

the softening and detexturising of tissues due to prolonged exposure to moistness

Risk assessment

Use a risk assessment tool to provide a framework for professional judgement when assessing Mrs Rosen's level of risk of pressure injury. The initial risk assessment must be completed as soon as possible after admission so that preventative measures can be taken. Some areas have particular quality standards relating to the prevention and management of pressure injury, and these will often specify the timeframe within which risk assessment should take place.

Assessment in wound management can be summarised thus:

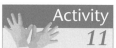

Activity 11

Try to locate the quality standard(s) for the prevention and management of pressure injuries in your workplace. How many of these assessment criteria are reflected within them?

Discuss your findings with your colleagues.

- Assessment is an ongoing process
- The nursing diagnosis is arrived at via an assessment
- The role of the nurse is to gather sufficient information to facilitate the identification of actual and potential problems, to formulate a nursing diagnosis and to provide the knowledge base for planning care interventions
- The client is recognised as the primary source of information and is involved in information-sharing
- Secondary sources of information include relatives, carers, friends, other members of the multidisciplinary team, documentation and electronically stored data
- The primary aim is to assess the client and his or her environment (local and general) in terms of conduciveness to wound healing
- The secondary aim is to establish and record wound status, including any factors that may complicate or impair the healing process
- A risk assessment should form part of the process.

Planning nursing care in wound management

Having made a thorough assessment using the previously described criteria and having developed a series of nursing diagnoses for Mrs Rosen, you will now be ready to enter the planning stage of the nursing process.

The two stages of planning have been described in Chapter 1; within the field

Chart 10.2 ● Wound status

Wound 1

- Cavity wound, located over left ischial tuberosity
- Diameter 6 cm, depth 6 cm
- Pressure sore grading of 4.0 (Reid and Morison, 1994; *UK consensus of pressure sore severity*) – full-thickness skin loss with extensive destruction and tissue necrosis, extending to underlying bone, tendon or joint capsule
- Wound bed composed of 70 per cent slough, 30 per cent eschar
- Moderate exudate level
- No signs of clinical infection
- Surrounding skin excoriated and poorly perfused
- Expected mode of healing – secondary intention

of wound management, it is important to ensure that, whenever possible, you involve the client in:

- Identifying the broad aim(s) of nursing care in the wound management plan
- Setting specific objectives
- Devising the appropriate intervention
- Identifying other members of the multidisciplinary team who can provide input for care-planning.

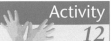

Activity 12

Review your assessment and nursing diagnoses for Mrs Rosen.

Select one of the actual problems identified and discuss how care may be planned, explaining how each nursing intervention will affect wound healing and identifying which other members of the multidisciplinary team may be involved.

You will now be starting to understand the complexity of nursing care in wound management. The interventions that relate directly to the wound itself form only part of a range of activities that are vital to supporting wound management. It is, however, useful to describe and analyse a specific plan of nursing care for the direct management of one of Mrs Rosen's pressure injuries.

Chart 10.2 describes Mrs Rosen's wound status on admission to hospital. It is now possible to design a nursing care plan for the management of this wound, based upon an assessment of the information, and informed by a sound knowledge base of the principles of wound management. Following the previously outlined stages, the care plan will develop as follows.

Identifying the broad aim will be carried out in conjunction with Mrs Rosen, asking her what she hopes will be the outcome of her stay in hospital and carefully establishing how realistic these hopes may be. It will also be necessary to find out the extent to which Mrs Rosen is willing to participate in her care and how keen or reluctant she may be to contribute to certain interventions. In this case, the broad aim may be identified as:

> To create a local environment that will be conducive to and promote wound healing. The expected outcome is that the necrotic tissue will be removed and the formation of granulation tissue will commence.

Specific objectives to be set should be negotiated with Mrs Rosen. They will include:

- Relieving pressure on the wound site
- Cleansing the wound to encourage the **autolysis** of necrotic tissue and its removal from the wound bed
- Controlling exudate to avoid leakage
- Keeping dressing changes to a minimum, changing them only when strike-through or soiling occurs
- Protecting the surrounding skin to prevent further breakdown.

Next, *appropriate interventions* should be devised. Having already established that each objective is a statement of intention, or a 'what we want to do', the next step involves designing nursing interventions, the 'how we are going to do it'. This can be done by reviewing each objective and:

- Describing the action to be taken
- Identifying the personnel who will be involved
- Identifying the equipment and resources that might be required.

Here is an example:

- Relieving pressure on the wound site (specific objective or 'what we want to do')
- Nursing intervention ('how we are going to do it')
  Action to be taken:
    Install a pressure-reduction airwave mattress and wheelchair cushion
    Encourage Mrs Rosen to move from side to side while in bed
    Mrs Rosen to agree to participate and use the prescribed equipment
  Personnel involved:
    Named nurse
    Mrs Rosen
    Equipment officer
    Physiotherapist

---

autolysis

the natural breakdown of dead, or foreign, organic material

CONNECTIONS

Chapter 8 deals with pressure sore prevention in more detail.

Activity

13

Work through this activity with the support of your clinical assessor/supervisor.

Select any one of Mrs Rosen's other specific objectives and, following the framework illustrated in the example in the text, design a nursing intervention to enable you to meet that objective.

Equipment/resources required:
    Airwave mattress and cushion
    Trapeze pole.

Implementing care

The implementation stage of any wound management plan is critical in that:

- You put your planned care into effect
- You delegate elements of planned care appropriately
- You actively involve the client and other members of the multidisciplinary team
- You record which elements of the care plan have been carried out, when and by whom
- You begin to evaluate *as you implement care*, noting the length of time taken to complete an intervention, the ease with which it was undertaken, the degree to which the client was able (or willing) to participate, any associated teaching, helping or educational activities and any changes that occurred while you were implementing care.

If we examine the implementation of two specific objectives in Mrs Rosen's care plan – cleansing the wound and controlling exudate – we can take a step-by-step approach to analysing how this intervention may be implemented:

1. On admission, the dressing in place is found to be unsuitable, that is, it does not conform to any of the criteria for an ideal dressing. It is now necessary to *implement* the planned nursing intervention.

2. The nurse selects the appropriate dressing, documenting the selection and giving a rationale, for example:

   Hydrogel selected to instil into wound bed to rehydrate the wound and promote the removal of necrotic tissue by autolysis. Adhesive foam dressing selected to cover the hydrogel in the wound bed and absorb excess exudate.

3. The use of the dressing is explained to Mrs Rosen, who has an opportunity to examine the dressing and ask any questions.

4. Mrs Rosen is prepared and made ready for the dressing to be applied. She is encouraged to participate in this in anticipation of future dressing changes. She is also encouraged to make any comments throughout the dressing

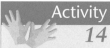

Activity

14

With your clinical assessor or supervisor, and following the local guidelines for aseptic technique, select a hydrogel and a polyurethane foam dressing from the treatment room of your clinical area.

Using the principles outlined in Chart 10.3, prepare everything you would need to implement the wound dressing element of Mrs Rosen's care plan.

Chart 10.3 ● The principles of aseptic technique

Aseptic technique is a method of carrying out procedures in an environment that is rendered as free from micro-organisms and contaminants as possible. Bree-Williams and Waterman (1996) suggest that this may be achieved by:

● Effective hand decontamination – cleansing (using soap and water, followed by thorough drying) and disinfecting (using a chemical disinfectant or antiseptic solution, followed by drying)
● Creating a sterile field – using a sterilised surface
● The exclusive use of sterilised equipment
● Ensuring that the outer wrappings of any sterilised equipment do not come into contact with either the sterile contents or the sterile field
● Using a 'no-touch' (forceps) or sterile-gloved handling technique
● Being aware of sources of contamination (used dressings, bodily contact – especially clothes, skin and hair – contact with non-sterile surfaces, contact with body fluids and aerosol contamination)
● Avoiding the introduction of contaminants into the sterile field
● The safe disposal of contaminants, away from the sterile field
● Achieving competency in aseptic technique, in accordance with evidence-based policy guidelines

change (for example to describe any pain or discomfort and to suggest ways in which she may assist).

5. The nurse prepares for the dressing change following the aseptic technique (Chart 10.3).

6. The nurse decides that the wound needs to be cleansed to remove any loose debris and particulate matter in the wound bed. An appropriate cleanser is selected and used to irrigate the wound bed (Pudner, 1997).

7. The dressing is applied according to the manufacturer's instructions.

8. The area is cleared. Mrs Rosen is made comfortable and given an opportunity to comment or ask any questions.

9. The episode is documented as soon as possible.

Evaluation of care in wound management

CONNECTIONS

Chapter 1 identifies ways of evaluating nursing care.

You have already discovered that evaluation is concerned with the effectiveness of nursing interventions. At this stage, it is necessary to pose the series of questions described in Chapter 1.

By focusing and reflecting upon what is happening, both during and after the implementation of a nursing intervention, and then recording your findings, the nursing documentation not only serves as a record of events, but also becomes a dynamic, working tool. The description of interactions between client and nurse will provide additional information. This may lead to:

- Further assessment
- Revisions to the care planned.

The key to success in making a care plan a 'working' document is your ability to evaluate the effectiveness of the nursing interventions you have designed. In the management of wounds, you will need to:

- Review the factors affecting wound healing and evaluate the prescribed nursing interventions
- Review the wound status and evaluate the prescribed nursing interventions.

■ Chapter Summary

The effective nursing management of wounds is a complex area of activity involving integrated and systematic assessment, the identification of problems, the generation of nursing diagnoses and the planning, implementation and evaluation of nursing interventions. This chapter has given you an overview of the elements underpinning the principles of the nursing management of wounds, highlighting the importance of ongoing, evidence-based education to inform decision-making in practice, the value of reflection as a way of evaluating your experiences, the varied nature and assortment of tools, frameworks and guidelines available to assist in making a professional judgement and the central role of the nurse in managing care.

Activity 15

Consider the wound dressing element of Mrs Rosen's wound management plan. List any possible information you might acquire from Mrs Rosen and your observations.

Describe how you might revise the care plan as a result of your findings. Discuss this with your clinical assessor or supervisor.

Activity 16

Undertake an Internet search using the search field 'wound management'. Make a note of the search engine used (how efficient was it?) and the search field (how productive was it?; did you need to widen or reduce it?).

Post your findings on the student notice board and invite comments.

● **Test Yourself!**

1. What are the different accountability relationships within which professional practitioners are required to discharge their duty of care to the client?

2. What do you understand by the term 'wound'?

3. How may wounds be classified?

4. What different types of risk assessment may be undertaken?

5. The skin is the primary organ of the integumentary system. What are its components?

6. What are the four main phases of wound healing?

7. The factors affecting wound healing have been described in terms of the *person* and the *context* in which they exist. How many of these factors can you list?

8. What are the elements required to provide the optimum environment for wound healing?

9. What are the assessment criteria for wound management?

10. What is the purpose of a nursing care plan in wound management?

11. What do you understand by the term 'aseptic technique'?

12. What do you need to consider when you are evaluating nursing care in wound management?

Addresses of Professional Associations

European Tissue Repair Society
Wound Healing Institute
Department of Dermatology
Churchill Hospital
Old Road
Headington
Oxford OX3 7LJ
Tel: 01865 228264

European Wound Management Association
PO Box 864
London SE1 8TT
Tel: 020 7872 3496
email: ewma@kcl.ac.uk

Tissue Viability Society
Glanville Centre
Salisbury District Hospital
Salisbury
Wiltshire SP2 8BJ
Tel: 01722 336262
email: tvs@dial.pipex.com
Website: www.tvs.org.uk

Wound Care Society
PO Box 263
Northampton NN3 4UJ
Tel: 01604 784696

Further Reading	DoH (Department of Health) (1998) *A First Class Service. Quality in the NHS.* Stationery Office, London.

References

Allison, J. (1995) The effect of continuing education on practical wound management. *Journal of Wound Care* **4**(1): 29–31.

Bale, S. and Jones, V. (1997) *Wound Care Nursing: A Patient Centred Approach.* Baillière Tindall, London.

Bree-Williams, F.J. and Waterman, H. (1996) An examination of nurses' practice when performing aseptic technique for wound dressings. *Journal of Advanced Nursing* **23**: 48–54.

Carpenter, D. (1993) Key working and primary nursing: accountability and professional practice. In Giddey, M. and Wright, H. (eds) *Mental Health Nursing. From First Principles to Professional Practice.* Chapman & Hall, London.

Cullum, N. and Dealey, C. (1996) Presentation given to the all party group on skin at the House of Commons. *Journal of Tissue Viability* **6**(1): 20–3.

Davis, M.B., Austin, J. and Partridge, D.A. (1991) *Vitamin C. Its Chemistry and Biochemistry.* Royal Society of Chemists, Cambridge.

DoH (Department of Health) (1991) *The Patient's Charter.* HMSO, London.

DoH (Department of Health) (1997) *The New NHS: Modern, Dependable.* Stationery Office, London.

DoH (Department of Health) (2000) *The NHS Plan.* Stationery Office, London.

Edwards, M. (1995) Healing practices. *Nursing Times* **91**(11): 62–4.

Hallett, A. (1995) *Guidelines for Practice: Prevention and Management of Pressure Sores.* Portsmouth Health Care NHS Trust, Portsmouth.

Leaper, D. (1996) Antiseptics in wound healing. *Nursing Times* **92**(39): 63–8.

Lewis, B.K. and Harding, K.G. (1993) Nutritional intake and wound healing in elderly people. *Journal of Wound Care* **2**(4): 227–9.

Marks-Maran, D. (1993) Accountability. In Tschudin, V. (ed.) *Ethics, Nurses and Patients.* Scutari Press, London.

Morgan, D.A. (1994) *The Formulary of Wound Management Products.* Euromed Communications, Haslemere.

Morison, M. (1991) *A Colour Guide to the Nursing Management of Wounds.* Wolfe, London.

Nelson, E.A. (1997) Consensus statements. *Journal of Woundcare* **6**(3): 107.

NMC (Nursing and Midwifery Council) (2002) *Code of Professional Conduct.* NMC, London.

Norton, D., McLaren, R. and Exton-Smith, A.N. (1975) *An Investigation of Geriatric Nursing Problems in Hospital.* Churchill Livingstone, Edinburgh.

Plummer, E.S. and Albert, S.G. (1995) Footcare assessment in patients with diabetes: a screening algorithm for patient education and referral. *Diabetes Educator* **21**(1): 47–51.

Pudner, R. (1997) Wound cleansing. *Journal of Community Nursing* **11**(7): 30–6.

Reid, J. (1994) Towards a consensus: classification of pressure sores. *Journal of Wound Care* **3**(3): 157–60.

Reid, J. and Morison, M.A. (1994) Towards a consensus: classification of pressure sores. *Journal of Woundcare* **13**(3): 157–60.

UKCC (United Kingdom Central Council for Nursing, Midwifery and Health Visiting) (1989) *Exercising Accountability.* UKCC, London.

UKCC (United Kingdom Central Council for Nursing, Midwifery and Health Visiting) (1994) *The Future of Professional Practice – the Council's Standards for Education and Practice Following Registration.* UKCC, London.

Van Der Kerkhof, P.C.M., Van Bergen, B. and Spruijt, K. (1994) Age related changes in wound healing. *Clinical and Experimental Dermatology* **19**: 369–74.

Waterlow, J. (1988) Calculating the risk. *Nursing Times* **38**(9): 58–60.

Wells, L. (1994) At the front-line of care. *Professional Nurse* **9**(8): 525–30.

Chapter

Social Behaviour and Professional Interactions

11

Contents

Learning outcomes

This chapter, concerned with one-to-one and group interactions, is divided into three sections. After reading through it, you should be able to:

- Describe the core qualities of therapeutic communication

- Identify six therapeutic interventions and suggest ways in which these might be implemented in your practice

- Describe the difference between primary and secondary groups

- Describe the interdependence of team, task and individual needs

- Discuss the importance of assertiveness to nursing practice

- Describe the process for refusing requests and handling criticism

- Reflect on further areas of study to enhance your own therapeutic communication skills.

The first section of this chapter examines therapeutic communication, or the therapeutic use of self. It will start by exploring the meaning of these terms before asking what qualities are required to enhance communication beyond just conveying information. The last part of this section will examine in more detail some of the tools available to start the process of developing good therapeutic skills that can be used with patients, families and colleagues.

Nurses seldom work in isolation but are more usually part of a team. Groups tend to have their own dynamics, and an understanding of how groups function can help in developing happier and more efficient teamwork. Nurses may work with a variety of diverse groups, for example support groups for patients, therapy groups, commonly found in mental health settings, and families, which form a special kind of group. The second section will examine some of the issues important to group dynamics. What constitutes a group? What sort of group are you likely to encounter? What is the role of nurses as group members? What makes effective teams and good leaders?

The third part of this chapter will examine a more specific aspect of interaction, building on some of the issues raised in the first section. Nurses are at the forefront of care and have an important role in liaising with an extremely wide range of people. In doing so, they sometimes have to deal with difficult situations. This section will examine how, through developing assertiveness, nurses can develop greater self-confidence and work more effectively towards positive working relationships and patient outcomes.

therapeutic

aiding an individual's well-being

Throughout this chapter, the term 'nurse' will be used for the person who is the provider of the **therapeutic** communication. The nurse may be from any branch – mental health, learning difficulties or adult nursing. The terms 'client' and 'patient' are often used interchangeably, some branches using the term 'client' more freely than others. To avoid any confusion, the recipient of the therapeutic exchange will be referred to here as the client.

Finally, this chapter is not intended to be a training manual or a comprehensive guide to social interactions. Instead, it offers some signposts on which to base further study, investigation and development.

■ Therapeutic Communication

therapeutic communication

purposeful communication aimed at enhancing an individual's well-being

The term 'therapeutic communication' has been chosen rather than 'interpersonal skills' or 'counselling'. We all use interpersonal skills all the time whenever we are relating to another person, sometimes constructively, sometimes destructively. To be therapeutic, however, means to aid the well-being of an individual; thus, therapeutic communication has the intention of assisting or helping others.

There is evidence to suggest that the communication exchange between nurses and clients, including relatives, is not always as good as it might be (Ley, 1988; Brereton, 1995). There are many diverse and complex reasons for this. Perhaps the fact that we are all communicating all the time results in a feeling that we do not need to learn how to do something we have been doing all our lives: it seems to be common sense. Perhaps nurses have become complacent about communication. Furthermore, there is a tendency for some nurses to see themselves as people of action rather than words. Many nurses are not comfortable unless they are 'doing', a stance influenced by the ethos of today's clinical environment and the pressures of work. Hewison (1995) found support for the fact that many nurse–client interactions continue to be task orientated, routinised and often superficial.

Nevertheless, nurses do express a desire to communicate well with clients; Buckroyd (1987) found that paediatric nurses wanted to be able to help children in distress but often felt ill equipped to deal with these emotional and difficult interactions. Skilled therapeutic interventions can, as Nichols (1989) points out, minimise the psychological morbidity associated with ill-health, and nurses are ideally placed to provide this kind of care to clients. Therapeutic communication is an essential and central aspect of nursing whichever branch nurses specialise in, and it should not be seen as just the domain of those in mental health settings. Is, then, therapeutic communication the same thing as counselling?

It is difficult to avoid the term 'counselling' when discussing therapeutic communication, but it has unfortunately become something of a misused term. Indeed, the *Oxford Dictionary* defines counselling as 'to advise, to give advice to people professionally on social problems'. We will look more closely at the notion of advice-giving later in the chapter, but some people, such as financial counsellors and legal counsellors, do just that: they give advice. Other counsellors would never give advice. Some people call themselves counsellors following a very brief training, whereas others undertake years of preparation. According to the British Association for Counselling (1996):

> The overall aim of counselling is to provide an opportunity for the client to work towards living in a more resourceful way... Counselling may be concerned with developmental issues, addressing and resolving specific problems, making decisions, coping with crisis, developing personal insights and knowledge, working through feelings of inner conflict or improving relationships with others. The counsellor's role is to facilitate the client's work in ways which respect the client's values, personal resources and capacity for self determination.

There are, within this statement, some important elements that have signifi-

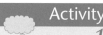

Activity 1

Identify, from the British Association for Counselling quote, the elements that you feel are important to your chosen branch of nursing. Think of how you might apply these to three or four clients you have had contact with.

cant implications for nursing practice. Nurses will therefore aim to apply these elements in the care of their clients, regardless of their chosen branch, so it may appear from this that nurses are engaged in counselling. However, the British Association for Counselling (1996) also states that 'Only when both the user and the recipient agree to enter into a counselling relationship does it become "counselling" rather than the use of "counselling skills".' As Burnard (1995a) cautions, counselling and the use of counselling skills are not the same thing. Although they may share many common features, they are different and require a different sort of relationship. Most nurses are engaged in the use of counselling skills rather than in counselling, and to avoid confusion the term 'therapeutic communication' will be used. It is important to stress, however, that although nurses may not by definition be counselling, the outcomes they achieve may be the same, and the value of their contribution should certainly not be underestimated.

The next section will focus primarily on the core qualities that underpin therapeutic communication and some of the skills that can assist in the process and practice of therapeutic communication.

■ Core Qualities

Three particular qualities have been identified as playing an important part in any therapeutic alliance:

1. Empathic understanding
2. Genuineness, or **congruence**
3. Unconditional acceptance.

congruence

a matching of inner feelings and outer behaviour

The requirement for these attributes was first identified in the context of counselling by Carl Rogers, the father of person-centred therapy. Rogers identified these three qualities as being necessary and sufficient to enable constructive personality change (Rogers, 1957). In other words, no other forms of therapeutic intervention are needed. This approach has had a considerable influence on nursing because of the control it gives back to clients, empowering them to make their own decisions and enabling their psychological growth. Nurses are however, rarely in a position to use these interventions exclusively – to do so risks ignoring many other helpful strategies (Burnard, 1995b) – but the three core qualities are considered to be important components in the therapeutic relationship and lay the foundation on which other skills and strategies can be built. They are thus worthy of further explanation.

Empathic understanding

Empathic understanding is essentially a sensitivity for *what* another person is feeling but not for *how* he or she is feeling. You can never feel exactly the same as other people as their construction of the world will always differ from yours in some way. You can, however, be sensitive to what they are feeling and convey this to them in a way that helps them to feel someone has a valid insight into their world: they feel understood. Rogers (1980) describes empathy as 'a way of being with another person, entering into their world, communicating their sensings'. Nevertheless, it remains a difficult concept to understand and to practise as it is more than just a communication process.

Egan (1994) defines two types of empathy: 'primary empathy' and 'advanced empathy'. The former is much more straightforward, although not necessarily simple. It involves listening carefully to what clients are saying and responding in a way that indicates an understanding of what they are saying from their perspective. The latter is a deeper kind of empathy more akin to reading between the lines, picking up not only what the client says, but also what lies behind it. As Rogers (1980) suggests, it is 'sensing meanings of which the client is scarcely aware'. This might usefully be compared with being a musician. Some musicians can read the score and play the notes in the correct sequence, but the highly skilled musician sees behind and beyond the notes, understanding the full expression of the music as intended by the composer. Developing these sensitivities appears to come more easily to some than others, but empathic understanding can be enriched with careful reflection on how you respond to clients. What is not required is some sort of phoney understanding. It is important to be genuine.

empathic understanding

a capacity to sense accurately the feelings and personal meanings of another person

Activity 2

Think of someone you know well, and, in your mind, try to become that person. As that person, write a character sketch of yourself. In other words, try to see yourself through someone else's eyes.

Genuineness

Genuineness is about being open and honest, and is sometimes referred to as congruence or authenticity. This is not to suggest that carers are being dishonest, but it is possible to be deceived about your feelings towards others. The professional mask often worn by nurses can distort the way of being with a client. Genuineness is less to do with telling untruths and more to do with having an openness, an attitude that conveys congruence between what you are thinking and feeling, and what you are saying. It is not hiding behind a uniform or a professional role: the very process of professionalisation can result in taking on a role that hides the self. Unfortunately, such a lack of genuineness often shines through to clients like a bright light, causing them to withdraw into themselves. Egan (1994) offers some guidance on developing an attitude of genuineness:

genuineness

the ability to show oneself without putting on a façade

CONNECTIONS

Chapter 12 looks at the development of self concept and self-awareness.

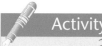

Activity
3

Draw a life line similar to the one in Figure 11.1 and identify the positive and negative influences in your life. Think about how these events have helped to mould and create you, and how they might influence your relationship with your clients.

● *Not overemphasising the helping role:* and thus avoiding being patronising and condescending
● *Being spontaneous:* this is not the same as overtly expressing all your current feelings, but it does mean not being afraid to express them when appropriate
● *Not being defensive:* as a nurse, you will not always find that you are able to help, but getting to know your own strengths and weaknesses will enable you to be less defensive
● *Being open:* when appropriate, do not be afraid to use your own life experience (see Nelson-Jones, 1997, for guidance on appropriate self-disclosure).

Much of being genuine is about having a better understanding of ourselves. Activity 3 and Figure 11.1 will give you some insight into your own experiences. If, for example, you have experienced a loss, this might help you to understand a client better, but it might also make you less tolerant of an angry client who reminds you of your own undealt-with anger.

Unconditional acceptance

unconditional
acceptance
_____
an attitude that values
the worth of another
person

Unconditional acceptance or unconditional positive regard is a frequently misunderstood quality. It can appear as if you must like everyone, regardless of what they have or have not done or who they are. Indeed, if you accept the statements above about genuineness, pretending that you like everyone means that you are not being genuine. Unconditional acceptance, however, is about accepting clients as fellow humans entitled to care and respect, which is not the same as liking them as you do your friends or accepting their behaviour and value systems, which may be at odds with your own. As Mearns (1994) comments, 'Don't confuse unconditional positive regard with liking'. You may not like certain individuals, or their behaviour, but it is not for you to judge them, especially from your position as a carer. Developing the skill of acceptance

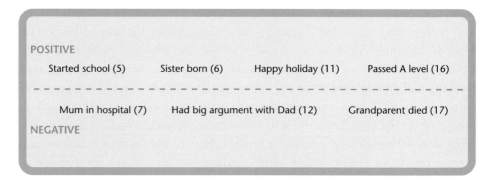

Figure 11.1 ● Example of a life line (with age in brackets)

depends very much on your ability to accept yourself. Fromm (1975) notes that to love others, we must first love ourselves.

None of the above qualities is easy to develop or to execute, although some nurses will find this easier than others. What is of concern is the way in which individuals often assume that they possess these qualities just because they have read about them, as if they develop through some osmotic process. These are qualities that take time to develop and must be practised. In reality, they are never fully available to us, so we can only aspire to them. One way to start the process of developing them is to begin reflecting on our interactions with clients and colleagues.

Therapeutic Skills

Heron (2001) has devised a simple but comprehensive model for therapeutic communication that is referred to as six-category intervention analysis. Within the six primary categories lie a wide range of more specific interventions; although the categories are considered to be exhaustive, the interventions are not and have the capacity for great flexibility. Heron (2001) emphasises that the categories are not a model of counselling but instead a set of analytical and behavioural tools. Many of the interventions are not uniquely identified by Heron, but he provides an effective framework within which all six interventions, including those related to giving information and advice, can be used in one-to-one interactions. Figure 11.2 illustrates the six categories.

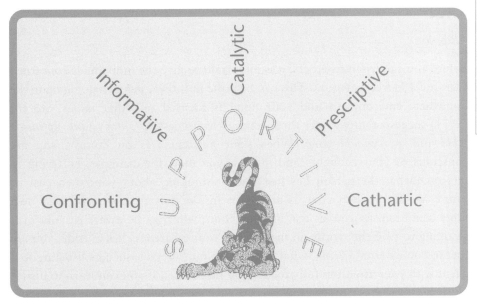

Figure 11.2 ● Six-category intervention analysis (after Heron, 2001)

CONNECTIONS

Chapter 13 provides some guidelines on how to reflect on your practice.

Activity

4

Make a list of clients who might be very difficult to accept because their value system, beliefs or behaviours are very different from your own, for example a drug addict.

Think of a client or someone you know whom you do not really like. Write down five positive qualities about that person.

Discuss with a colleague how you might better manage working with a client you do not like or whose values and behaviour are opposite to your own.

The first three categories – confronting, informative and prescriptive – are authoritative in that the nurse is taking greater responsibility for guiding the client's responses. The facilitative interventions are catalytic, cathartic and supportive; with facilitative interventions, the authority remains primarily with the client.

No single intervention is more important than any other, and none of the interventions seeks to control or take autonomy away from the client. The emphasis is instead on developing an enabling relationship in which clients can explore their own worlds and make appropriate decisions for themselves.

Catalytic category

catalytic interventions

a set of basic interventions that assist the client with self-discovery and learning

Although there is no hierarchy to the six categories, the catalytic category will be outlined first because it probably contains the most frequently used interventions. Heron describes **catalytic interventions** in terms of learning and problem-solving. These interventions enable clients to explore their thoughts and feelings, thus gaining insight and enabling them to be in a better position to make decisions about their future. The skill lies in effective listening and responding in ways that help clients to move on, but at their own pace and with their own agenda. This category requires the nurse to identify which intervention from the toolkit is most appropriate for assisting clients in this exploration. The following interventions will be outlined here: listening; simple and selective reflection; paraphrasing; open and closed questions; logical and empathic building; and checking for understanding.

Listening

Before you can listen to others, it is important to give the individuals concerned your full and free attention. This can be difficult if there is much going on in the immediate environment and your mind is focused on other issues. Stevens (1971) suggests that we have three zones of awareness; a *fantasy zone*, an *inside zone* and an *outside zone*. When your awareness is on fantasy, you are conscious of your thoughts and images; you may, for example, be trying to interpret what the person has just said or thinking about your own past or future agendas. When your awareness is inside, you are aware of your own inner sensation: as you sit reading this book, you may be aware of your eyes straining to read the words on the page. If your awareness lies outside, you are focused on external events, what is going on outside you, such as listening to a client with your attention fully focused on him or her. If you can learn to distinguish between these zones of awareness, it is possible to use them much more effectively, thus keeping your focus out and with the client, fleetingly changing the focus to fantasy to check out your own thoughts and occasionally being aware of your own internal sensations.

One way in which you can demonstrate your attention and interest in clients is by giving them quality time. Even if this is only a couple of minutes, it can be devoted to the client as quality time rather than being a rushed and haphazard event with you distracted by your surroundings and what is going on in your head. This, of course, takes practice, but giving quality time to others is one of the most important skills you can offer. In addition, your body language should convey the message that you are listening with interest to the client. Maintaining good eye contact, a relaxed open posture and a friendly and interested facial expression invites the client to talk to you. The occasional appropriate nod of the head indicates that you are listening and interested. Once you are giving clients your full attention, it is necessary to demonstrate that you are trying to understand their world from their frame of reference. In other words, you are being empathic rather than imposing your world, values, beliefs or judgements on the client. Some of the more common interventions you can use to facilitate this process are described below.

Simple and selective reflection

Simple reflection, sometimes known as echoing, is helpful when the client appears stuck. It involves repeating the last word or few words back to the client with the same intensity of expression used by the client. The client may, for example, end the sentence saying, 'and I feel very unhappy'; you respond, 'You feel very unhappy', and the client is encouraged to continue the story, 'Yes, ever since…'. The difficulty in using this intervention is in deciding when it is appropriate and beneficial, as inappropriate use will simply annoy the client.

Selective reflection is similar, involving listening carefully for issues that seem to stand out as being significant and then feeding them back to the client without changing the content: 'You commented a moment ago about how angry you were with your mother.' This gives the client the opportunity to continue to develop this theme. Care must be taken not to direct the client down avenues of your own choosing rather than of the client's choice. It is easy to think that you know what the client's problem is, but in reality you will often be misguided in your assumption. In both simple and selective reflection, you should be listening for the emotionally charged words the client uses.

Paraphrasing

Paraphrasing is one way of conveying to clients that you have listened to them and have tried to grasp an understanding of what they are saying to you. When paraphrasing, you rephrase what the client has said in your own words. An example of this type of intervention might be:

Client: I'm very worried about my daughter. This problem has been going on for so long, I wonder if she will ever be the same again.

Nurse: It seems like there is no end to your daughter's problem and you're worried she will never be the little girl you used to know.

Open and closed questions

dichotomous

divided into two separate groups

These **dichotomous** interventions are relatively simple but take practice to master. Open questions invite an open answer, whereas a closed question invites a closed answer. 'Do you have pain?', as an example of a closed question, invites a yes or no response, whereas 'How are you feeling?' invites a response much more of the client's choosing. Although it is rather simplistic, the 'who', 'what', 'where', 'when' and 'how' questions tend to elicit a more open response. The important word to be remembered here is 'invites': a closed question may instead receive an open response and an open question a closed one.

These questions are more appropriately seen as lying on a continuum of being more or less open; the more open they are, the greater the opportunity for client self-direction. Closed questions are more frequently asked by the compulsive helper who tends to try to maintain control of the interaction. They can, however, be useful in eliciting specific information such as a name or telephone number. 'Why' questions should be used cautiously as they may alienate clients by forcing them to introspect inappropriately. After all, if they knew 'why', they would very often not need help.

Logical and empathic building

Logical building helps to develop a scaffolding for the client by bringing together salient points from the dialogue. Clients are often confused and appear to be rambling as they try to express their feelings; the nurse can assist by periodically marshalling the various points into some coherent order. You might, for example, say, 'It seems as if these are your main concerns, Mr Jones. You are worried about how you will cope if you return to work and about who will take care of the children.'

Empathic building is rather like reading between the lines. As you carefully listen to what the client is saying, you are attempting to understand the feeling behind the words. It is important to use other cues such as tone of voice, eye contact and facial expression to help you to understand what the client might be experiencing. Your empathic understanding is then relayed to the client in the form of a statement: 'It sounds as if you are really hurting about...' or 'You are really frightened because...'.

Checking for understanding

It is very important to check periodically that you are, as fully as possible, understanding what the client is saying. This is especially important if you feel that you are becoming confused or if the client is giving contradictory messages. Clarifying the situation can prevent much misunderstanding and helps you to stay within the client's frame of reference.

Cathartic category

As a baby and during infancy, the tendency is spontaneously to give vent to emotions, be they of joy, grief, anger or fear. As you grow older, the responses become modified through modelling, learning or choice as you decide the best way to master life. You learn perhaps that it is wrong to cry and bad to express anger, that to be fearful might show weakness, or even that it is *not OK* to have fun and enjoy yourself. This may make it difficult to express yourself, particularly at times of crisis. The difficulty with helping others with their emotions is that you may not yet have come to understand your own repressed emotional world. It is one thing to intellectualise and say to the client that it is OK to cry, but if you are sitting there feeling uncomfortable with your own emotions, this may well be conveyed to the client. It is also unhelpful to coerce someone into expressing emotions, such as insisting on a bereaved person crying. Given time, space and permission, clients can choose when and how they want to express their emotions.

Working with emotions can be difficult and often requires specific training, but becoming more responsive to people's emotional needs does not require in-depth training. What it does require, however, is for you to become sensitive to your own emotions and those of your clients. The angry client may awaken memories of an angry parent in your life, or a dying client may provoke memories of an earlier loss. What makes you laugh, cry or get angry? Do you close down your emotions because it is easier that way and you stand less chance of getting hurt? The best way to help clients with their emotions is to be accepting of them and give them permission – permission to be angry parents when they find that their new baby has learning difficulties, permission to be afraid when they find out they have multiple sclerosis or cancer, permission to cry when old hurts are uncovered in a group therapy session, permission to feel relief when someone they love dies as their loved one has been released from suffering and they themselves from the burden of caring.

cathartic interventions

interventions that seek
to enable clients to let
go of painful emotions
including anger, fear,
love and grief, thus
releasing tension that
has built up within them

Touching, eye contact, listening, being with someone and giving permission
are all ways of using **cathartic interventions**, but it is also important to be
conscious of the cultural perspective. Touch may not be acceptable in some
cultures, and eye contact may offend. Do not be afraid to check these things out.
Does your eye contact cause the client to withdraw or become more responsive?
Ask whether clients would like you to hold their hand.

Confronting category

confronting
interventions

interventions that
directly challenge and
heighten the client's
awareness of restrictive
attitudes, beliefs or
behaviours of which he
or she may be unaware

Confronting interventions are involved with informing clients of what they
are unaware of. Because of the nature of confrontation, the intervention may be
received by clients with some degree of shock as they come face to face with
issues that they were either not aware of or not acknowledging. For the nurse,
the process of confrontation can also be uncomfortable. He or she is to some
extent making an informed judgement that the client will benefit from the
confrontation, but the nurse's fear of being wrong or managing the confrontation poorly can lead to anxiety about how to deliver the information. Furthermore, the nurse may become aware of feelings related to previous
confrontations in his or her own life. These anxieties can lead the nurse to avoid
the issue and 'beat around the bush' or alternatively take a very direct and
heavy-handed approach. A more appropriate approach is to take control of
these inner feelings and get the confrontation right in order to convey the
confrontation clearly and supportively.

What sorts of issue might be seen as confrontations? There are many potential examples, such as breaking bad news or raising awareness of attitudes and
behaviours. The examples below give some indication of how confrontations
can be used:

- In a group session, John appears to avoid talking about his feelings:
  *'You have explained what you were thinking John, but what is it you are
  feeling?'*
- Mr Patel does not appear to be taking responsibility for looking after his
  recently fashioned colostomy:
  'I notice you are always asking Nurse Radley to change your colostomy bag'
- Fasia is a young woman with Down's syndrome who is preparing for her first
  job:
  'Fasia, are you aware that whenever someone speaks to you, you look away?'
  (The nurse demonstrates what Fasia may be unaware of)
- You notice that the parents of 3-month-old Stephanie, admitted with a chest
  infection, are irregular visitors:
  'It seems you are unable to visit Stephanie very often.'

Breaking bad news is a further example of a confronting intervention. Maguire and Faulkner (1993) make the point that you cannot soften the impact of bad news as it remains bad news however it is broken, but you can break the news in a way that is supportive and gives the client a chance to absorb what is happening. There is insufficient space here to discuss in detail the problems of breaking bad news, but the following (Buckman, 1993) are useful guidelines:

- Prepare clients for the news, offering them privacy and ensuring that they are sitting down
- Inform them that you have bad news, and then give them the facts in a simple, informative and unambiguous manner
- Allow them time to take in the news, giving them the choice of being alone or having someone remain with them
- Finally, be supportive throughout the interaction and offer follow-up help.

> **CONNECTIONS**
> *Chapter 9 deals with end-of-life issues.*

Informative category

Why do you need to give information? Clients clearly require information so that they can understand their illness or health problem. Without information, they are left groundless and are not in a position to make reasoned decisions about their care. It is important that information is given to help clients to understand and maintain control rather than this just being a duty of the health-care professional. It appears that most people want information about their illness, even if it is bad news (Ley, 1988). It also seems that clients are reluctant to seek out information in health-care settings, often being afraid of wasting nurses' time, being unsure of whom or what to ask, or sometimes not being sure whether they *can* ask for information. It therefore falls to the health-care professional to ensure that quality information is delivered appropriately and in the client's best interest.

Prescriptive and **informative interventions** are often seen as the easiest to master. Most people feel that they are capable of providing information, but it is perhaps this confidence itself that results in a poor delivery of information. Although clients want and need information, it must be delivered at the right level in the right quantity and at the right time. Too many clients fail to understand the information given to them or forget what they have been told, especially if this is bad news (Ley, 1988). You may be able to remember occasions on which a lecture has been overloaded with information or delivered at a depth or in a manner that leaves you confused. The good lecture provides the right information at the right depth and at the right time in the course, perhaps leaving you to find something out for yourself. This last aspect is often important in mental health nursing, where you may wish to encourage clients to find out some information for themselves and take responsibility for doing so.

informative interventions

interventions that seek to impart new knowledge, information and meaning that are relevant to the client's needs

Prescriptive category

Prescriptive interventions, such as suggesting a course of action the client might take, attempt to redirect the client's behaviour. One pitfall of this intervention is that it can be too prescriptive, thus removing control from the client. What health-care professionals believe is in the clients' best interests does not always relate to how clients themselves see the situation. Nevertheless, the nurse is in possession of much knowledge and may feel that a certain action really will be best for the client, therefore suggesting, recommending or proposing some action to the client and leaving the situation open for its acceptance or rejection. On other occasions, the nurse may be even more consultative, suggesting a number of options to clients and discussing these in a way that gives them maximum control and choice. At other times, the nurse may be very directive, for example when stopping a diabetic client accidentally overdosing with an insulin injection.

CONNECTIONS

*Chapter 3 discusses
safety issues.*

Supportive category

Supportive interventions underpin the use of all other interventions. Whatever intervention is being used, it should be used in such a way that supports the individual and is not in any way destructive. Heron (2001) identifies three ways of using interventions. The first is a valid way that is appropriate to the needs of the client. In other words, it is the correct intervention delivered in the right way at the right time and in the correct manner. The second interventional style is degenerative, in which, despite good intention, intervention is used poorly because of a lack of skill, experience, self-awareness or a combination of all three. Finally comes a perverted intervention in which the intervention is used in a deliberately perverse way, to the detriment of the client.

CONNECTIONS

*Chapter 12 looks at
the development of
self-awareness.*

Although the supportive category underpins all other categories, it is also a category in its own right. The interventions it encompasses involve the affirmation of others, being with them and demonstrating in a genuine way a care and concern for them. It may involve appropriate touch or appropriate self-disclosure. You demonstrate support for your clients when you willingly do things for them, when you greet them welcomingly and celebrate their achievements, however small these may appear to be. This should be conveyed in an unpatronising way, and you must resist becoming overly nurturing, which may deny clients their independence. The three core conditions identified above are central to the supportive category.

Activity
5

For each of the six categories discussed above, give two or three examples of how you might constructively use them when interacting with actual clients or colleagues with whom you have worked.

The above interventions provide a useful framework within which therapeutic communication can be developed. What has been presented here is an outline on which you can build. All the interventions can be developed and extended, requiring practitioners to research their use and practise their application if they are to be successfully employed.

■ Working Together – People in Groups

As social animals, people tend to live in groups or be members of a group. There are a whole variety of different groups to which you might belong: you probably belong to a family, have a group of friends, perhaps belong to a club and maybe are a member of an organisation such as the Royal College of Nursing. You will belong to a large group called 'nurses', you may be a committee member, you are part of a work group in your clinical area, and, as a student, you are part of a particular intake. Other groups you may come across may be study groups, rehabilitation groups and therapy groups. Nursing involves working as a team with other nurses and working with other professionals as part of a multidisciplinary team; the more effective the teamwork, the better the client care and the better your satisfaction with your work role.

Belonging to a group has many benefits, such as a feeling of belonging, having a shared identity and the benefits of the support you receive from the group. There is a degree of security from being part of a group in which attitudes and values are similar and in which learning can take place. There is, however, also some cost to belonging to a group. You are expected to conform, and you may feel that you are surrendering some of your own personal identity.

The study of groups has interested psychologists and sociologists for a long time and has generated considerable research. This section will confine itself to some of the core issues of groups as a platform for further study.

> **Activity 6**
>
> Think of all the groups that you belong to, both in and out of work. Choose two or three of these and consider what role you play in the group.
>
> Make a list of all the people that might go to make up a multidisciplinary team in your area of practice.

What is a group?

Most people have a common concept of what a group is, and few of the examples above will be difficult for readers to identify as groups. It should also be evident that groups are very diverse and can vary considerably in their size and function, some being more formal than others. Because of this, definitions are not always helpful, and it is more productive to focus on some of the central characteristics of groups than on definitions. A principal feature of a group is that individuals believe themselves to be members of the group, there being some degree of interdependence and interaction.

Groups can be divided into primary and secondary groups. Secondary groups are usually considered to be larger, and their members have less direct contact. The hospital in which you work is a larger group, and you may never have contact with many of its members. Nursing as a profession is a large secondary group, as is a political party.

Primary groups tend to be closer and more intimate, all the members having face-to-face contact. Such groups might be family groups, friendship groups or small work groups. If you belong to a group, you probably have some expectations of that group, for example the way in which members are likely to behave, some of the attitudes you might expect them to hold and perhaps a code of conduct, be it explicit or implied. Nurses will be expected to have an attitude of caring and of working in a manner that is in the best interests of the client. These expectations are known as norms and are attained through observation, experience and learning. Although there is invariably a degree of flexibility, it is also expected that all members of the group will more or less conform to these norms. Without some conformity, it would be very difficult to operate in a social world. We would be left with a sense of 'anomie', a bewilderment with no frame of reference. Imagine what would happen if, each time you came to work, your group of nursing colleagues behaved radically differently, one day caring, the next not, sometimes wearing a uniform and sometimes casual clothes.

The group you work with in your clinical area is a formal primary group, and this group will have established a set of informal norms and expectations related to the group's behaviour. The degree to which members of the group uphold these norms is an indication of the cohesiveness of the group. Other, more formal, norms may be imposed by the hierarchy, and these would also be expected to be adhered to. Needless to say, these two sets of norms may on occasions clash, causing some discontent.

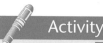

Activity 7

Make a list of the norms for your clinical area. A simple example may be whether or not you wear a uniform. What might the consequences be if the group ignored these norms?

Leadership of groups

Various research studies have identified different styles of leadership and their effectiveness (Lewin et al., 1939; Sayles, 1966; Fielder, 1971). These styles reflect the divide between being autocratic, when one person makes the decisions; democratic, when a consensus of opinion is sought; person centred, in which the leader places greatest emphasis on people; and task centred, in which the focus is on completing the task. These dimensions are probably best viewed as a continuum rather than as definitive styles of leadership. Good leaders, although they may have a predominant style, will adjust their leadership according to the situation (Bass, 1990). It is, for example, often important to be autocratic in a cardiac arrest situation, everyone needing to know exactly who is in charge and what needs to be done. On other occasions, such as when deciding on a new policy, a more democratic, person-centred style may be more productive, allowing for open discussion and the sharing of ideas.

Leaders may be emergent, elected or appointed. Emergent leaders are common in crisis situations or when no leader has previously been identified; elected leaders are common in political situations or on committees. In the case

CONNECTIONS

Chapter 6 provides guidelines on the management of a cardiac arrest.

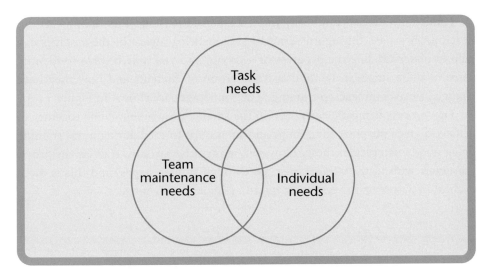

Figure 11.3 ● Three circles model (after Adair, 1988)

of a clinical area, there is usually an appointed leader, someone given the position because of their skills and qualifications. Although you may currently be a student, you will in due course become a staff nurse and will be expected to have some responsibility as an appointed leader.

Adair (1988) identifies three broad areas of need to be considered by the leader in order to maintain good teamwork. These are the 'team', the 'task' and the 'individual', each being equally important and interrelated, as shown in Figure 11.3.

Maintaining the team

A team is made up of individuals and as such takes on its own personality distinct from that of its individual members. One of the responsibilities of the leader is to form a cohesive group that will together go forward to meet the agreed objective without diminishing the individuality of its members. One of the difficulties often expressed by new staff nurses is how to effect an appropriate distance from the group, one that is neither overfamiliar nor too distant. Adair (1988) suggests that distance should be emphasised if the nurse was known to the staff before adopting the new position, if the nurse feels that staff are becoming overfamiliar and taking advantage of the situation, or when the leader is responsible for implementing unpopular decisions. Distance should be minimised when trying to establish and build trust, and if all members are roughly equal in knowledge and experience. The assertiveness skills referred to in the next section of this chapter should help in this respect.

Teams take time to establish, and Tuckman (1965) suggests that, as groups develop, they pass through a series of stages. Being aware of these stages can help in understanding the progress of a group, and you may be able to identify some of these stages in relation to your group of students and how they have changed since commencing training. The four stages are shown in Figure 11.4.

This process is most clearly seen in the smaller groups that come together to achieve a given purpose, the groups and subgroups formed during nurse training being good examples of these. However, many other groups, such as the group you work with in the clinical area, go through similar stages, and this is often cyclical in nature as the environment and personalities change.

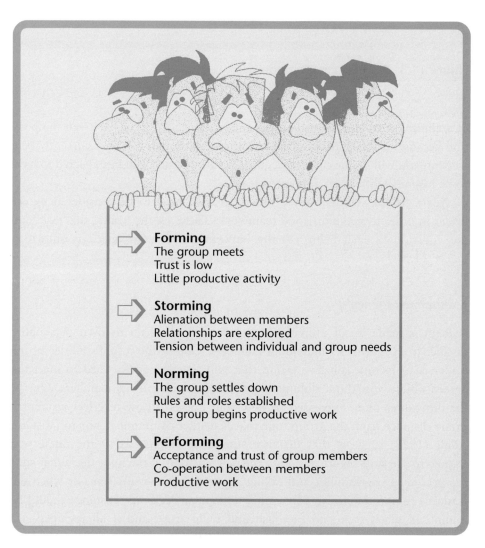

Forming
The group meets
Trust is low
Little productive activity

Storming
Alienation between members
Relationships are explored
Tension between individual and group needs

Norming
The group settles down
Rules and roles established
The group begins productive work

Performing
Acceptance and trust of group members
Co-operation between members
Productive work

Figure 11.4 ● Group processes (after Tuckman, 1965)

Maintaining the task

The task is the objective to be achieved by the group. Such objectives may be very varied, from the day-to-day care of individuals to establishing new **protocols** for working practices. The success of such endeavours may depend heavily on the team working together and will require clearly defined objectives. Imagine working with a team and trying to achieve some very ill-defined goal. This will be not only inefficient, but also very frustrating for the team members. When all the team members understand what is required of them and what their role is in achieving the aim, morale and enthusiasm for the task will remain high.

protocols

regulations or patterns of working

Activity 8

Think of a particular task you might want to achieve as a team, such as implementing a new ward procedure. Using Figure 11.3 above, blank out the Task area of the three circles. How will this influence achieving your objective? Now blank out the Team area. How will this influence reaching your goal? Finally, blank out the Individual area of the three circles and carry out the same exercise.

Maintaining the individual

All groups consist of individuals and as such have individual needs and individual skills. The leader must be careful not to undermine these needs but to encompass them; in this way, individuals can be valued and their skills used to maximum effect within the group. Meeting members' needs may be as simple as ensuring regular meal breaks or valuing them as individuals, providing security, trust and a sense of autonomy.

Leaders do not always of course select their own team members, and some members will need more support than others. Harkins (1987) has identified a phenomenon called social loafing in which some members of the group may do as little work as they can get away with. It is a bit like one member of a tug-of-war team appearing to pull but in fact not exerting any effort at all, the task then becoming far harder for the other members. By identifying each person's role, encouraging and monitoring progress, and encouraging group support, social loafing can be minimised.

■ Being in Control rather than Controlling

Assertiveness is sometimes confused with aggressiveness, arrogance and getting one's own way. It is not, however, about controlling others but about being in control of yourself. It is about respecting yourself and others, recognising that you have rights, including the right to be listened to, while remembering that others also have the same rights. It is about good, positive and equitable communication and negotiation so that both people in the interaction feel respected. It is working towards a win–win situation rather than a win–lose or lose–lose scenario. Some people find that being assertive comes quite naturally to them, others feel less confident and sometimes intimidated, whereas others become aggressive.

assertiveness

a positive way of behaving in relationships that is based on honesty, openness and a respect for all parties

There are many reasons why people behave in the way they do, often related to learned behaviour during childhood. Some of the messages commonly conveyed by parents, teachers and the media are shown in Chart 11.1.

Chart 11.1 ● Behaviour messages

- Be strong
- Be successful at any cost
- Don't let people walk over you
- Don't be weak
- Stand up for yourself
- Be in control

- Be gentle
- Be kind
- Don't argue
- It is wrong to be angry
- It is selfish to think of yourself

CONNECTIONS

Chapter 7 explores gender issues.

transactional analysis

a theory of personality and an approach to communication that promotes personal growth and change

Those in the first column have traditionally been the messages conveyed to boys and those in the second column the messages to girls. Men traditionally strive to win and see compromise or giving in as weakness and failure. Women have tended to acquiesce, being afraid to speak out, especially on their own behalf. The young are often told not to answer back, to have respect for authority, but although this may be valid, what they are not told is how to be heard while still being respectful to others, whoever the others may be. The messages in either of the columns may of course apply to either sex, and not all women become passive or all men aggressive.

The 'I'm OK, you're OK quadrangle', taken from **transactional analysis** and shown in Figure 11.5, gives us a picture of the different ways in which people may have learned to respond as a result of childhood experiences. In quadrant 1, the aggressive person does not really care about the rights or feelings of the other person: the 'I'm all right Jack' syndrome. In quadrant 2, the person puts himself down; he may be fearful of hurting or offending others and tends to believe that others are better, echoing the 'children should be seen and not heard' approach. This person may be liked but not respected, or may be seen as weak and used by others. In the third quadrant, the person is deceitful. He may be very complimentary to others or be full of excuses and apologies; before you know where you are, you are doing something for him that you did not really want to do. You suddenly feel cheated and not quite sure how you got into that situation. The assertive person, shown in quadrant 4, cares both about himself and about others. He speaks clearly about his wants and needs in an unambiguous way but also listens to the needs and wants of others. Although some people's behaviour very obviously matches one of these quadrants, it is more common to take something from each of the four quadrants. It is more usual for us to be able to be assertive in some situations and not others. Some people are assertive at home or

Activity 9

Try to identify situations in which you find it easy to be assertive and ones in which you find it difficult. Ask yourself what it is about these situations that makes it easier or harder.

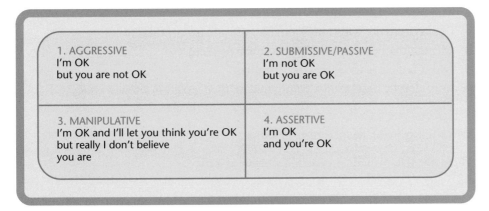

Figure 11.5 ● The 'I'm OK, you're OK' quadrangle

with their friends and relations but not assertive at work. Others may be assertive at work but struggle to be assertive in their private lives.

Why assertiveness?

Although assertiveness is important for any group, nurses have been identified as a group that finds being assertive difficult (McCartan and Hargie, 1990). This might be attributable to being a profession whose principal purpose is to care for others. Furthermore, nursing has historically had a tradition of duty and subservience. Becoming more assertive is, however, important for two main reasons. The first is to promote mental health in that non-assertive behaviour can lead to being pushed aside and not listened to, or to being labelled aggressive. Indeed, these have been some of the common stereotypical portrayals of nurses: the submissive, dutiful carer and the dominant, matronly figure. Both these approaches can lead to increased stress and loss of confidence for the nurse, whereas being assertive earns respect from others and an increase in self-confidence.

Second, it is important for the sake of those for whom the nurse is caring and for colleagues and staff working alongside the nurse. Being assertive enables the nurse to be in a position to be an advocate for the client, be this in relation to a client's direct care or indirectly by challenging working practices. Staff working relationships can be one of the greatest stresses for health-care workers, but by caring for one another, by being open and respectful, working relationships will be enhanced. Hargie et al. (1994, p. 273) identify seven functions of assertiveness that will help individuals to:

● Ensure that their personal rights are not violated
● Withstand unreasonable requests from others

- Make reasonable requests of others
- Deal effectively with unreasonable refusals from others
- Change the behaviour of others towards them
- Avoid unnecessary aggressive conflicts
- Confidently, and openly, communicate their position on any issue.

Enhancing your assertiveness skills

There are five principles central to being assertive:

1. *Listen carefully to what the other person has to say:* this immediately shows some respect for the other person's opinion and feelings. Furthermore, you have the information you need rather than defensively jumping to conclusions.
2. *Say what you think and feel:* your feelings and thoughts are as important and relevant as anyone else's. You have the right to be heard.
3. *If appropriate, say what you want to happen:* without this, the other person is left guessing what you want. It is important here to be specific.
4. *Be persistent:* do not be side-tracked or wrong-footed but stay with the issue in hand, repeating it if necessary until the issue has been satisfactorily addressed.
5. *Be prepared to compromise:* this must be done from a position of choice to bring about a satisfactory conclusion for all involved rather than because of coercion or 'just for a quiet life'.

Non-verbal communication

non-verbal communication

communicating without the use of spoken language, for example by gestures, body posture and facial expression

In addition to these central aspects, it is important to project yourself in a positive manner using your body language and **non-verbal communication**. It is no good saying the right things if your body language does not complement your words. Birdwhistell (1970) estimates that up to 70 per cent of social interactions are conveyed via a non-verbal channel; therefore, if your non-verbal communication conveys aggression or passivity, that is what the receiver will be aware of no matter what you are saying.

Positive communication requires positive non-verbal communication. It is of course important to take into account cultural differences in body language, in which eye contact, proximity and touch may be very different. In principle, eye contact should be direct and appropriate rather than aggressive staring or passive avoidance. Good eye contact demonstrates that you are interested in the other person and have nothing to hide. An individual's personal space is also important. We usually stand closest to those with whom we are most intimate and furthest away during normal social encounters (Hall, 1966). Standing inappropriately close can be threatening, whereas standing too far off can be interpreted as withdrawing. Your posture should be upright and open, with an absence of any gestures that could be interpreted as being aggressive, such as finger-pointing, folded arms or the hands on the hips. The tone of voice should be firm but relaxed and gentle. A good understanding of non-verbal communication can enhance interactions, and it is worthwhile taking the time to consider how you use non-verbal communication and to observe how others use it.

Assertiveness techniques

Two aspects of assertiveness will be outlined here – responding to criticism and turning down a request or demand – both of which can be potentially difficult to manage. They also contain many of the central elements of assertion, in particular listening and responding, and three useful techniques: the broken record, fielding the response and fogging (see below).

Saying no

Saying no can be particularly difficult for some people. It often raises old anxieties, reminders of when people have said no to us, particularly as children. There is often an underlying fear of hurting or offending others. Furthermore, if you say no, they may not like you, and the feeling of rejection can be painful and frightening. Simply agreeing to a request when you do not want to can, however, mean being taken for granted and used by others. It can also mean not respecting the other person's ability to accept the refusal. Remember that you have the right to say no without feeling guilty. It is the request rather than the person that is being turned down. Nevertheless, some people do seem to have difficulty in understanding that no means no, so it is unfortunately sometimes necessary to be persistent and explicit in saying no.

Before saying no, take time to consider the request. You may, for example, say, 'Can I come back to you in five minutes?' or 'Can I consult my diary before I give you an answer?' If you really do want to say no, say it clearly and unambiguously. You do not have to give a reason, but if it helps then do so, providing that it does not undermine your decision. Remember that it is your choice whether to say yes or no. It is the act of choosing that is so important; you do not then feel you have been railroaded into a decision or have backed down when you really wanted to say no. Once you have made your decision, then is the time to stick to it; two techniques can help in sticking to the point.

The broken record

This really is just repeating what you have already said. If, for example, your manager asks you to do an extra shift but you already have a prior appointment,

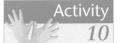

Activity
10

If you find it difficult to use your voice assertively, choose a range of scenarios and try verbalising your response to yourself until you get a feel for the right manner and tone of voice. If possible, stand up and speak into a tape-recorder.

you may, after careful consideration, say, 'No, I can't do that shift; I have already made other arrangements.' But your manager persists. You can respond by saying, 'As I said, I have made other arrangements and I am not able to do that shift.' Remember that this should not be conveyed in an aggressive manner but in a firm and respectful one. In some cases, it may be necessary to repeat yourself several times to reinforce the message, and you should try to use some of the same words each time so that you do not become diverted.

Fielding the response

This is in some ways similar to the above, but it involves a summarising technique as well as sticking to and repeating your statement. This summarising can be very important because it conveys to others that you have heard them and that you understand their point of view. In the following example, you acknowledge the other person's difficulty and indicate that you would be willing to help if you could, but you also make it clear that you have needs of your own and that these, too, should be respected:

> 'No, I can't work that shift. I realise that you are short of nurses for this shift and if I could help I would, but as I have said, I have made other arrangements.'

Managing criticism

Managing criticism is included here because nurses, along with many other professionals, receive criticism as part of their everyday lives. Criticism can be positive if handled well but a source of hurt and anger if it is not constructively imparted. Given constructively, criticism can help you to reflect on your practice and, if appropriate, modify and enhance it.

There are basically three possible responses to criticism. First, the criticism may be *invalid*, in which case you can reject it. Second, it can be *valid*, in which case you can accept it. Third, it can be *partly valid*, in which case you can accept the valid aspects and reject the invalid ones (Bond, 1986). Before any judgement can be made, you must, however, listen to the criticism. Do not reject it immediately; if necessary, ask for time to think about what you have been told.

Some examples may help to illustrate the three responses.

- **Valid**
  Staff nurse to student: 'Nurse Kahn, you have forgotten to attend to Mrs Walmsley's dressing'
  Student: 'Yes I have, I'm sorry. I will go and do it as soon as I have finished this'

- **Partially valid**

  Staff nurse to student: 'Nurse Reid, you're always late for these meetings'

  Student: 'I am late for this meeting and I apologise, but in fact I have been here on time for all the other meetings'

- **Invalid**

  Staff nurse to student: 'You don't attend any of the ward rounds'

  Student: 'I do; in fact I have been on every ward round that has taken place when I have been on duty.'

Fogging

A useful technique to use when you feel that you are being attacked is that of fogging. Fogging tends to slow the other person down and gives you time to formulate a response. There is often an expectation on the part of the person attacking you that you will immediately disagree, but if you agree in part with what they are saying, this tends to draw them from their critical parental stance to a more adult one. An example may help to illustrate this. After you have been in the difficult situation of breaking bad news to a client, the charge nurse sees the client crying and appears to blame you: 'What have you said to Ms Bland? You have obviously upset her.' You might respond by saying, 'Yes, she is very upset; I have just explained to her ...'. Here, you are not agreeing that it is your fault, but you do agree that Ms Bland is upset. The scene is then set for more constructive dialogue to take place between you and the charge nurse.

Conclusion

The very notion of assertiveness can alienate some people. This may be because of their misunderstanding of assertiveness or because of their observations of people who claim to have been on an assertiveness course. It is, in essence, just good, caring communication, communication that respects one's autonomy and the autonomy of others. The techniques involved in being assertive are relatively straightforward, but changing your behaviour may be less easy. What assertiveness training rarely does is address the archaic reasons why you as an individual communicate the way you do. This is not to say that you cannot improve your communication skills through being assertive, but this needs to be carried out alongside developing your own self-awareness. It may, however, take time and practice to adjust the way in which you present yourself. Taking small steps in situations you can cope with will be more rewarding than trying to change overnight. Use your reflective practice to examine your own behaviour, and consider situations in which you were assertive and in which you wish you had been more assertive.

> **CONNECTIONS**
>
> *Chapter 13 reviews how to reflect on your practice.*

◼ Chapter Summary

In the author's recent experience, a client who was about to die commented that the nurse caring for him seemed to have chosen the wrong profession. It was not her knowledge or technical skills that concerned him but the poor way in which she communicated with him and the other clients around him. Fortunately, there are many examples of good communication to counter this rather sad tale. Clients need more than scientific intervention as part of their care. During your nurse education, you will learn many facts and gain expertise that will undoubtedly be of benefit to the clients in your care. Whatever your chosen branch, your skills must include an expertise in open and caring communication with clients, families and colleagues; without this, you will be failing in your duty of care. It is possible to enhance your communication style and develop good therapeutic communication skills supported by research-based theory. This chapter has only allowed a glimpse into the world of social and professional interactions but provides a basis for further study, reflection and practice.

● Test Yourself!

1. Name the three core qualities that are necessary for personal growth and change.

2. Name the six categories of Heron's six-category intervention analysis and give examples of how these may be used in your area of practice.

3. Give five interventions that could be used in the catalytic category.

4. List seven members of the multidisciplinary team in your area of practice.

5. Describe what is meant by a 'primary group' and a 'secondary group'. Give two examples of each.

6. Describe the elements of the three circles model.

7. What are the four stages that Tuckman suggests groups move through as they establish themselves?

8. There are four ways to respond in an interaction, one of which is by being manipulative. What are the other three?

9. What are the five principal stages of being assertive?

10. Criticisms may be 'valid', 'invalid' or 'partially valid'. What are the recommended methods of responding to these types of criticism?

11. How are you going to develop the themes described in this chapter?

Further Reading

The following books will help to develop the themes referred to in this chapter.

The core conditions

Mearns, D. and Thorne, B. (1988) *Person-centred Counselling in Action*. Sage, London.

Rogers, C.R. (1980) *A Way of Being*. Houghton Mifflin, New York.

Therapeutic interventions

Culley, S. (1991) *Integrative Counselling Skills*. Sage, London.

Heron, J. (1990) *Helping the Client: A Creative Practical Guide*. Sage, London.

Egan, G. (1994) *The Skilled Helper*, 5th edn. Brooks-Cole, Monterey, CA.

Groups

Adair, J. (1988) *Effective Leadership*. Pan Books, London.

Niven, N. and Robinson, J. (1994) *The Psychology of Nursing Care*. Macmillan – now Palgrave Macmillan, Basingstoke.

Assertiveness

Bond, M. (1986) *Stress and Self-awareness: A Guide for Nurses*. Heinemann Nursing, London.

Other useful texts

Buckman, R. (1993) *How To Break Bad News*. Papermac, London.

Hargie, O., Saunders, C. and Dickson, D. (1994) *Social Skills in Interpersonal Communication*, 3rd edn. Routledge, London.

Nelson-Jones, R. (1997) *Practical Counselling and Helping Skills*, 4th edn. Cassell Educational, London.

Stewart, W. (2001) *An A–Z of Counselling Theory and Practice*. Nelson Thornes, Cheltenham.

References

Adair, J. (1988) *Effective Leadership*. Pan Books, London.

Bass, B.M. (1990) *Handbook of Leadership: Theory, Research and Managerial Applications*, 3rd edn. Collier-Macmillan, London.

Birdwhistell, R.L. (1970) *Kinesics and Context*. University of Pennsylvania Press, Philadelphia.

Bond, M. (1986) *Stress and Self-awareness: A Guide for Nurses*. Heinemann Nursing, London.

Brereton, M.L. (1995) Communication in nursing: the theory–practice relationship. *Journal of Advanced Nursing* **21**: 314–24.

British Association for Counselling (1996) *Code of Ethics and Practice for Counsellors*. BAC, Rugby.

Buckman, R. (1993) *How To Break Bad News*. Papermac, London.

Buckroyd, J. (1987) The nurse as counsellor. *Nursing Times* **83**: 42–4.

Burnard, P. (1995a) Counselling or being a counsellor? *Professional Nurse* **10**(2): 261–2.

Burnard, P. (1995b) Implications of client-centred counselling for nursing practice. *Nursing Times* **91**(26): 35–7.

Egan, G. (1994) *The Skilled Helper*, 5th edn. Brooks-Cole, Monterey, CA.

Fielder, F.E. (1971) Validation and extension of the contingency model of leadership effectiveness: a review of empirical findings. *Psychological Bulletin* **76**: 128–48.

Fromm, E. (1975) *The Art of Loving*. Unwin, London.

Hall, E.T. (1966) *The Silent Language*. Doubleday, New York.

Hargie, O., Saunders, C. and Dickson, D. (1994) *Social Skills in Interpersonal Communication*, 3rd edn. Routledge, London.

Harkins, S. (1987) Social loafing and social facilitation. *Journal of Experimental Social Psychology* **23**: 1–18.

Heron, J. (2001) *Helping the Client: A Creative Practical Guide*. Sage, London.

Hewison, A. (1995) Nurses' power in interaction with patients. *Journal of Advanced Nursing* **21**: 75–82.

Lewin, K., Lippitt, R. and White, R. (1939) Patterns of aggressive behaviour in experimentally created 'social climates'. *Journal of Social Psychology* **10**: 271–99.

Ley, P. (1988) *Communicating with Patients*. Croom Helm, London.

McCartan, P.J. and Hargie, O.D.W. (1990) Assessing assertive behaviour in student nurses: a comparison of assertion measures. *Journal of Advanced Nursing* **15**: 1370–76.

Maguire, P. and Faulkner, A. (1993) Communicating with cancer patients: 1. Handling bad news and difficult questions. In Dickenson D. and Johnson M. (eds) *Death, Dying and Bereavement*. Sage, London.

Mearns, D. (1994) *Developing Person-centred Counselling*. Sage, London.

Nelson-Jones, R. (1997) *Practical Counselling and Helping Skills,* 4th edn. Cassell Educational, London.

Nichols, K.A. (1989) Institutional versus client-centred care in general hospitals. In Broome, K.A. (ed.) *Health Psychology: Processes and Applications*. Chapman & Hall, London.

Rogers, C.R. (1957) The necessary and sufficient conditions of therapeutic personality change. *Journal of Consulting Psychology* **21**(2): 95–103.

Rogers, C.R. (1980) *A Way of Being*. Houghton Mifflin, New York.

Sayles, S.M. (1966) Supervisory style and productivity: review and theory. *Personnel Psychology* **19**(3): 275–86.

Stevens, J.O. (1971) *Awareness: Exploring, Experimenting, Experiencing*. Real People Press, Moab, UT.

Tuckman, B.W. (1965) Development sequence in small groups. *Psychological Bulletin* **63**(6): 384–99.

CATHERINE THROWER

Chapter

Understanding Ourselves

12

Contents

Learning outcomes

The main aim of this chapter is to stress to all those working within the health-care profession the importance of understanding the self. After reading the chapter, you should have a greater understanding of:

- **Self concept:** the development of self concept, models of self and self-awareness

- **Stress:** models of stress and modifiers of stress

- **Attitudes:** attitude formation and the relevance of attitudes for health-care practice.

'Understanding ourselves' may seem a self-evident concept; after all, who should know better about what goes on in our heads than ourselves? How often do we think that others do not understand? Why else would we need to put our point of view in to the public arena but to enable others to understand our perspective? The self is a private world that may in everyday life need little exploration, and there are circumstances in which an exploration of understanding the self may seem like luxury, if not indulgence. Do the homeless, the hungry or those in war-torn areas of the globe need to understand their motivation for their behaviour? A model proposed by Abraham Maslow places these questions in context.

Maslow's hierarchy of needs (Figure 12.1) is a framework that orders the needs of life. It predicts that there is an order in which needs have to be satisfied to enable individuals to reach their full potential. The lower levels identify the requirement to satisfy physical needs such as hunger and warmth, with a progression through needs such as love and esteem to aesthetics and the final need of self-actualisation (Maslow, 1968). Maslow's theory of growth and development will be further discussed later in this chapter.

As nurses, there is a need to maximise our potential as carers not only to understand what it is to be a professional carer, but also to understand our own motivation for wishing to care and to be able to disentangle our own thoughts and emotions from those of the people we look after. The nature of caring dictates that the people with whom we are in the most intimate contact are the most vulnerable. If we make assumptions about behaviour based on our own past

Maslow's hierarchy of needs

a pyramid, with basic needs (physical, safety) at the lower levels, which the person has to satisfy, before progressing to achieve higher order needs (love, esteem, cognitive, aesthetic), culminating in self-actualisation at the pinnacle

CONNECTIONS

Chapter 4 provides more information on satisfying the basic need for food.

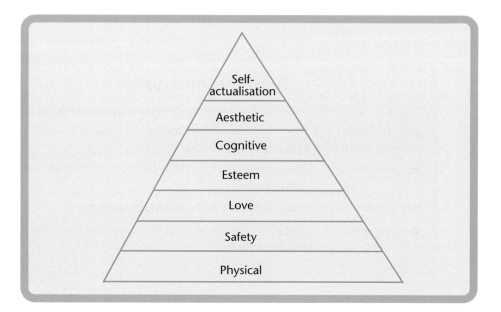

Figure 12.1 ● Maslow's hierarchy of needs

experience and feelings, we may be doing our patients a grave disservice. When a nurse is, for example, faced with the death of a patient and grieving relatives, is her distress a sharing of those people's distress and loss, or has it more to do with unresolved issues of grief or mortality in her own life? Thus, an understanding of our own thoughts, feelings and behaviour is essential so that we can give the best possible care and reach our maximum potential as excellent carers.

CONNECTIONS

Chapter 9 explores bereavement.

Activity
1

Before reading on, try this brief exercise. Write down 20 answers to the following question: 'Who am I?'

■ Self Concept

Self concept is the knowledge that a person has about himself. It is information chiefly acquired by interactions with others (Baron and Byrne, 1997). It is a schema, an organised set of beliefs and feelings that are self-referent. The self concept influences how we process information about the external social world and its relationships to 'me'. The schema holds information about motives, emotions, self-evaluations, abilities and so on (Baron and Byrne, 1997), and we access this self-schema every time we use self-referent information.

self concept

the knowledge that a person has about him- or herself

Research into the self concept frequently uses the 'Who am I?' approach, sometimes known as Gordon's phenomenological approach (Gordon, 1968), as a method of study. Rentsch and Heffner (1994) used this methodology to explore self concept with a group of student subjects. The researchers asked the question, 'Who am I?' of 230 subjects. Their analysis confirmed Gordon's eight broad categories of the self, reflecting a combination of social identity and personal attributes. These are (Rentsch and Heffner, 1994):

● *Existential aspects:* for example I am unique, I am special, I am attractive
● *Self-determination:* for example I can achieve my educational goals
● *Interpersonal attributes:* for example myself in relation to others, I am a student nurse, I am a daughter/son
● *Ascribed characteristics:* for example I am a woman/man, I am 19 years old, I am British
● *Interests and activities:* for example I enjoy football, I like dogs
● *Internalised beliefs:* for example I am a socialist, I am opposed to fox-hunting
● *Self-awareness:* for example my beliefs are well integrated, I am a good person
● *Social differentiation:* for example I am poor, wealthy, I am gay.

The self concept is, however, more than the sum of the answers to 'Who am I?' The schema for self contains information about our past experiences; it encompasses our memories and our expectations of the future. Baron and Byrne (1997) maintain that the self is a sum of everything a person knows and what he imagines he can be.

To conceptualise this schema as a fixed structure is, however, misleading as there is change over time: the self concept alters with life events and new learning. It may be that it is vulnerable to change in a short period of time; for example, if a woman loses her job, her self concept will undergo a redefinition from being a person who is employed to one who is unemployed. The opposite can of course occur when a person gains employment, passes a driving test or achieves a goal. The concept of self is therefore not a rigid percept but one that is fluid and vulnerable to change.

It is important to understand the effects of change and why this change to the self-image occurs as a failure to do so may lead to psychological discomfort as the person resists the redefinition of or addition to self-knowledge. Change can be threatening, particularly if it is enforced rather than chosen.

■ Development of Self Concept

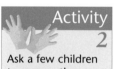

Activity 2

Ask a few children to answer the question 'Who am I?' What descriptors do the children use?

The sense of self develops as a function of growing older. The child learns about the environment and her relationship to the people and objects within that environment by being in the world. The child learns that she is a separate entity within the world rather than symbiotic with the caregiver and the external world. She learns that objects exist independently of her; that is, the child comes to understand that when she cannot see a toy, it still remains in the world rather than no longer existing. Similarly, the child learns that she exists independently of her environment and that she can act and have an effect on the world, particularly on other people. As a result of interactions with caregivers, friends, teachers and so on, children learn about an 'I' separate from other people and objects (Mischel, 1986). Consequently, they establish a **self-schema**. In early infancy, this is knowledge about the self existing as an independent entity, but as the child matures, the schema enlarges. During middle childhood, there is a shift in the self-descriptors from concrete, physical descriptions to social comparisons and psychological descriptors (Brooks-Gun and Paikoff, 1992). Montemeyer and Eisen (1977) asked a group of young people aged from 10 to 18 years to answer the question 'Who am I?' They found that there was an increase in the use of self, ideology and belief references with age and a decrease in physical categories as descriptors.

self-schema

your mental representation of understanding about yourself

Erikson's theory of personality development

at each of the eight stages of development, from the first years of life to the ageing years, there are special issues that must be confronted before personal development can succeed. His ideas were developed from psychoanalytic theory

■ Erikson's Theory of Personality Development

One theoretical framework that places the establishment of the self-schema within a developmental context is Erikson's eight-stage psychosocial theory of development (Erikson, 1959). Each stage has a task of transition or crisis, the resolution of each crisis influencing the subsequent stages. The task is to resolve the conflict between two opposing choices and to balance in favour of a positive or negative outcome. A positive resolution will result in the acquisition of an adaptive strength that will sustain the individual's progress through the next stage of life span development. Each life crisis gives the individual more knowledge about the world and his relationship to it (Erikson, 1959):

- *Stage 1 – Trust versus mistrust*
  Trust is about learning what to expect from the world. This is not just that the world is a safe place with consistency and nurturing, but also that dangerous people can be trusted to be dangerous. Irregularity and inconsistency will, however, lead to mistrust, and the child experiences anxiety and insecurity
  Adaptive strength: Hope
- *Stage 2 – Autonomy versus shame and doubt*
  This is a stage of gaining mastery over the world and, particularly for the young child, over the body. If the child is encouraged to explore her body, there will be a growth of self-confidence, enabling an exploration of the physical and social worlds. If constantly criticised, the child will feel ashamed and come to doubt herself
  Adaptive strength: Will
- *Stage 3 – Initiative versus guilt*
  The child will begin to ask questions to further her knowledge and skills, realising that she has some influence over her environment and the people in it. The child may become successful at manipulating her surroundings, but if reaching out to the world is met with disapproval and reproof, the child will feel inept, resulting in an emerging sense of guilt
  Adaptive strength: Purpose
- *Stage 4 – Industry versus inferiority*
  The child is learning about accomplishment and task completion. A sense of industry will feed a sense of achievement, whereas failure to complete or accomplish will result in a sense of inferiority, which may be lifelong
  Adaptive strength: Competence
- *Stage 5 – Identity versus role confusion*
  This was viewed by Erikson as crucial stage of development. **Identity** is a structure within an organised set of values and beliefs about oneself. These may be expressed in a variety of ways – occupation, politics, religion and relationships, for example. Erikson maintains that an integrated identity cannot occur before adolescence because of immature cognitive, physical and social development, but a failure to integrate during this stage will result in role confusion
  Adaptive strength: Fidelity

identity

a structure within an organised set of values and beliefs about oneself

- *Stage 6 – Intimacy versus isolation*
  This stage presents the young adult with the task of forming intimate relationships with others. It encompasses a sense of connectedness, a fusion of one's identity with someone else's safe in the belief that you will retain your sense of self intact. The opposing resolution is isolation, a feeling that occurs when a person is threatened by the behaviour of others
  Adaptive strength: Love

- *Stage 7 – Generativity versus self-absorption*
  The positive aspect of this task is generativity: an interest in the next generation. The primary interest is in nurturing offspring but, for those without offspring, energy may be directed into creative and altruistic concerns. The opposite of this outwardly directed interest is self-absorption, an indulging of the self as though it were a child, one's one and only child
  Adaptive strength: Care

- *Stage 8 – Integrity versus despair*
  This is the final life task in which the individual is faced with integrating the life cycle, an acceptance of one's life as being one's own responsibility
  Adaptive strength: Wisdom.

generativity

an interest in the next generation

Erikson's theory outlines a framework of growth and development that is inevitable and irresistible. Erikson (1959) hypothesised a ground plan for growth, each stage having its time of ascendancy until all aspects of personality are fully developed to form an integrated personality.

Resolution in a negative direction means that individuals become restricted in their development and fail to benefit from the adaptive strength associated with each life task. Working with the vulnerable, nurses need to have insight into the self, some understanding of how life tasks have been resolved. Nurses need to access their own thoughts, feelings and motivation for behaviour to be able to have an awareness of how they may respond to the thoughts, feelings and behaviour of others. There is an acknowledgement within the field of health care that we need to demonstrate positive regard; nurses aim to promote a sense of value in their patients, but to be successful, we need to have an understanding of the self in terms of our own values, attitudes, thoughts and feelings. We need to be comfortable with ourselves before we can understand others.

Self-awareness

self-awareness

the condition of being able to analyse motives for behaviour

Rawlinson (1990) defines self-awareness as:

bringing into consciousness [those] various aspects of our understanding of ourselves.

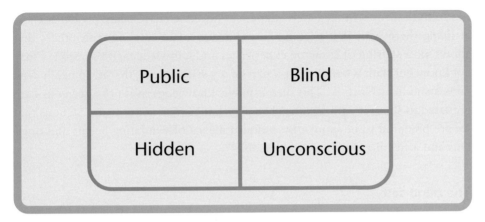

Figure 12.2 ● The Johari window – four facets of the self

The 'various aspects' refer to the components of self. Rawlinson differentiates self-awareness from self-consciousness, which, rather than being a constructive appreciation of the self, is a concern for others' perception of our own self.

Self-awareness is a condition of being able to analyse the motives underlying our behaviour. Most of the time we act and interact giving scant attention to why, the focus being the consequences or achievement of our goals. Self-aware-ness is the antithesis of self-consciousness, the latter being a concern with others' opinions and the former a concern with the motives for and effectiveness of one's behaviour.

A model of self that illustrates the importance of self-awareness in the growth and development of a confident, effective person is the Johari window (Luft and Ingham, 1955). This model is depicted as a window with four panes, each repre-senting a facet of the self (Figure 12.2).

The Johari window is useful in understanding the nature of self-awareness. The aim is to enlarge the **public self**. The more comfortable we are with what others know about us, the easier it is to understand pain at times of change for ourselves and for others. But this is just one model of self; others offer different frameworks in which to strive for self-knowledge.

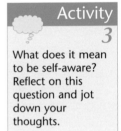

Activity
3
What does it mean to be self-aware? Reflect on this question and jot down your thoughts.

public self

the things we know about ourselves and are comfortable for others to know

The public self

This part of self is that information which we know about ourselves and are happy for others to know. This may include name, occupation and marital status. It may also include age (although some people prefer to keep their age a secret), background and personal details. If, for example, I meet anyone from Norfolk, I am, as a person who lived there for many years and has happy memories from that time, immediately prepared, indeed keen, to share my experiences of living there with that person. This is a way of interacting with others that allows me a sharing of common experiences and knowledge with someone I may not know but with whom I share a part of my self concept, that is, someone who knows and likes Norfolk. This then is public knowledge; it is not a secret as I am prepared to share it with anyone. These exchanges are not only interactions that we are prepared to be known by, but also means of validating beliefs and opinions and affirming the status of 'person'.

blind self

things known about us by others, but not known to us

The blind self

This is knowledge known to others but not known to the self. It is an area of knowledge that can be threatening. What is it that others are not telling us? It could be that a woman's dress is tucked in the back of her knickers or that a man's fly is undone. More often, however, it is the psychological, behavioural or social equivalent. The 'other' is able to form a totally different perspective on our behaviour, habits and mannerism of which we are totally unaware. Do you know what you look like from the back view? Do you know what your walk looks like? Others may find our presence pleasing but, conversely, they may find it unpleasant. The more information that we are given about the blind self, the greater the degree of self-awareness that is allowed to develop. If I am given information about my behaviour of which I have previously been unaware, I have the choice to change or to continue with the knowledge of the effect that this behaviour may have on others.

Giving an example of knowledge in the blind self is not easy as I do not know what others know about me to which I am not privy. When I was sister in a day hospital, however, I was asked by a member of staff whether I would be willing to allow a health-care support worker to be flexible with her time as she had family problems. As part of my self-image was kind and caring, I had no hesitation in agreeing, provided that the day hospital was safe for patients and the care was delivered as it should be. I was curious to know why this woman had not asked me herself. The reply from the staff nurse to this query was that I was unapproachable. This came as new knowledge to me and challenged my existing self concept as a kind, caring and considerate manager. I could have responded in two ways. First, I could have been defensive. When the self concept is threatened or challenged, there is a shift to mobilise defence strategies to protect the status quo. Hostility is one means of defence: I could have become angry, projecting my feelings of threat on to the other person. A second response is to accept that this was how I appeared to this member of staff and the person on whose behalf she was speaking. These responses will be discussed below.

CONNECTIONS

An incident of this kind would respond to a structured approach, as outlined in Chapter 13.

Defensive response

A **defence mechanism** is a protective strategy employed when the self is under threat. When information is threatening, the self rallies a defence mechanism to maintain an equilibrium. The psychodynamic view proposes that the human organism is unable to tolerate anxiety, and we deal with this state by developing defence strategies that protect against this painful state. Defence mechanisms arise from the unconscious as a way of distorting reality in order to exclude feelings of anxiety from consciousness (Pervin, 1984). Being given information about yourself that is unacceptable will produce a state of anxiety, and one way of dealing with this is projection. Projection occurs when internal, unacceptable feelings are projected externally; thus, feelings of internal hostility are projected outwards, leading to the perception of the other person as hostile. In the example above, I held the view that I was an approachable manager, but this view was under threat. A hostile response would have shifted this internal hostility from the self externally to the staff nurse, invalidating her opinion.

defence mechanism
a protective strategy employed when the self is under threat

Acceptance

An alternative approach is to acknowledge the state of anxiety produced by this incongruous information, choosing to alter the image of self conveyed to the world. By accepting the 'other's' perspective, not necessarily as truth but as a valid opinion, there is a growth in self-awareness. So in my example, I could not accept the truth of being unapproachable, but I did accept that this was how I was perceived by others.

The hidden self

This is the part of the self that is hidden from public gaze. This corner of the window hides that of which we are ashamed, frightened and embarrassed; here lie unacceptable thoughts and feelings. A disclosure of information from this area is threatening and can elicit great anxiety. As an example of the hidden self, we can draw on the literature on carers. Caring for a dependent relative can be a pleasure and enjoyable: it can bring meaning to life and a new perspective to a relationship. However, it is not unusual for carers to feel hostile and angry towards their charges. Admitting that we have these thoughts is a frightening exercise. The dependent person cannot help being ill or disabled; the crying, sleepless baby is vulnerable and helpless. Disclosing feelings of bitterness, resentment, anger and hostility may bring criticism and hostility on the carers themselves, the logic being that, 'If I admit that I feel like hitting X, I will be reviled and ostracised.'

hidden self
the things we hide from others

The reality may, however, be that, by disclosing these fears, the person will find warmth, understanding and support. Revealing secrets may bring a realisation that others feel like you do and behave like you do, and that behaviour, thoughts and feelings that leave you feeling guilty and ashamed are common to others in a similar situation. It is no accident that self-help groups are a popular means of offering support for people caring for dependent relatives. Affiliation with other people in a position similar to our own is an effective way of easing anxiety and lessening our sense of isolation. These groups provide a forum for people to disclose unacceptable thoughts and feelings, facilitating a growth in understanding of the self as carer. There are times when this hidden part of the self needs help to facilitate disclosure, but accepting this part of the self concept helps the individual to feel more comfortable with the self and as such enables a growth in self-understanding.

unconscious self
_____

things not known to
ourselves or others

The unconscious self

This is an interesting but enigmatic area of the self. This is knowledge not known to the self or others, and the question 'Does it exist?' has to be asked. The psychodynamic theory of personality maintains that the unconscious drives behaviour and can be revealed by free association and within dreams. However, the antithesis of this is of course the behavioural perspective. If it cannot be observed, it cannot be studied, but behaviour can be observed and can therefore be attributed to the consequences of action. This is not necessarily to deny the unconscious but to deny the validity of being able to say that the unconscious is a cause of behaviour. Wittgenstein maintained that when an individual looks inside himself, he finds a beetle in a box, a beetle that only he can see and touch (Humphrey, 1984). We all have a beetle, but I do not know what your beetle is like and you have no access to mine. Therefore what can I say about how your beetle influences your behaviour? If so little of this section of the window is available to the world, the unconscious is a territory to be explored only by the intrepid and with experienced, expert guidance (Humphrey, 1984).

■ Maslow's Hierarchy of Needs

Maslow's hierarchy is usually depicted as a pyramid with basic needs, such as safety and hunger, forming the base and self-actualisation forming the pinnacle (see Figure 12.1 above). A more appropriate view may, however, be to see this structure in terms of a more fluid model. Maslow viewed basic needs as drives that, when they were met, enabled a move to a higher level of need. Not everyone chooses to move beyond a particular level of need; it may be that the rigidity of Maslow's framework provides a safe boundary for the self concept, but choosing to move on to a greater fulfilment of need is to expand self-knowledge, broaden experience and move towards a greater understanding of the courage and anxieties of others.

Rogers' Model of Self

Rogers' model of self consists of all the knowledge that we have about the self, all the constituents of 'I' or 'me' (Atkinson et al., 1993). The three dominant features of this model are the real self, the ideal self and the self-esteem. Rogers maintained that we tend to interpret events in the world in relation to the self. We all have a percept of how we are in the world, an image of the self and its relationship to others, objects and events. This image is modelled on the ideal self, the goal for which we strive, the perfect, the self without flaw. The difference between the image we have of the self and the ideal self is the measure of self-esteem, the worth that we attribute to the self. This self-image and level of self-esteem is not, however, necessarily a true reflection of the real self. It is possible for people who outwardly appear successful and competent to have a low self-esteem and to define their self concept as inadequate. This may be because people set themselves goals that are too high or unachievable, a consequence of which may be, for some, a need for therapy to assist with the attainment of psychological well-being (Atkinson et al., 1993).

Rogers' model of self developed from explorations of individuals' subjective understanding of their 'self', consisting of 'I' or 'me'

Self and Sources of Stress

When the self concept is threatened, the resulting discomfort is a manifestation of stress, so the relationship between stress and the self concept needs to be explored in order to achieve a better understanding of the self.

Selye (1980) maintains that stress suffers from being too well known and too little understood. Nursing is a pressurised occupation. Nurses are put under pressures of time and limited resources, daily facing the pressures of others' pain, discomfort and distress with little time to acknowledge the effect that this may be having on their own emotions and self concept. Self-esteem has certainly been implicated as a factor influencing our perception of stress. Stress occurs when the demands of the situation exceed an individual's personal resources, and whereas a degree of stress is thought to be useful in motivating us to action, there needs to be an awareness of how to maintain a balance between what is motivating (the degree of arousal necessary for the successful performance of a task) and arousal that exceeds an optimum level for effective performance. The experience of the latter is stress, which is unpleasant and anxiety-provoking.

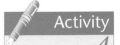
Activity 4

What causes you stress? Draw two columns, heading one 'Positive' and the other 'Negative'. List your answers according to whether you find the stressor motivating or threatening.

■ Models of Stress

Stimulus-based model

A simple model of stress is the stimulus-based model, which characterises the environment as providing a stressor and the person as experiencing stress or strain. But although this may offer a description, it does not elucidate the process by which people find themselves under pressure.

Response-based model

The response model offers a more detailed approach to understanding stress. The environment is the source of the stressor or stimulus, and the person's stress is the response. Selye conceptualised this as a non-specific response to excessive demands on individual coping resources. Selye believed that the response did not depend on the nature of the stressor and that the response was a protective mechanism (Cox, 1978). There are three identifiable stages to the response syndrome that form the **general adaptation syndrome** (GAS).

general adaptation syndrome

response to stress characterised by three stages; the alarm reaction, the resistance stage and, finally, exhaustion

Alarm reaction

This stage is related to a high level of physical arousal, which causes the release of adrenaline. It is during this initial stage that the organism's susceptibility to the specific stressor increases, and if the severity of the response is great enough, death may ensue. With less severe stressors but prolonged exposure, however, pituitary/adrenocorticotrophic hormones are released, and the resistance stage of the GAS is initiated.

Resistance stage

During this stage, physical arousal remains high. Adaption occurs as the parasympathetic nervous system attempts to counteract the effects of the sympathetic nervous system. The organism is therefore able to resist the debilitating effects of the stressor, although the threshold for eliciting the stress response has been lowered for further encounters with this specific threat or other non-specific stressors.

Exhaustion

If exposure continues, the final stage of the GAS is entered, that of exhaustion. Hormone reserves are depleted, fatigue results and the felt experience of this stage is frequently that of depression.

Interactional model

This approach to stress incorporates the stress response model with the demand placed on the individual and the subjective perception of that demand. There is an acknowledgement that the consequences of coping strategies will influence the perception of felt stress and that this provides feedback for future action when faced with a similar threat. Cox and Mackay (1978) proposed the man–environment transaction model, which they describe as eclectic, drawing on stimulus and response models. It, however, explicitly identifies that a stress system is an individual perceptual phenomenon (Cox, 1978).

The man–environment model has five identifiable stages:

1. Actual capability and demand.
2. Perceived capability and demand.
3. Psychophysiological changes.
4. Consequences of coping responses.
5. Feedback.

The last component is a particularly important feature of this model as it is the feedback the individual receives from the environment that determines the degree of felt stress and the perceived effectiveness of coping strategies.

> **CONNECTIONS**
>
> *Chapters 11 and 15 deal with teams, which may influence the level of stress we feel.*

Information-processing model

This approach emphasises the importance of cognitive and attentional factors. The individual selectively attends to stimuli and will interpret information as stressful or otherwise by comparing it with past experience (Figure 12.3).

Memory and decision-making therefore play a role in the processing of stimuli, and cognitive appraisal will elicit emotions, such as anxiety, anger, fear

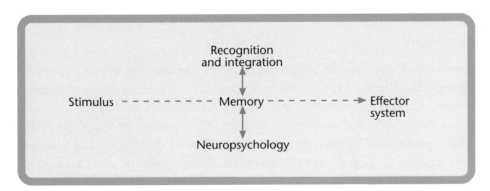

Figure 12.3 ● Information-processing model of stress

and sadness, previously associated with similar situations. This model proposes that stressors and stress responses can only be so if the individual's perception of the situation is that a threat exists. This view is in line with the premise that what one individual perceives as a threat, another may view as a challenge. Why is it that one individual will succumb to the debilitating effects of stress, manifest in illnesses such as peptic ulcers, coronary artery disease and depression, whereas another person in the same circumstances thrives on the motivation of the environment. Kobasa (1979) identifies challenge as a characteristic of the hardy personality, an individual whose susceptibility to illness is less than that of others who may perceive life events as stressful and have less than effective coping strategies.

■ Factors Affecting Stress

What acts as a source of stress will vary from one individual to another, but there are some events and encounters that have a shared effect; it is the interpretation of these as either a threat or a challenge that differs. The stressful life events model is one model delineating events as sources of stress (Holmes and Rahe, 1967). The Holmes and Rahe social readjustment rating scale was the outcome of research that asked people to rate the degree to which they found life events stressful. The resulting list covers a whole range of general life experiences such as the death of a spouse, marriage, childbirth, moving house, Christmas and going on holiday. But is the experience of a desirable event the same as that of one with negative consequences or connotations? Is the stress of preparing for Christmas a similar experience to that of losing a job? Although there may be emotional strain associated with positive events, there is an expectation of reward that provides a perspective different from that of events that may have negative connotations.

Why is it then that people vary in their response to events and encounters? There are several possible factors influencing this appraisal.

Personality

It seems that some people are predisposed to experience life events as stressful (Watson and Clarke, 1984); some individuals have a predisposition to negative affectivity, expressing distress and discomfort across a variety of situations rather than responding to specific situations. The corollary of this is the person who is predisposed to interpret demanding events as challenging and is able to cope effectively. Kobasa (1979) described this personality type as a hardy personality. The hardy personality has three constructs:

- *Challenge:* a willingness to accept change and to face novel situations as opportunities for growth and development
- *Commitment:* the tendency to involve oneself in whatever situations or events one encounters
- *Control:* the belief that one has influence over life events and the assumption of personal responsibility for those events.

Hardy individuals are mentally and physically healthier than others. They seem to appraise events more favourably than other individuals and have more effective coping strategies than non-hardy personality types.

Social support

Social support is the perceived comfort derived from a social network that includes significant others, family, friends, community organisations and professional practitioners. There are four broad types of social support:

1. *Emotional:* this is an expression of empathy, caring and concern towards a person. It provides a sense of belonging and being loved at times of stress.
2. *Esteem:* this support is expressed through positive regard. Esteem support enables the development of a sense of worth and competence.
3. *Tangible/instrumental:* this is support that comes from practical help. It may manifest itself in any way from the loan of money to someone doing the shopping or housework, or helping with personal care. This is the support given by someone when individuals are unable to perform a task or activity themselves.
4. *Informational:* this support is derived from advice, direction, suggestion and feedback. This support is manifest as information that allows an individual to make an informed appraisal or decision.

Social support reduces the stress that people experience. Stress has been demonstrated to have detrimental effects on health, and social support has been shown to be protective against these adverse effects. So how does social support protect against ill-health? Two theories have been proposed:

- The *buffering hypothesis* proposes that a good supportive network has a protective effect at times of high stress (Cohen and Hoberman, 1983)
- The *direct effect hypothesis* maintains that social support is beneficial regardless of the amount of stress experienced, influencing the appraisal of events as stressful or challenging (Cobb, 1976).

> **CONNECTIONS**
>
> *Chapters 11 and 15 discuss teams, which can be a useful source of social support.*

social support
the perceived comfort derived from a social network that includes significant others, family, friends, community organisations and professional practitioners

Emotion

Negative events have a greater potential than positive events to be interpreted as stressful, and our emotions will influence the appraisal of a situation. Common emotions associated with stress are fear and anger, whereas a similar event associated with a pleasant emotion may not be interpreted as stressful. If while travelling we are, for example, aroused to anger by delays, our interpretation may be that the journey is stressful, but if the delay in the journey is perceived as an opportunity for time out from a busy schedule, the journey may be described as pleasant.

Recognising stress in ourselves, being able to identify the feelings that indicate stress, is important as the effect that this has on our behaviour within the clinical area will affect the patients for whom we are caring. Similarly, we need to have an understanding of what our patients may be experiencing, not so that we are in position to say, 'Yes, I know how you're feeling and this is how I deal with it' or to be able to evaluate someone else's experience, but so that we, as nurses, can empathise with our patients and provide the support that may be necessary to reduce the adverse effects of their experiences.

We need to have some understanding of how stress can affect behaviour in order to understand our patients' behaviour. This may enable us to anticipate times when stress may be heightened and when it may be at a minimum. An understanding of how people may appraise a situation as stressful needs to be part of the nurse's repertoire of skills in order to provide care most effectively. Being there for people when the need for support is at its most pressing is one of the most valuable skills of caring. The practice of nursing requires prioritisation when delivering care and being able to anticipate possible stress for patients when making these judgements.

So, making judgements about patients' affect, behaviour and cognition requires skill in empathy and analysis. An understanding of the self is essential to begin the process of analysis. We need to understand our thoughts and feelings in order to tease out the rationale for the actions and reactions of self and others. We also need to have an understanding of attitudes in order to be able to suspend our subjective evaluations and account for the evaluative judgements of others.

Attitudes

As we grow from infancy to adulthood, we are influenced by a variety of different pressures from parents, family, friends, school and the media. These pressures form the basis of our **attitudes**, beliefs and opinions. Attitudes reflect our values, the worth we attribute to events, people and objects. Sharing values is a way of building relationships; we seem to have a natural rapport with those who share our perspective. The way we dress, the music we like, the political

attitude

the sum of one's beliefs and opinions

beliefs we hold all contribute to the development of friendships. But when we nurse, we cannot be that selective. Indeed, all human life is to be found in the health-care context. Nurses are charged with being genuine, being warm and demonstrating unconditional positive regard; these are Rogers' core conditions necessary to effect change within a therapeutic relationship (Rogers, 1959). How easy is it though for these conditions to exist? There are times when we are as nurses required to suspend judgement in order to give our undivided attention. In some cases, this is not difficult, but, in others, our attitudes, beliefs and opinions may block our ability to enter the 'other's' world perspective and give care at an optimum level. Making the effort to know someone's background may make the difference between treating someone as an object in receipt of a service and a person who requires nursing care.

As an illustration of this point, let us consider the experience of a student nurse asked to care for a man with **Parkinson's disease**. This patient had a reputation among the nurses for being difficult. The student said she did not like him because 'You can't like everyone, can you?' This statement requires challenging and analysis in the context of nursing care. When we acknowledge likes and dislikes, we are expressing an attitude. On what are these judgements based? Sometimes they are based on only limited information: our interactions with the patients and possibly the comments of our colleagues. Knowledge can be inaccurate and incomplete, and, as nurses, we need to be prepared to alter our opinions, to allow our knowledge of our patients to be fluid and flexible. How is this achieved? By being non-judgemental. A person-centred approach to care, an approach that starts with the patient before any judgements or decisions, is more likely to facilitate a rapport that will contribute to reducing the impact of the stress of being a patient.

> **Parkinson's disease**
>
> a slowly progressive neurological disorder with resting tremor, muscle rigidity and weakness, shuffling gait and a mask-like appearance

The gentleman with Parkinson's disease had been admitted for a review of his condition. He was slow when mobile and dependent when in bed. He had the typical mask-like expression seen in patients with Parkinson's disease and demonstrated the on/off syndrome when walking. He was perceived by the nurses as demanding because, when he asked for assistance, he was time-consuming and appeared ungrateful for the help. The nurses found him difficult to please, and he always insisted on having things done strictly his way. The student nurse interpreted his behaviour as difficult and hostile, and the consequence was that she judged him as an unpleasant man.

This may of course have been an accurate judgement, but an alternative explanation is that here was a man angry and frustrated at his loss of independence. He was pedantic about his needs; he wanted his way because he was no longer able to perform, without help from another person, activities that most of us take for granted. This patient's expectation was that others would substitute what he would like to do for himself. This nurse needed to develop her skill of

> **CONNECTIONS**
>
> *This scenario would benefit from a structured, thoughtful approach, as described in Chapter 13.*

empathy to see the world from his perspective. Nurses need to listen to the patients' stories – most people have a story if we can make the right connection – and see beyond the label of 'difficult to understand'. As nurses, if we label our patients as we do our friends and acquaintances, we fail to acknowledge the meaning of our profession, the meaning of care.

Part of this process is to understand attitudes, how they are formed and how they can be changed. Attitudes influence behaviour, and as such we need to have an insight into the effect of our own attitudes on our nursing practice. We also need to consider our patients' attitudes and how these may be influencing their compliance with treatment and their thoughts and feelings about being in a vulnerable, dependent position.

There are three components of an attitude:

1. *Affective:* the feelings held towards an object or event that is to some degree either positive or negative. This is the component that represents our likes and dislikes.
2. *Behavioural:* the observable translation of an attitude. If feelings are positive, we develop an approach tendency or behaviour that increases contact with the object or causes us to engage with that situation. If our feelings are negative, we tend to develop avoidance tendencies or behaviours that distance us from the object or event.
3. *Cognitive:* the rationale part of the attitude, defining the object or situation towards which the attitude is directed. This encompasses people and groups, and consists of knowledge about the object or situation even though this knowledge may be incomplete.

Activity 5

What is your opinion of smoking? How did you form this opinion? What do you think about people who smoke? What do you think about people who don't smoke?

This three-component model of attitudes is useful in trying to make sense of our experience, but it is based on the the assumption that all three components are consistent. If, for example, we hold positive beliefs about an object or event, this should elicit positive feelings and an approach tendency. But is this always the case? Try Activity 5.

Your opinion about smoking may be influenced by whether your parents smoked, whether your friends, the people with whom you wish to affiliate, smoke and whether you smoke. Perhaps you think that smoking in moderation is OK and that people who do not smoke are prudish and boring. You may, however, believe that smoking is a health hazard not just for those who smoke, but also for those of us who have to inhale the smoke from others' cigarettes, making smokers selfish and antisocial, if not downright dangerous. It may be that you hold strong beliefs about smoking because of your experience of its effect on someone you know, or you may have beliefs about smoking but not to such an extent that you object to others smoking in your presence.

An alternative model is the expectancy value model. This proposes that we hold attitudes according to what we expect of an object or event and the degree to which this event or object will contribute to our goals and values.

Attitudes are formed by both direct and indirect methods. Direct experiences tend to produce more accurate knowledge on which to form judgements, but indirect methods also have a great influence. These include vicarious experience as well as what others, for example parents, peer group, schools and the media, say and do.

Changing attitudes can be a difficult task, but it does have real relevance for nurses as it is people's attitudes towards health behaviours that influence risky health behaviours and whether they are likely to modify any behaviour that will lessen their susceptibility to ill-health. The relationship between the patient and the nurse can be an important factor in changing a person's attitudes. Some of the factors that contribute to a change in attitude include:

- Trust
- Like and dislike
- Credibility
- Perceived attractiveness
- Individual beliefs
- Self-esteem.

In other words, the relationship between the nurse and patient is important in influencing patients' attitudes. This highlights the importance of the nurse developing interpersonal skills and understanding how to establish and build a rapport.

What happens when our behaviour is inconsistent with our beliefs? When we behave in a way that is contrary to our beliefs, we are left with a feeling of psychological discomfort described as **cognitive dissonance**. This discomfort may arise, for example, when a person who smokes firmly holds the belief that it is harmful to the self and others, or one who drives a car on a regular basis believes that this is major form of pollution and therefore also harmful. Any behaviour that counteracts our beliefs can lead to a feeling of discomfort, which we try to reduce. Individuals, on the whole, strive for cognitive consistency. As nurses, an understanding of self and motives underlying behaviour can lead to an attitude change and a greater degree of objectivity when making an assessment of the patients in our care.

A further issue that needs to be addressed in a discussion of attitudes is that of **prejudice**. Prejudice arises from a faulty generalisation directed towards a specific person or group of people because they are members of a particular group. A prejudice ignores qualities or characteristics that would negate our

cognitive dissonance

a state of tension which occurs when an individual holds two or more thoughts/beliefs that are psychologically inconsistent

prejudice

the combination of negative beliefs, attitudes and discriminatory behaviour towards those in a particular target group

opinion, and whereas prejudice is generally thought of as being negative, we may equally well ignore negative qualities as well as positive ones (Oliver and Hyde, 1993). If, as nurses, we believe that people who are short-tempered and particular in the way in which their needs are met are difficult patients, we will adopt a prejudicial approach to people who fit these criteria. The cognitive component of prejudice is more commonly known as a **stereotype**. One definition of a stereotype is that it is a type of shorthand, a way of understanding without having to go to first principles each time we wish to communicate or understand an event or situation. The knowledge that we hold about the world is organised into schemata, clumps of knowledge that include stereotypes, but by using this shorthand in our professional life, we exclude a great deal of knowledge and information about people that will enrich our understanding and enhance our nursing care.

The student nurse described above who said she did not like the gentleman with Parkinson's disease had adopted an attitude about this patient based on her belief about how patients should behave and possibly about the nature of Parkinson's disease. This also suggests, however, that her knowledge about the condition was incomplete, and that her attitude towards the patient's behaviour was limited and prejudicial. Knowledge should be acquired as this student progresses through her training. Will an increase in knowledge widen her understanding? The expectation is that it will, and that it will in turn influence her attitude to patients with Parkinson's disease who remain expressionless, unable to give the usual feedback that helps us to understand our impact on another person.

Will this increase in knowledge also help to develop the individual's understanding of her action and reaction to patients who may be having difficulty coming to terms with a redefinition of self from independent to dependent? This requires an analysis not just of knowledge in terms of generalising neutral facts to the subjective human experience, but also of the nurse's own thoughts, feeling and behaviours.

stereotype

a form of cultural shorthand; shared knowledge or information about an object or event

■ Chapter Summary

This chapter attempts to explain why it is important for nurses to have an understanding of the self. It covers issues of the self concept and its development, self-awareness, stress, attitudes and prejudice.

Nurses need to have an understanding of the self in order to enable a greater understanding of the people for whom they care. A knowledge of the self will promote empathy by a growth in self-awareness and an insight into the factors that may threaten the self concept, such as stress and prejudice. By understanding our own motivations for behaviour, our own responses to stress, the origins of attitudes and prejudices we will better understand those of the people for whom we care.

● Test Yourself!

1. Define the self concept.

2. What is the difference between being self-aware and being self-conscious?

3. Can you define stress?

4. List the factors that may modify the impact of stress.

5. What are attitudes?

6. Why is it important for nurses to have an understanding of attitude change?

7. What are some of the factors in the nurse–patient relationship that contribute to attitude change?

▓ References

Atkinson, R., Atkinson, R., Smith E. and Bem, D. (1993) *Introduction to Psychology*, 11th edn. Harcourt Brace Jovanovich, Fort Worth, TX.

Baron, R. and Byrne, D. (1997) *Social Psychology*, 8th edn. Allyn & Bacon, Boston.

Brooks-Gun, J. and Paikoff, R.L. (1992) Changes in self feelings during the transition towards adolescence. In McGurk, H. (ed.) *Childhood Social Development, Contemporary Perspectives*. LEA, London.

Cobb, S. (1976) Social support as a moderator of life stress. *Psychosomatic Medicine* **38**: 300–14.

Cohen, S. and Hoberman, H.M. (1983) Positive life events and social supports as buffers of life change stress. *Journal of Applied Social Psychology* **13**: 99–125.

Cox, T. (ed.) (1978) *Stress*. Macmillan – now Palgrave Macmillan, London.

Cox, T. and McKay, C. (1978) Stress at work. In Cox, T. (ed.) *Stress*. Macmillan – now Palgrave Macmillan, London.

Erikson, E. (1959) *Identity and the Life Cycle*. International University Press, London.

Gordon, C. (1968) Self concept: configurations of content. In Gordon, C. and Gergen, K.J. (eds) *The Self in Social Interaction*, Vol. I: *Classic Contemporary Perspectives*. John Wiley & Sons, New York.

Holmes, T. and Rahe, R. (1967) The Social Readjustment Rating Scale. *Journal of Psychosomatic Research* **11**: 213–18.

Humphrey, N. (1984) *Consciousness Regained: Chapters in the Development of Mind*. Oxford University Press, Oxford.

Kobasa, S. (1979) Stressful life events, personality and health. An inquiry into hardiness. *Journal of Personality and Social Psychology* **37**: 1–11.

Luft, J. and Ingham, H. (1955) *The Johari Window: A Graphic Model for Interpersonal Relationships*. National Press, New York.

Maslow, A. (1968) *Toward a Psychology of Being*. Van Nostrand Rheinhold, New York.

Mischel, W. (1986) *Introduction to Personality*, 4th edn. Holt, Rinehart & Winston, Fort Worth, TX.

Montemeyer, R. and Eisen, M. (1977) The development of self conception from childhood to adolescence. *Development Psychology* **13**(4): 314–19.

Pervin, L. (1984) *Personality: Theory and Research*, 4th edn. John Wiley & Sons, London.

Oliver, M.B. and Hyde, J.S. (1993) Gender differences in sexuality: a meta analysis. *Psychological Bulletin* **114**: 29–51.

Rawlinson, J. (1990) Self awareness: conceptual influences, contribution to nursing, and approaches to attainment. *Nurse Education Today* **10**: 111–17.

Rentsch, J.R. and Heffner, T.S. (1994) Assessing self concept: analysis of Gordon's coding scheme using 'Who am I?' responses. *Journal of Social Behaviour and Personality* **9**(1): 283–300.

Rogers, C. (1959) A theory of therapy, personality and interpersonal relationships as developed in the client centred framework. In Koch, S. (ed.) *Psychology: A Study of Science*, Vol 3: *Formulations of the Person and the Social Context*. McGraw-Hill, New York.

Selye, H. (1980) The stress concept today. In Kutash, I.L, Schlesinger, L.B. et al. (eds) *Handbook on Stress and Anxiety*. Jossey-Bass, San Francisco.

Watson, D. and Clark, L.A. (1984) Negative affectivity: the disposition to experience aversive emotional states. *Psychological Bulletin* **96**: 465–90.

Chapter

Reflective Practice

13

Contents

Learning outcomes

This chapter seeks to enable you to gain familiarity with the key features of reflective practice. Specifically, you should become aware that reflective practice is not an isolated phenomenon but a process designed to assist us to learn from what we do, gaining knowledge and experience, not from conventional sources, such as textbooks, journals and study days, but from the richest source of learning – practice itself. At the end of the chapter, you should be able to:

- Identify sources and types of knowledge, and their potential shortcomings in the nurse education setting

- Contrast the media image of nurses against the reality

- Define reflective practice and its contribution to nursing practice

- Identify and utilise reflection-*in*- and -*on*-action

- Contrast ritualistic and reflective practice

- Formulate and use critical incident analysis as a means of reflection

- Identify the place that experience plays in developing knowledge

■ Discuss how reflection can influence learning in the practice setting.

Each theme within the chapter offers reflective activities to enhance the learning experience, some offering suggested responses for the activities. These are far from exhaustive, so record your own answers in a notebook in order to enhance your own reflective skills.

■ Reflection – Seeing Ourselves as Others See Us?

Students entering nursing today will naturally encounter many new, seemingly alien, concepts and experiences. They will frequently have entered with a ready-prepared mind-set of what will confront them and the role they will be expected to play. Many people in our society, and indeed those starting nursing, harbour stereotyped images of what nursing involves and what nurses do, but one has to become ill or actually nurse to truly see nursing at first hand. The majority of people do not, however, nurse or become ill, so most remain in ignorance of the true nature and realities of nursing. A distorted, idealised image of nursing and nurses, possibly perpetuated by the media, frequently remains unchallenged.

Few conversations with actual or potential clients will proceed very far without evidence of the stereotypical nurse image emerging, perhaps through traditional associations with activities such as temperature-taking, fevered-brow-mopping, back-rubbing and, sadly, within our seemingly elimination-fixated culture, even dealing with the ubiquitous bedpans and enemas. Perhaps those indefinable epithets of kind, dedicated, vocational, caring or even angelic will be applied. Thankfully, all these are far from reality and now hopelessly outdated with the emergence of today's research- and evidence-guided practitioner.

Students come from this lay-conceptual environment and can harbour similar anticipatory images of their perceived role, possibly originating years before. None of us will have escaped childhood without at least one encounter with a small girl proudly sporting her first 'little nurse' costume, complete with gaudily coloured stethoscope, thermometer and fob-watch. Nursing recruitment campaigns, even in recent years, have perilously focused on such question-able imagery.

On entry into nursing, conflict and dissonance can often result when the reality fails to meet the expectation. Once in the clinical setting, students strive to make sense of the maze of alien activities, roles and terminology encountered. They frequently attempt to understand it all by striving to fit the newly encoun-tered reality to the previously anticipated public image. As a result, practice can

CONNECTIONS
Chapter 15 offers a detailed explanation of the concept of professional socialisation.

CONNECTIONS
Chapter 12 offers an explanation of stereotype.

CONNECTIONS
Chapter 12 explains cognitive dissonance.

become hesitant, rigid and unimaginative. Unthinking task orientation is frequently the most comfortable approach as this often best fits the image they believe to be accurate. Such a haven offers security not only to students. Even for veteran practitioners, Street (1991) observes, survival involves many nurses, midwives and health visitors switching to autopilot, attempting to meet increasing demands by mechanistic practices. Perhaps reluctantly, thoughtful, imaginative, individualised care is not valued as time-economical but is seen more as diverting the practitioner from 'getting the work done'.

Melia (1987), citing Menzies (1960), explains that resorting to routine or ritual is the most common way of coping with stretched resources. Dividing patient care into an array of disjointed, routine tasks is a means of protecting the nurse from the pressures of work. Naturally, the holistic needs of clients are not met, but the carer achieves solace by striving to maintain expert performance, unfortunately, however, only of routines and tasks.

At first glance, this may appear to paint a rather bleak picture of nursing, but it is not meant to. Numerous exciting initiatives have addressed many of these traditional problems. Not least of these are the establishment of the patient allocation and primary nursing approaches to care. Such initiatives are laudable, and students working in such progressive environments are fortunate. Few students will, however, be so lucky as to work within such enlightened practice settings in *every* clinical placement. It is when we are less fortunate that the above propositions will, unfortunately, be all too familiar. On these occasions, reflection can offer a lifeline towards achieving more meaningful practice and learning, even if nurses are compelled to work within a task-orientated care environment.

■ Reflection – Thoughtful Practice

When considering mechanistic approaches to care, most thinking students will immediately realise the flaws. By addressing only the immediate tasks, as such systems do, the work may seem to get done and the routine tasks completed, but by failing to consider care thoughtfully and critically, *individualised* patient needs are not met. This is because it seems to make life easier to standardise the care given. Everyone receives the same, irrespective of need, and the resulting care demands little thought that might interfere with the primary purpose of finishing the work on time.

Does, however, detached, unthinking care really save time, energy and resources? Enlightened practitioners would immediately be dubious of any form of battery nursing. Routine-driven, standardised care can superficially appear to get the work done faster, but it ignores one essential fact: it frequently results in the repetition of unnecessary procedures.

Activity 1

Reflect on your experiences of the stereotypical images of nurses and their work. How are we seen by the media, in films and so on?

Consider your personal impressions before entering nursing of what you would encounter and what the work would involve. Think about the advice and comments of parents, friends and so on when you announced your decision to enter nursing.

Jot your thoughts down, and, in retrospect, consider how accurate they actually were and whether they truly prepared you for the reality of nursing.

CONNECTIONS

Chapter 1 cautions on the merits and pitfalls of common approaches to managing care.

CONNECTIONS

Chapter 2 discusses
the healthy
partnership.

CONNECTIONS

Chapter 4 covers
the imperatives of
meeting nutritional
needs.

CONNECTIONS

Chapter 16
contextualises the
notion of quality in
clinical interventions.

Activity
2

Think about the last
week you spent in
practice and
critically assess the
care you were
involved in.

Make a list of the
care interactions in
which you were
involved that
required little or no
thought. From this
list, try to identify
those which could
be seen as
'ritualistic'. Now
consider those
occasions when
time allowed you
to sit and talk to
your client, perhaps
giving advice or
reassurance, or just
explaining their
care in your own
way.

Not everyone will actually *need* 4-hourly clinical observations, daily fluid balance monitoring, hourly neurological observations, preoperative shaving and a daily bed bath. Moreover, the time spent in giving this unnecessary care could be better utilised in undertaking *quality* interventions with those who really need them, which result in more clinically effective and lasting outcomes.

Put another way, the time saved by *not* bed-bathing the whole of bay 6 before coffee-break could be utilised in, for example, giving precise dietary advice to elderly, postoperative patients. *We* may understand how vital dietary protein is in assisting the healing process, but does the client? It takes time to educate or re-educate such clients, like most people socialised over years into fixed dietary patterns. Yet for their fullest and quickest recovery, additional and possibly expensive dietary changes or supplements will be needed, and clients need to understand this fully in order to comply.

Information-giving or re-education requires time, skill and patience on the part of knowledgeable carers. If lifestyle changes are to be successfully achieved, the new information needs to be carefully and empathically packaged and sold. It is, however, the courageous nurse, let alone student, who has the audacity to sit down and quietly educate the client when what is perceived as *real* work is going on around. Despite high ideals such as supernumerary status for students, many will still be pressured by their peers into conformity with outdated working practices.

Quality interactions such as patient education are time-consuming and intellectually demanding, seditious concepts to those who recognise only physical labour as having any real, intrinsic value in the care setting. Can we then be surprised by the increasing number of media scandals illuminating the plight of malnourished, dehydrated or similarly neglected clients? Management responses to such crises frequently involve expensive, knee-jerk reactions – changes in catering arrangements, dietetic consultations, even another charter or mission statement – whereas in reality, all that is probably necessary is the fostering of a climate or work ethic that cultivates the provision of 'thoughtful, quality nursing'.

This thoughtful element, nurturing the desire and creating the opportunity to provide and modify care in terms of the individual rather than the task, forms the embryonic roots of reflective practice. When being thoughtful, even critical, about our practice, we start to consider not just what we are doing but how it is being done, why it is being done in this way rather than another, and even whether it needs doing at all. Just because it was done yesterday, is it still needed or justifiable today? Has the client's condition changed or improved, altering his or her care needs? Has new evidence emerged that now challenges a care activity or procedure? Through a thoughtful, questioning process, the minute aspects of care are repeatedly re-analysed to confirm their continuing validity. Without such a reflective approach, task-orientated practice would dominate.

Jarvis (1992) cautions that all care activities constantly run the risk of degenerating into habitualised, presumptive and ritualised actions. Superficial, mechanical approaches should have no place in an activity as sensitive as nursing, dependent as it is on the quality of its interpersonal interactions. People are unique and respond best when treated as individuals in a unique and humanistic manner. Even though many nursing actions may be repeatedly performed, they must always be individually planned and monitored. A change in a client's condition, either deterioration or improvement, can be subtle and easily missed when masked by rigid adherence to an unthinking ritual.

Danger exists when people start to be just viewed as cases, virtually becoming dehumanised by their carers. When this happens, clients and patients run the risk of being seen as merely the passive recipients of care, and the danger of care moving from the carefully planned to the 'taken-for-granted' is increased.

Palmer et al. (1994) suggest that reflective practice has emerged as a means of overcoming the potential alienation of nurses from their clients brought about by today's 'high-speed' care. Although they justifiably caution that reflection should not be perceived as a universal panacea for all the ills of nursing, it does offer practitioners a means by which to interrogate their care, thus avoiding the pitfall of Jarvis's presumptive and ritualised practice. For the student, reflection offers the tools for meaningful learning within the practice setting. The concept of reflection as a means of enhancing practice is, however, nothing new, perhaps first being considered as early as the 1930s by Dewey (1933). Many others since have contributed to its understanding, among them Habermas (1977), Van Manen (1977), Mezirow (1981), Schön (1983), Kolb (1984) and Boud et al. (1985).

Perhaps anticipating the notorious nursing impasse in relating theory to practice, Dewey postulated that, in order for theory to be linked to practice, the process of utilising experience by reflection should be adopted. Dewey contrasted routine and reflective human action. Routine actions he saw as being driven by impulse, tradition and authority. We can perhaps risk drawing parallels here with the disciplined origins of nursing, for example, within the religious orders and the military; more recently, this might be applied to the traditionalist, media images of rigid nursing hierarchies. Visions of tyrannical, matronly figures and obediently compliant student nurses quickly emerge. Within such 'routinised' actions, everyday practice is taken for granted. Providing the routines have been followed, the outcomes can be safely assumed. Process is subordinated to product, the end justifying the means.

Conversely, Dewey (1933) defines reflective action as an:

Activity

3

Now challenge the two approaches in Activity 2. Which gave you most satisfaction? Which afforded the most learning? Which was directly most beneficial to your client? Pause and reflect on your conclusions.

CONNECTIONS

Chapter 1 provides a fuller exploration of task-orientated or allocated care.

CONNECTIONS

Chapter 11 explores the subtle and often delicate constructs of therapeutic interaction.

CONNECTIONS

Chapter 16 outlines a definition of holism.

CONNECTIONS

Chapter 16 offers a detailed explanation of the theory–practice debate.

active, persistent and careful consideration of any belief or supposed knowledge, in the light of the grounds that support it, and the further consequences to which it leads.

Essentially, reflective action demands an open mind, responsibility and the commitment to consider all the possibilities and implications, not only to achieve an objective, but also to seek learning from the experience, thus enhancing future practice.

The Reflective Process for Lifelong Learning

Reflection is:

> [the] process of internally examining and exploring an issue of concern, triggered by an experience, which creates and clarifies meaning in terms of self, and which results in a changed conceptual perspective. (Boyd and Fales, 1983)

> a process of reviewing an experience of practice in order to better describe, analyse and evaluate, and so inform learning about practice. (Boud et al., 1985)

CONNECTIONS

Chapters 2 and 9 also touch on spirituality.

When the term 'reflection' is used, it can often evoke almost spiritual connotations, but in practice reflection should be seen as a learning tool and not merely a random, passive process. Rather than being a form of quiet contemplation, it is very much active. It can be learned and taught, and, within reason, controlled and guided. In practice, it should be regarded as a *conscious* process, not happening automatically but with a definite purpose in response to an experience.

In nursing, reflection seeks to identify the true value and meaning of our actions in order to quantify, augment, enhance or discard them, and to enable us to replicate them appropriately to their best effect in future interactions. Each situation reflected on must be treated as a unique event if the maximum learning is to be gained. Nurses constantly meet unique and challenging situations yet frequently fail to acknowledge them as learning opportunities essential to professional growth. Given the pace of today's practice, it becomes all too easy to lapse into presumptive or habitualised care.

Although the conditions we care for and the nursing care we give may frequently appear repetitive, they are for the client a new and unique experience. Unlike nurses, clients are not exposed to such events on a daily basis. When we lapse from viewing the experience from the client's perspective, we close down our ability to function empathically and thus stop interrogating what we do. Pain, anxiety, fear and ignorance become just detached descriptors for problems in the care plan rather than the very real human experiences that they are. When this happens, we are just a short step from becoming presumptive in our anticipation of the outcomes of our care.

CONNECTIONS

Chapter 11 gives a greater insight into the need for and nature of empathic understanding.

Berger and Luckman (1967) caution that, left unchecked, all human action is subject to habitualisation. They see human actions hierarchically (after Jarvis 1992):

1. *Creative/experimental actions:* new experiences that are being worked out in practice.
2. *Repetitive acts:* acts that are thoughtfully repeated during the normal process of living.
3. *Presumptive acts:* actors presume upon the situation and its outcomes and act almost unthinkingly.
4. *Ritualism:* where participants mindlessly go through the motions.
5. *Alienation:* when the need for the action has become lost through mindless repetition, thus losing its purpose.

In habitual or ritualised care, there is frequently an expectation that the client will conform to a prescribed outcome, and it is not uncommon for clients to be penalised when they fail to do so.

In her seminal work, Stockwell (1984) provided an insight into this sinister side of caring and where it can lead. She gives disturbing examples of the rewards and deterrents that carers will use to impose clients' conformity to the care regimen. Individual needs are subtly suppressed in deference to the need for compliance and order. Yet, in reality, when the views of the client are not fully explored, an essential component of realistic, effective care-planning is missed. The resulting conformity is achieved by a power-coercive imperative rather than the much more desirable normative-re-educative approach. This is only a short step from anticipating or assuming outcomes, carers possibly going to extraordinary lengths to ensure compliance.

At its simplest, a presumptive interchange might be:

Mr Brown, you can't possibly still be in pain, you only had your pain-killers an hour ago. Mr Wilson and Mr Adams had exactly the same operation and analgesia as you, and they're not complaining.

CONNECTIONS

Chapters 1 and 6 proffer much more desirable approaches to pain assessment.

In this case, the strong signal being given to Mr Brown is to *conform*! Such a scenario might seem far fetched, but it will nonetheless be familiar to many. We all know what we should do, but when we work in an ethos that forces us to

Chart 13.1 ● Atkins and Murphy's (1994) reflective framework

- Be aware of uncomfortable feelings or thoughts
- Describe the situation, including thoughts and feelings
- Analyse the feelings and knowledge relevant to the situation
- Evaluate the relevance of the knowledge
- Identify any new learning that has occurred
- Put it into action in a new situation

ration our resources, coercion to comply can seem justifiable as the most time-economical means of providing care. Conversely, when we nurse reflectively, we maintain responsiveness to the *actual* rather than the *assumed* needs of the client.

No-one is suggesting that we try to reflect on each and every situation or event we encounter: reflection is a demanding and often disturbing activity, and we would soon burn out. Instead, a simple commitment to developing the skills is enough. If we are clear on the advantages that reflection can bring to our practice, there should follow a readiness to develop our reflective skills. Over time and with practice, the reflective process gets easier and the skills essential to its use become integrated into what we do. We need, however, to be clear on the potential benefits. Reflection on our care opens the mind, ensuring flexibility and creativity, rather than merely making our interventions fit predetermined expectations and assumptions.

Although reflection can frequently be spontaneous, a structured development of the relevant skills is much more desirable. Atkins and Murphy (1994) offer the reflective framework shown in Chart 13.1. A closer exploration of the stages of this process will help to illustrate the nature and potential of reflection.

Be aware of uncomfortable feelings or thoughts

It is all too easy to coast along in our practice, frequently oblivious to the need for minor adjustments or changes. Left unchecked, presumptive and anticipatory action can follow. Conversely, when in tune with our actions, we will often detect a shift from that which is confidently and competently known into areas that are new, untested or uncertain.

Such a deviation may generate feelings of insecurity, our actions no longer being guided by what is implicitly known through teaching or experience. Outcomes may seem risky, uncontrollable and unpredictable, and a sense of uncertainty results. Boyd and Fales (1983) speak of this as being 'a sense of inner discomfort', whereas Schön (1983) calls it 'the experience of surprise'. It is these sensations which best act as triggers for reflection, as it is on such occasions that the potential for learning from a situation is at its highest. The experience need not be unpleasant or apply merely to negative situations: heightened awareness can equally be triggered by a positive or fulfilling event, such as being praised or thanked for our care. The secret of meaningful reflection is to recognise this sense of heightened awareness as a learning opportunity holding great potential for professional growth. Whether these are good or bad experiences, the practitioner and certainly the student determined to develop reflective skills should not allow such events to pass unexplored.

CONNECTIONS

Chapter 12 provides more information on self-awareness.

There is a great temptation, especially for students, to assume that most events met in practice are common and encountered again and again as we progress through our placements, but in reality every care situation is a one off or has aspects unique to its construction. If the maximum learning is not immediately gained from every situation, an invaluable opportunity for improving knowledge, professional growth and insight is lost, possibly never to be repeated. The next similar opportunity may lie far in the future, perhaps when the nurse is qualified – and it may then demand immediate, *accountable* action. Sadly, responses then may be delayed or inadequate because the opportunity was not taken to learn from it when it was first encountered, perhaps years before.

Care interactions, successful or otherwise, cannot be taken for granted. We grow professionally only by considering why events went well or badly, and not simply by accepting their outcome as being inevitable. To do this, we must be in tune with our feelings and recognise the occasions on which we experience doubt or uncertainty as being powerful triggers for learning through reflection and not, as frequently happens, as occasions when we must dig our heels in and hope to bluff it out.

Reflective and professional practitioners are those who welcome every opportunity to test, analyse and interrogate their practice in the pursuit of excellence, currency and validity, or better still, to have their practice appraised and challenged by their peers, even if they are junior. This holds the truest potential for professional growth and nurtures the seeds of clinical supervision.

Describe the situation

If the maximum learning is to be gained from any event, it is essential that every single aspect of it must be examined. It is not enough just to gain a superficial overview: all of its characteristics, even the most sensitive and disturbing, need to be explored.

CONNECTIONS

Chapter 12 offers more on the development, influences and challenges associated with attitude and prejudice.

In nursing, where all of the extremes of life and the human condition are encountered, this can frequently be a painful process. In illustrating the student's difficulties in reflecting critically, Palmer et al. (1994) speak of the plethora of emotions to which practice exposes us: despair, fear, suffering, disgust, distress and even ecstatic relief. Each should be analysed if the maximum potential for growth and learning is to be achieved. Williams (1996) suggests that such growth may emerge as problems are discovered, solutions proposed or attitudes, assumptions and prejudices challenged.

Analyse the feelings and knowledge relevant to the situation

The critical interrogation of a practice situation will require meaning to be drawn from a variety of domains if reflection is to be maximised. Such knowledge may already be possessed or, alternatively, the situation may prompt its being sought. For a student reflecting on a challenging care interaction, this may mean reading up on the salient features or seeking advice from a senior colleague, mentor or tutor. This facilitates the opportunity for shared exploration, airing anxieties and testing perceptions.

This process of analysing an experience is central to the quality and accuracy of reflection. Through it, attitudes, even prejudices, that might otherwise obstruct the process of healthy and impartial reflection can be confronted and overcome. It is this interrogation of our feelings that determines how we should respond to events, how we can learn from them and what personal changes will result, be these perceptual or behavioural. Boud et al. (1985) suggest that this self-interrogation process has four distinct features:

1. *Association:* ideas and feelings arising from the experience being reflected on being tested against perceptions from previous events, experience or attitudes.
2. *Integration:* savouring the information and knowledge, and identifying links between different parts.
3. *Validation:* checking to ensure that impressions emerging from the reflective experience are legitimate.
4. *Appropriation:* once the validity of the new knowledge or perception has been verified, assimilating the knowledge or belief into one's own value system.

Evaluate the relevance of the knowledge

After analysis, a clearer understanding of the key features of the event or phenomenon should emerge. As stated above, this may involve a change in perception or behaviour in anticipation of our future management of a similar situation. Equally, however, the outcome may corroborate a previously held view. Thus, the reflective process tests a belief or personal 'given', validating its authenticity.

In a practising profession such as nursing, testing the currency of belief is healthy as it forces the questioning of one's professional values, a process of critical analysis. This is a central feature of all adult learning. We learn best when we are made to rationalise rather than dogmatically accept some long unchallenged concept, perhaps sometimes even despite its being awarded validity by having achieved the lofty status of a competence. Palmer et al. (1994) see such challenging as the emergence of humanistic ideology in clinical practice, rightly confronting other traditional outcomes of learning. It acknowledges the primacy of the *process* rather than the *product* of learning.

The achievement of learning from a reflective episode is, however, not the end of the process: the learning experience is not complete until its relevance has been weighed against its implications for our practice. When we reflect and learn from a new event, we store that learning in our professional armoury for use in a future setting. It may never occur, but the mere process of reflective learning will have brought about a dynamic reappraisal of our beliefs – the essence of professionalism.

CONNECTIONS

Chapter 12 proffers an explanation of belief and belief systems.

Identify any new learning that has occurred

Even when learning has been achieved, the process continues. It is possible that the reflective event might have only partially equipped us for practice. The process of learning is not static: it must be continually refined and polished. This may demand further action on the part of the reflective practitioner, for example evaluation by a trusted mentor, further reading or plans to undertake an appropriate continuing education programme or study day. All of these and more may be necessary in maximising and consolidating the learning.

Put it into action in a new situation

Like it or not, the process explored here has in reality illustrated a reflective journey stimulated by real practice experiences. Like any journey, however, either it can be used to achieve a greater understanding of the scenery passed through or, conversely, the richness of its staging points can be allowed to erode. The journey's end is very much the learning we have achieved, but this becomes redundant if we do not act upon it and allow it to influence our future practice. One journey along this path will never be enough if we are to become seasoned reflective travellers, but it does get easier. Like all travel, every time we wander along a route, the more familiar and less threatening the terrain becomes.

Activity

4

The reflective framework (see Chart 13.1 above) passed through six stages. Choose a significant learning event from your own recent practice and try to relate it to the framework, if possible identifying each of the stages.

■ Reflection – Taking Control

By now, you should be starting to see the potential advantages that reflection brings not only to your practice, but also, more importantly, to your perceptions of learning. Several authors (Dewing, 1990; Jarvis, 1992; Coutts-Jarman, 1993) have stressed the importance of reflection as a learning tool. Today's students, because of their supernumerary status, enjoy a particular opportunity to develop in this way. Driscoll (1994) points out that it is, in contrast, a sad reality that traditionally trained nurses were not routinely encouraged to question their practice. Reflection offers a means of adding structure to our questioning, a commodity to be highly prized in the culture of nursing (Powell, 1992). Perhaps bound by traditional, authoritative perceptions of low status, student nurses still, however, frequently enter training programmes unaware that they can now enjoy such freedom in modifying the ways in which they learn.

During their education programme, junior nurses frequently spend much of their time seeking 'rule-book' solutions. This, the technical-rational imperative, presupposes that there is always a prescriptive answer to everything. For many years, nurses bound themselves to the notorious Procedure Book, which went far in perpetuating this restrictive, unthinking approach to professional practice, but similar current professional issues will still be familiar to nurses today. Running parallel with moves to reduce junior doctors' hours, nurses are once again looking for rules to guide what they can do. If we are not careful, new, expanded roles may once again restrict the activities of professional practice to an array of carefully compartmentalised skills.

Few could argue with the necessity for policing and auditing one's practice against defined protocols and standards, but practitioners would be well advised to break away from self-imposed boundaries as these can, in reality, generally control only the macro-elements of nursing. No protocol can ever be devised that guides our practice in the micro-interactions of expert, professional nursing. Schön's (1987) much-quoted 'swampy lowlands' of professional practice are where nursing's most intricate and complex decisions must be made. Often messy and confusing, they frequently defy resolution by formal protocols or traditional types of knowledge. The United Kingdom Central Council for Nursing, Midwifery and Health Visiting's (UKCC) *Scope of Professional Practice* went some way towards offering guidance for professional decision-making without the need for too many defined rules (UKCC, 1992). It is with each individual practitioner that the potential for professional artistry and growth truly lies.

In the course of our work, we are frequently confronted by problems for which no solutions exist in the literature or through formal guidelines. On these occasions, we are expected to 'think on our feet'. All practitioners will readily agree that nursing practice frequently takes place without the benefit of true evidence. But, although the refinement of evidence should always continue, its temporary absence need not hold any anxieties. Providing we critically appraise what we do through reflection, we are likely to remain safe even in 'the swampy lowlands'.

Benner (1984) alludes to the intuitive characteristic of nursing as being the bench-mark of expert practice. Nurses accrue clinical knowledge over the course of their careers yet lose track of the exact circumstances in which that knowledge was gained. Benner further refers to the frustration that many expert nurses frequently feel when trying to pass this expertise on to their students. So much of it has been obtained from the myriad of sources to which individual practitioners have been exposed over their careers that it is impossible to isolate the exact circumstances in which the knowledge was obtained. Polanyi (1967) refers to this as 'tacit knowing'.

Mentors naturally try to guide students using sound, theoretically correct sources, but they are frequently left frustrated. The exact mechanisms underlying their expertise are complex and unique to each individual. Everyone learns differently, assimilating and distilling the experience of their practice in their own way. Such a process cannot be replicated on demand, as its theoretical constructs, and the conclusions drawn from them, may have been lost in the mists of time. The frustration all too frequently results in an authoritarian dismissal such as 'Because it is' or 'That's the way we do it around here' or 'Sister prefers it this way', sadly all too familiar to most students. Both parties are left frustrated, and potentially rich learning opportunities are left incomplete. Mentors feel they have failed students in not being able to deliver a more professionally robust response, and students feel injured because they have been 'fobbed off' with something dangerously close to an authoritarian demand for unquestioning compliance.

So if students are to avoid confrontations and frustration in attempting to gain the maximum information to facilitate their learning, how can progress be made? It is here that reflection truly comes into its own. Learning nursing can be achieved providing we realise that it is not the *quantity* of nursing knowledge that is at issue but the *quality*, not the *breadth* but the *depth*. The distillation of this is within the grasp of every student.

Few could argue that, when learning something new, it is best to learn every aspect of it in order to gain the most complete interpretation. Yet how many of us truly do so? The impetus is quite often merely to gain a cursory familiarity and to hope that the rest will somehow fall into place or take care of itself. When we buy a new TV set, video or hi-fi, for example, how many of us can truthfully say that we read the instruction manual from cover to cover before plugging it in? Few of us have the time or the inclination to be so thorough.

Activity 5

Think back on your last week in practice and identify a simple procedure in which you were involved that demanded little thought. Remember that this care may not have appeared 'routine' to the client. Identify the domain of care involved. Was it:

● Physical or mechanical (psychomotor) – performing a procedure
● Psychological – knowledge, understanding
● Social – implications for family, significant others, work, home
● Emotional or spiritual – fear, anxiety, relief.

Activity 6

Refer back to Activity 5 and reflect on the implications for the client, identifying what additional care might be given related to the remaining domains. Finally, consider how you might next approach a similar care activity, meeting all of the care domains.

Learning nursing can be similar for many students. There appears to be so much to learn that it frequently seems sufficient merely to gain a working knowledge in order to 'survive' in the clinical setting without drawing attention to our 'newness'.

Most nurses can cite an example from their training of when the TV analogy applied. Many will remember the early days of a first clinical placement, having been exposed to the vagaries of the sphygmomanometer and blood-pressure taking. What agonies such a simple procedure produced! For most, all that seemed to matter was that they appeared proficient, yet a simple clinical measurement seemed to take on the intensity of complex brain surgery.

But even when the technique was apparently eventually mastered, how many could honestly have accurately recited in full the implications of peripheral resistance or cardiac output for the reading, let alone have listed the psychological, non-verbal cues to watch out for during the procedure? These might have drawn attention to the patients' acute anxiety at the possibility of suffering hypertension, the implications of this for their lifestyle and their need for reassurance. To be perceived as acting expertly, one would naturally hope to be able to link all aspects of practice: the pathophysiological, the psychosocial and the nursing characteristics. Yet, sadly, many are merely satisfied with obtaining the reading accurately and continuing to replicate it ad infinitum. Thus, much of the richness of a potential learning experience in seemingly simple practice activities can remain underdeveloped.

Now do Activity 5. Remember that all care, regardless of the domain within which it takes place, has implications for all the other domains if if it is to be achieved to its maximum potential and, of greater importance to the student, if the maximum learning is to be achieved. When you have completed Activity 5, move on to Activity 6.

Activity 5 required you to think of the widest implications of your care. This is where the maximum learning from even the simple nursing events lies. Your mentor or supervisor may find time to tell you the basics of the care to be carried out, the quantity of learning, but you control its breadth – the quality. It is in this extension of each learning event that reflection offers the best opportunity for expanding knowledge and professional growth. Jarvis (1992) suggests that reflection should cause practitioners to 'problematise' their practice, thus constantly extending the knowledge, skills and attitudes demanded by the event.

■ Types of Reflection

When incorporating reflective processes into our learning and practice, it is prudent once again to stress that reflection is an active rather than a merely passive or random process. As Jarvis (1992) cautions, reflective practice is not simply thoughtful practice. Furthermore, reflection is not a unidimensional event but manifests itself in many different forms.

The much-popularised work of Schön (1983, 1987) acknowledges the reality that much in professional practice fails to conform to the positivist, technical-rationalism of traditional, professional education. As Palmer et al. (1994) interpret, that approach is suited best to problem-solving in the set-piece, contrived world of the laboratory rather than the complex, urgent and often surprising arena of professional nursing practice.

As we discussed earlier, much of our practice is implicit and, albeit familiar, often impossible to describe in words. Even more frustrating to the positivist is that much of what we do is so complex that it defies rigid control. To attempt to control it would eradicate the responsiveness of the interaction and with it much of its richness. Yet much of the effectiveness of our care goes unheralded simply *because* it is so complex and geared to the uniqueness of the moment. As such, it is difficult to replicate our actions when a similar situation occurs in a future interaction, and we once again risk resorting to unthinking ritualisation.

Reflective practice is seen by many as a means of encapsulating the 'essence of practice'. Linked to what we do, Schön postulates that reflection should be operationalised at two points – during and after an intervention – his much-cited reflection-in-action, and reflection-on-action (Schön, 1983).

reflective practice
professional practice guided by structured reflection on feelings, experience and empathy in order to make practice robust and enhance learning

Reflection-in-action

Reflection-in-action is the process whereby the nurse identifies learning in a new situation as it is encountered and thinks about it while still acting. This is the 'active reflection' that Darbyshire (1993) describes as 'thinking on your feet' or 'keeping your wits about you' rather than working on autopilot. It not only involves thinking about one's practices as they are actualised, but also demands a quantity of preparatory thinking – Van Manen's 'anticipatory reflection' (Van Manen, 1977). This relates to the manner in which the care situation is approached, making a tacit comparison with previous experience to ensure that we are not already equipped in some way to deal with what is being met.

reflection-in-action
reflection on an event as it is being experienced

It is during the reflection-in-action phase that Atkins and Murphy (1994) see practitioners appraising their range of skills and experiences, and, if appropriate, adapting or modifying them to meet the new situation. As practitioners move towards expert practitioner status by the accumulation of experience, it is this examination of our practice that Cervero (1988) sees as the true artistry of nursing, described by Powell (1989) as 'flexible experimentation' in problem-solving.

Reflection-on-action

CONNECTIONS

*Chapter 16,
covering nursing
praxis, can be read
to round off your
coverage of
reflection-in- and
-on-action.*

reflection-on-action
_____

in-depth reflection on an
event after it has finished

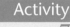

Activity

7

During your next
clinical practice,
identify an occasion
on which you have
to force yourself to
reflect while
carrying out a
nursing activity. As
this proceeds,
consider how it is
going and how it
relates to your
knowledge and
beliefs.

Afterwards, ask
yourself: How did it
go? How did I get
there? Could I have
done it differently?
What other
knowledge would
have been helpful?

critical incident analysis
_____

a learning technique
that breaks an event
down into its main
components for the
purposes of reflective
analysis

It is naturally not enough to content oneself with being in tune with one's actions simply as they unfold. There is perhaps too much of a tendency to look back on our actions in a matter-of-fact manner, especially when they have been successful. Sensing that an event has gone well obviously infers that similar situations have occasionally gone badly.

It could be argued that, when a nursing action has gone especially well, this is not the time for smug satisfaction but should instead create more of an imperative to extract exactly which features caused it to be so successful. If one can distil the quintessential features that led to its success – one's approach, mood, knowledge-base, experience and so on – something very meaningful has been gained that can be taken forward into the next, similar care intervention. In every sense, it is this which will again truly constitute professional growth.

Greenwood (1993) describes **reflection-on-action** as a cognitive post mortem. Outcomes are reviewed in order to explore the approaches that the practitioner brought to the interaction, their degree of success and thus concrete evidence for adjustment, augmentation or even rejection. As Atkins and Murphy (1994) put it:

> reflection on action is a very necessary retrospective analysis and interpretation of practice in order to uncover the knowledge used and the accompanying feelings within a particular situation.

One should especially note the importance of feelings in this process, considering them as a stimulus or catalyst for further, deeper reflection – Boyd and Fale's (1983) 'sense of inner discomfort' and Schön's (1987) 'experience of surprise'.

■ Critical Incident Analysis

The value of reflective practice, and the positive influence it can have on learning, is hopefully becoming clearer. One technique that formally requires you to focus your attention on a practice event for reflective purposes is **critical incident analysis**. You may not have come across this process before, but it is rapidly growing as a reflective learning tool, not just in nursing, but in all fields of professional practice.

Crouch (1991) sees the critical incident as 'an observation or activity which was sufficiently complete in itself so as to permit inferences and predictions to be drawn from it'. If the maximum learning is to be gained, and/or a nursing activity validated, the activity must be subjected to further, formal analysis.

When significant events occur in our practice, be they positive or negative, the maximum learning is often denied because of their complexity. All of the salient features blend into one, and we are simply left with the outcome and any residual feelings on it. Critical incident analysis dissects the event into a 'snapshot in time'. It allows the exploration of just one aspect of the event, preferably the moment that determined its outcome and prompted our conclusions on it. The simplest, daily nursing activities can be subjected to this process, and, as Crouch (1991) suggests, the effects of care on our clients can be seen or interactions between us and our colleagues illuminated.

Parker et al. (1995) acknowledge the importance of meaningful reflection to the critical incident analysis. They advise using the process to focus on the experience (a parallel with Schön's reflection-on-action) and to identify one's feelings about it. The salient features should be documented, extrapolating which domains of learning were influenced or involved during the incident. Were they affective (emotions, values and attitudes), cognitive (knowledge, facts and givens) or psychomotor (practical skills)? Through such an analysis, the abstract concepts involved in complex nursing interventions can broken down into meaningful factors for use in future practice.

Examples of critical incidents and their analysis might help here.

Incident One

This incident took place in a psychiatric assessment unit in the small hours of a night duty and involved Deborah, a second-year mental health branch student. Her description of the incident is given in Casebox 13.1.

Analysis

The analysis is given in Deborah's own words.

My feelings

'On reflection, I realised I was completely out of my depth and had lost control of the situation. It further occurred to me that I had put myself at considerable risk and had possibly irretrievably alienated myself from John. This was *my* environment, not John's. How could I have been so arrogant as to believe that John, possibly feeling abandoned by society, should passively conform to its values and rules?

'I had allowed myself to let my perceptions of status alone control the situation, foolishly feeling I had the right to impose authority over him. I had been blinkered by my determination to stick to the rules. Most of all, I felt guilty that I had not shown the caring or empathy that might have helped John and prevented the situation from escalating.'

Casebox 13.1

John had been admitted during the previous day. He was a 50-year-old, homeless man with a psychiatric history and had suffered facial injuries following an assault while on the streets. I had had the opportunity to talk to John before the unit was settled for the night, and he had presented as a confused, lonely man, although he was reasonably calm and lucid.

At about 1 am, I got up from the nursing station in response to a noise in the unit and saw John smoking in a part of the ward designated as a no-smoking area. I approached him, advised him that he shouldn't be smoking there and asked him to put the cigarette out and return to bed. He did this without complaint.

About 2 hours later, I again became aware of movement in the same part of the ward and went to investigate. I found John once again smoking in the no-smoking area. Perhaps confident with my previous handling of the situation, I again, this time more forcefully, asked him to put the cigarette out and return to bed. It was then that I realised John was crying and starting to become more agitated. Not really knowing what to do next, I attempted to take the cigarette from him, at which point John physically pushed me away and became abusive. I was confused and frightened, realising I was in an isolated part of the unit and perhaps about to be physically assaulted.

John became progressively more abusive and agitated, but thankfully a trained member of staff came to investigate the disturbance and calmly managed to coax John to a ward annexe, where he calmed down; he eventually returned to bed.

The official view

'Although my trained colleagues applauded my alertness and readiness to respond to the situation, I was advised of the dangers of isolating myself with a disturbed patient without first seeking trained support.'

What have I learned?

'After discussion with my mentor, I felt clearer about the incident. I gained an invaluable insight into ways of dealing with disturbed psychiatric patients, particularly with regard to communication. I have sought more information from my tutor about the management of aggression, and have learned how important factors such as proximity, posture, eye contact, touch and voice tone are to interactions. Most of all, I've learned that it's all right to make mistakes. That, as a student, I learn from getting it wrong occasionally, providing I look back on the events objectively and carefully.'

Incident Two

This incident involved Alan, a child branch student on his first placement, an acute paediatric ward, and is described in Casebox 13.2.

Casebox 13.2

I had been on the ward for about 4 weeks. I'd had to think very hard about coming into nursing, but the time on the ward had convinced me I'd made the right decision. Furthermore, I'd found nursing children especially rewarding.

By the end of the first month, I'd found my feet and was beginning to feel more confident in my practice: taking more responsibility, voicing my opinions, suggesting changes in care regimes, that sort of thing. Acorn ward is brilliant, and the staff really encourage you. The work is not too taxing, and the children are in general not too ill, so not having been really stretched, I began to think I'd seen it all. Then **Timmy** came in.

Timmy was a loveable 3-year-old. He'd come up from A&E after suffering a pulled shoulder and was naturally very distressed. However, he soon quietened down when he was prescribed analgesia. The problem was, as I began to deduce, that the staff were a bit concerned about the circumstances of his injury. Something about the A&E staff not being happy with his mother's explanation. This was the first time I'd heard the term, 'non-accidental injury'.

Nothing was obvious. He seemed clean, well-dressed and cared for. However, though never previously admitted, Timmy had been seen in the A&E department on two or three other occasions, and this had set the alarm bells ringing.

My problem came when I met Timmy's mother, Tina. Although she seemed perfectly normal, albeit concerned for Timmy, I found myself unable to interact with her as comfortably as I normally do with other parents. Try as I might, I could hardly even make eye contact with her, and I even found I was almost spying on the woman. You know, watching her when she was with Timmy, yet pretending to be doing something else. I feel sure she must have noticed, as it must have been obvious that I was uneasy when she was about.

It all came to a head when I was helping Timmy with his supper. She volunteered to do it, but I made some excuse that it was better that I did it or something. She suddenly blew up, exclaiming, 'For God's sake, I'm not going to kill him!' She got very upset and accused me of treating her like a criminal. The awful thing is, I suspect I probably had been.

I was too embarrassed to go near her again, and naturally my confidence took a nose dive. Whenever Timmy needed care, I found some excuse to be doing something else.

The upshot was that the paediatricians and, I think, the social workers eventually decided that there was nothing suspicious about Timmy's injury. He has four other brothers and sisters, and they were all playing together when the injury happened. His mum, Tina, is a lone parent and can't be watching them all the time. The A&E staff were probably just being cautious.

It's amazing how rational you can be when the facts are known, but having alienated myself from the mother and having made her feel like a child abuser, I felt pretty wretched. It took all of my courage to go to work the next day, and it made me start to doubt my ability to continue with the course.

Analysis

Alan's analysis is given below.

My feelings

'I'd always considered myself to be quite open minded, without too many obvious prejudices. In this case, though, I'd allowed myself to be judgemental before all the facts were known. This had alienated me from Timmy and made his mother feel I was accusing her. Reflecting afterwards, there were so many clues I'd allowed myself to miss. There was obviously a genuine love between them. Timmy showed no signs of hesitation or concern with his mother. Despite obvious hardships, the children were clean, happy and well cared for.

'All right, there was some suspicion on admission, but nowhere near concrete enough for me to act in the way I did. Despite the pressures at home, the other children and so on, Tina still found some way to be with Timmy while he was in hospital. Hardly the action of an uncaring mother.

'After Timmy was discharged, I talked it over with my assessor. She started off by telling me how well I'd been doing, and even cited a couple of examples when I'd correctly used my initiative. She reassured me that, in circumstances like Timmy's, there is naturally an element of concern. But it is not for us, the staff, to pass judgement. On the contrary, alienating ourselves from the parents can be the worst thing if any further suspicious actions are to be observed. She was very understanding and reassured me that judgement gets better with experience. Considering I'd made such a fool of myself, her patient explanation and confirmation of my satisfactory progress helped to restore my confidence.'

What have I learned?

'From the incident, I've learned to think thoroughly before forming any opinion, even when there are apparent grounds for it. My assessor was right. If Timmy had been abused, what good would I have been to him by making it so obvious that I was suspicious of his mother. Even if she had been hurting him, it's a time for help and support not recrimination. I've resolved to learn more about non-accidental injury, and my tutor has arranged for me to spend a couple of days with the child protection team during my community placement. Most of all, it's made me grow up and refrain from being too blinkered and idealistic. Accidents, even in the best family circumstances, will always happen. Tina was under great pressure, but despite all the hardships, she was doing her best for her children.

'I have learned much from this incident, but most of all I learned something about myself. I feel I will be a better nurse because of it and, through my assessor's example, ultimately a better staff nurse.'

> **Activity 8**
>
> During your next clinical practice, identify an event that went either very well or very badly, or which simply epitomises the norm for that setting.
>
> Subject it to critical incident analysis, perhaps using the following headings: context, key players, objective description of the events, why the incident is critical, your concerns and feelings, what was most demanding and most satisfying about the incident, and how it might influence your future practice.

Deborah and Alan both correctly identify the learning that took place, but it could have been very different had they been content merely to walk away after the incident, lick their wounds and try to put it behind them. As it was, they utilised critical incident analysis to explore their respective experiences, painful as they were at first, seeking guidance in the process to test their understanding.

The result was that they learned and grew from their situations and will be far better equipped to deal with similar situations in the future. Especially notable is the way in which the incident prompted them to seek further sources of formal learning. In essence, the analysis directed their learning while allowing them to retain control, one of the most significant features of the technique. This is so much more constructive that merely feeling bad or being admonished for getting it wrong. Equally, Deborah and Alan alone owned their feelings, and the learning that resulted from reflecting on these was unique to them both and thus all the richer.

Nurses are increasingly being formally asked to explore reflective aspects of their practice. Initiatives such as Post-registration Education and Practice (PREP) require this to be carried out formally using instruments such as the professional portfolio. Nurses should try to perfect these explorations through approaches such as critical incident analysis, but the technique should equally be used during clinical placements in order to extract the maximum learning from them.

> **Activity 9**
>
> From Activity 8, try to highlight: the reflective learning experience; the pre-existing skills you employed in the situation; any skills you acquired to meet the situation; and what new skills or knowledge you will need in order to meet a similar incident in the future.

▮ Learning from Experience

For the student entering nursing, learning can quite often be seen as a rigid process, out of the control of the recipient. In recent years, however, the values of the students' own experiences and their own interpretations have increasingly been correctly seen as being of great worth in the process of gaining knowledge.

Burnard (1987) has proposed that the potential for knowledge lies in three complementary domains. **Propositional knowledge** is that which is associated with more traditional sources, such as formal lectures, textbooks and so on. **Practice knowledge** is that achieved through a 'hands-on', skills acquisition mode. Of equal and possibly greater value, however, is **experiential knowledge**, gained through a direct, personal encounter with a subject, person or event. In the past, much emphasis was placed on the first two sources of knowledge in the preparation of nurses; as Warner Weil and McGill (1989) state, a recognition of the value of the student's experiential or experience-based learning was not fully accepted until fairly recently.

Burnard (1987) defines experiential knowledge, although personal and subjective, as 'a process in which a particular experience is, on reflection, translated into concepts which in turn become guidelines for future experiences'. It always begins with the experience itself, which is then subjected to reflection,

propositional knowledge
knowledge acquired from lectures, textbooks and formal sources

practice knowledge
knowledge acquired from practical experiences

experiential knowledge
knowledge acquired through lived experience

analysis and evaluation. For Parker et al. (1995), experience is attending to and organising information in order to make sense of a real-world event. Experiential learning can be viewed as synonymous with meaningful discovery through personal involvement in a human experience.

The phenomenon of experiential learning was considered by Kolb (1984), who saw it as offering a model of learning and adaptation. It is consistent with the structure of human cognition and the stages of human development and growth, perhaps again paralleling theories of adult learning. Kolb conceives that experiential learning passes through a four stage cycle:

1. An experience.
2. Observation and reflection.
3. The formulation of abstract concepts and generalisations out of that reflection.
4. Testing the implications of concepts learned on new situations.

Jarvis and Gibson (1985) suggest that the experience can occur within the cognitive, affective or psychomotor dimension. Although it might be facilitated by a teacher or supervisor, it might equally be an everyday event or a spontaneous or vicarious learning opportunity. It is essential that, when such methods are used, the pace must be set by the learners as it is their experience and their learning.

Jarvis and Gibson further caution that if experiential learning is stimulated externally, by teacher or mentor, the following ground-rules must apply:

- Learners must be allowed to think things through for themselves and at their own pace
- They must be allowed to ask enough questions to stimulate the process of reflection
- It is not essential that a conclusion be reached – it's the process that matters
- Don't expect student and mentor to reach essentially the same conclusions – whose learning is it anyway?

Let us attempt to gain a greater understanding of Kolb's experiential learning cycle by applying it to a clinical scenario. Attempt to answer the questions posed in the activities below, placing yourself in the part of the subject. Possible responses are given at the end of the scenario.

The cast

- *Student nurse:* Bridget, mother of two, very enthusiastic but a bit apprehensive. First week, first placement

- *Supervisor:* Debbie, E grade staff nurse. Very experienced
- *Link tutor:* Peter. Reasonably 'visible' in the clinical area
- *Patient:* John, 18 years old, stable high cervical neck fracture following a motorcycle accident.

The setting

An acute trauma ward, a six-bedded bay close to the nurses' station, with five elderly male patients, chronically ill and restricted to their beds, and John. Debbie and Bridget were giving care to John, who was completely immobilised in rather threatening cervical traction following a spinal injury, a condition with which Bridget was unfamiliar. There were cords, pulleys and weights, and John was being nursed on a very complex-looking turning bed. Bridget was acutely aware of the potential dangers involved in mishandling this intricate array of equipment. The ever-present risk of dislocation resulting in death or permanent paralysis or disability was all too apparent.

On initial interview, Bridget revealed her sense of insecurity to Debbie. She told her that she felt threatened by the clients with their unfamiliar diagnoses and the strange terminology employed by the staff, and felt overawed at their familiarity with and confidence in administering care. Now carry out Activity 10.

Bridget supported Debbie and was by now feeling free to question all aspects of the care being given. By the end of the shift, having frequently returned to John to give additional support, she was beginning to feel more confident in her abilities. She allowed him to talk at length about his perceptions of his care, his fears and his hopes for a successful recovery. She in turn questioned him and colleagues about different aspects of the care being provided.

The following day Peter, the link tutor, visited the ward. He welcomed Bridget and asked how she was getting on. He asked if there was anything he could offer that might assist her in gaining understanding and confidence in her role during the clinical placement. Refer now to Activity 11.

By the end of the third day, Bridget was giving John's care with minimal supervision. She informed Debbie that the cord on his traction was too long (the weights being in danger of trailing on the floor). Debbie shortened the cords, explaining the need for non-slip knots, and showed Bridget how to tie them.

Bridget was concerned that John was somewhat isolated and perhaps lonely. In the next bay, there were two other patients of John's age. She suggested to Debbie that perhaps John could be moved there, and this was done. Bridget recorded this in her reflective diary and the following day discussed it with Peter. Peter congratulated her on her forethought, and for reflective purposes asked her to analyse the factors that prompted her proposal to move John.

By the end of the week, Bridget was much more confident and was being

Activity
10

In order to allay Bridget's fears, what might Debbie do or tell her that might make her more confident in dealing with this threatening and alien scenario?

Activity
11

Such an offer of help frequently occurs, although its purpose is sadly often missed or misconstrued. What might Bridget and Peter identify as opportunities to assist in this process, with particular regard to her care of John?

Activity
12

What additional things might Bridget do to improve the accuracy of her perceptions of this care scenario?

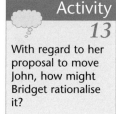

Activity

13

With regard to her proposal to move John, how might Bridget rationalise it?

allowed to play a greater part in her contribution to care. She even proposed a similar movement of patients according to age and condition, and her rationale for the changes was enthusiastically endorsed by her mentor. Now do Activities 12 (above) and 13.

Suggested responses to Activity 10

Debbie should:

- Advise Bridget of the need to be able to talk to John about his condition and perceptions of his care
- Encourage Bridget to be honest about her limitations to her client and, more importantly, to herself
- Carefully consider all aspects of John's care and the equipment involved, and provide Bridget with the opportunity to familiarise herself with the concepts involved
- Encourage Bridget to voice her anxieties, hopes and fears honestly
- Reassure her that reticence and anxiety are normal and indeed healthy
- Suggest that her maturity will convey credibility and empathy to a younger patient
- Explore the elements of Bridget's past experience that might be brought to bear on her care of John
- Advise her that Debbie will be on hand to offer support and advice, and confirm her readiness to do so
- Emphasise the need to discuss and reflect with other students on their care
- Allow Bridget to support Debbie in care provision, gently allowing Bridget to gain familiarity and confidence, while continuously testing for depth of understanding, in essence providing a role model.

Suggested responses to Activity 11

Peter, with Bridget, should:

- Go through and check Bridget's understanding of the aims and objectives set for the placement
- Identify any immediate anxieties and set additional short-term goals to overcome them
- Relate relevant care to the theory already covered in the course
- Check Bridget's understanding of the pathophysiological aspects of John's condition, perhaps through ward tutorials and using the ward and school library

- Guide Bridget through John's case and nursing notes, with a particular emphasis on his care plans
- Talk to Debbie to gauge Bridget's progress and ensure that she has realistic expectations of her placement
- Reassure Debbie of Peter's availability to visit the ward to assist and support throughout the placement, and give her licence to ask for this freely as required
- If he has access to any formal sessions on spinal handling, invite Bridget to attend them.

Suggested responses to Activity 12

Bridget could:

- Consult the case notes and care plans to see how care is recorded
- Under supervision, enter her care in the care plans
- Use ward and library reading resources to determine the optimum care for this type of patient
- Discuss her care with John and his relatives
- Discuss and compare her care and her understanding of it with other students on the ward
- Take up Debbie's and Peter's offers and consult them whenever clarification is required
- Maintain up-to-date entries of her care experiences in her reflective diary and check its accuracy with Peter, Debbie or her group tutor.

Suggested responses to Activity 13

Bridget can support her proposal thus:

- John's anxiety will accentuate his sense of isolation
- If the position in which John is being nursed restricts his ability to communicate, this too will add to his anxiety
- John has little in common with his fellow patients, who may be too ill to communicate
- The staff cannot be with John all the time
- Younger, perhaps fitter patients might help to keep John occupied and allay his sense of isolation
- Such patients could help to alert staff to any of John's needs, or give support and encouragement.

Looking more closely at this scenario, you will see that it is possible to relate Bridget's experience to Kolb's experiential learning cycle as follows.

The experience
Bridget meets a patient with a spinal injury for the first time and is given the task of contributing to his care.

Observation and reflection
Bridget told Peter that, as John was substantially younger than herself, she felt an ability to project empathy and understanding that was similar to what she experienced with her children, who were of a similar age, and that this eased the ability to communicate. Bridget was in effect correctly utilising her extensive life experience and maturity to gain an insight into John's anxieties, perhaps in a way that a more senior yet younger colleague might not be able to do.

Formulation of abstract concepts and generalisations out of the reflection
Although perhaps not entirely acceptable to the purist, such a strategy enabled a conceptualisation of the patient's anxiety state and stimulated theory development on how Bridget might help him. The following day, John looked visibly more relaxed, and with the noisy, expectant approval and encouragement of his peers, was becoming quite cheeky. John's improved mood acted as a reinforcement for Bridget's interventions.

Testing the implications of concepts learned by applying them to new situations
Later that shift, Bridget conferred with Debbie and was, as a result, allowed to make two other moves around the ward, matching patients by age, condition and mobility state.

Experience is a much-cited commodity in professional practice but remains a notoriously difficult factor to quantify. By using the experience of everyday practice events, combined with the principles of formal reflection, students can develop their knowledge in what is, after all, the richest domain of learning, nursing practice itself.

Reflection in the Practice Setting

As was stated earlier, students entering practice can frequently be overawed by the alien nature of every new environment to which their programme dispatches them. We try to assimilate the skills necessary to demonstrate an affiliation to our colleagues so that we will not stand out. There is often an overeagerness to achieve merely the basic skills and thus acquire just enough knowledge for immediate survival. Superficially, this may be acceptable, but by utilising our reflective skills we can start to cope with our newness and immediately develop ownership of our learning. Reflecting on every single aspect of our practice experiences from day one of each placement can help to broaden our learning and help us to start taking charge of our development needs from the outset.

The richness of the practice setting can be enhanced in so many ways if the minute features of personal experience are explored more thoroughly. In an excellent personal account of the positive influence that reflective practice can have, Palmer et al. (1994) cite reflection being used in helping the practitioner to ensure that behaviour remains congruent with professional values and attitudes. Reflection is thus a means for self-monitoring performance against one's aspirations for best practice. For the student, this might mean ensuring that the maximum potential learning is extracted from every experience, right from the start of training. Equally, it should be tempered by what we already know and bring into nursing. Reflection will facilitate this, as shown in the following scenario, taken a few years ago, from a student in the learning disabilities branch (Casebox 13.3).

With perhaps a few variations, this scenario is likely to be familiar to many students entering clinical practice for the first time, regardless of their chosen branch. The experiences of the first day, or even the first week, often merge into one, individual interactions and events being difficult to recall even when pressed. The overall impressions, such as whether it went satisfactorily or disastrously, will be retained, but minute features, each a potentially rich source of learning, are usually lost in our quest for acceptance by our colleagues.

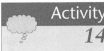

Activity
14

Imagine you are Emma. How do you think she felt? What preparation should she have received prior to arrival? How could the ward staff have contributed to this preparation?

Students will quickly learn that anxieties and apprehension are not confined to their first placement. Such feelings are highly necessary and, although less acute, usually stay with us regardless of how often we change our place of employment. Those all-important first few hours are, however, vital in easing our passage to becoming a useful member of the occupational group we seek to join. Reflection, both in and on action, can help in this process.

Using these strategies, look back on the scenario just portrayed and reflect on the questions posed in Activities 14 and 15 (below), checking your answers against the text below.

Suggested responses to Activities 14 and 15

● *How do you think she felt?*
Fearful, anxious, self-conscious, superfluous, a 'spare part', a spare 'pair of hands', threatened, out of her depth, uncertain, unsupported

Casebox 13.3

Prior to starting the course, **Emma** had had no previous experience of working with people with learning disabilities. Although lacking first-hand insight, she had experience of other voluntary and caring work, and she knew that this was a field in which she could function well. After the introductory block, Emma's set were scheduled to work one shift a week in their practice area. Emma was placed in Grove Villa, a nearby facility for children with severe physical and learning disabilities.

Arriving on the unit at lunchtime on the first day, it was immediately apparent that staffing was a problem, and there was an air of intense activity about the place. Although supernumerary, Emma felt that she should show willingness and help where possible. The Villa was quite old and the centre was imminently due to move to a more modern facility. For now, however, the accommodation consisted of a lounge–diner, a small ward kitchen for making drinks, an L-shaped dormitory and a

small bathroom with two baths, six cubicle toilets and six hand-basins. Although the Villa was light and cheerful, ventilation was a little poor, and the building was showing its age.

On arrival, Emma felt acutely aware of her lack of experience and was actually starting to feel a bit nauseated. Lunch had just finished and the lingering smell of food combined with the rather disagreeable odour coming from the lavatories, which were quite close to the door, was unpleasant. Having finished their lunch, the children were being taken to the bathroom area to be washed and use the toilet. The senior member of staff was dispensing medication from the drug trolley.

Everyone was very welcoming when she introduced herself, and, taking her cue from this, Emma asked what she could do. The charge nurse asked whether she would help to wash some of the children, take them to the toilet and,

if necessary, help to change their clothes. When she asked whom she should start with, she was assigned to Mark. Mark was aged 7, wheelchair bound and with physical and learning disabilities. She approached him, introduced herself and was greeted with a beaming smile, which she found tremendously reassuring.

After an embarrassing few seconds while she worked out the intricacies of the wheelchair, Emma took Mark through to the bathroom area. Other staff were there with about six other children. The smell in the toilet area was overpowering, and Emma felt quite sick, but she was reassured by one of the staff that she would get used to it. It was a rather tight fit in the bathroom, so a member of staff suggested that Emma should 'do' Mark at his bedside. Feeling a bit clumsy at first, as Mark had been incontinent, Emma finally coped satisfactorily with this, her first exposure to practice.

- *What preparation should she have received prior to arrival?*
  Orientation with the client group, a familiarisation visit to the Villa, an insight into ward 'routines'

- *How could the ward staff have contributed to this preparation?*
  The production of an orientation pack, the assignment of a mentor whom Emma could shadow for the first few days, teaching resources, a formal introduction to the staff and clients, assurance that she was supernumerary and had time to find her feet

- *What potential learning resulted from this brief experience?*
  THE SPECIFIC LEARNING
  Successfully washing and drying a 7-year-old with physical and learning disabilities
  THE PERIPHERAL LEARNING
  The location of the Villa
  The mealtime environment and 'routines'
  The responsiveness of her colleagues
  Mark's responsiveness to her
  The time of the medication round
  The operation of the wheelchair
  The location of Mark's bed

- *What pre-existing skills were utilised in the situation?*
  How to find things in a strange environment
  How to wash and dress dependent people

- *What new skills and knowledge are needed to maximise Emma's learning?*
  Theoretical input on dignity and privacy
  Methods for maximising client independence
  Theoretical input on skin care, cross-infection and so on
  Incontinence needs and aids.

Activity
15

What potential learning resulted from this brief experience? What pre-existing skills were utilised in the situation? What new skills and knowledge are needed to maximise Emma's learning?

Although the outcomes of Emma's care of Mark would seem at first glance to be simplistic, it must be remembered that it is usually the simple things that cause the most anxiety, and act as obstacles to learning, when one is new.

This was just one snapshot during one shift, perhaps only 15–20 minutes in time, yet Emma's real learning achievements, which might otherwise have gone unheralded, can clearly be seen following reflection. No matter how small or seemingly insignificant the event, a potential for learning and professional growth will exist. Real effort is needed, however, at least at first, to ensure that the breadth and depth of our development and learning are fully accredited. The development of effective, reflective powers will greatly ease this process.

■ Reflection and Clinical Supervision

clinical supervision

a blend of education, support and management

Earlier we briefly touched on a relationship between reflection and the increasingly in vogue system for professional support – **clinical supervision**. Mentored, supported or shared reflection is a natural progression once the basic concepts of self-reflection have been embraced. This might involve reflective discourse with a mentor, preceptor or supervisor, but it could equally well be with a colleague, peer, fellow student or even subordinate. The most important element is the quality, honesty and intimacy of the partnership. To this end, the selection of the supervisor is usually best left to the reflectee. Serious truths may be unearthed, a level of commitment and trust, one invariably beyond that which is possible merely within a friendship, being central to the relationship.

CONNECTIONS

Chapter 12, in its exploration of the defence response, illustrates this discomfort when challenged.

By this stage of the chapter, it should have emerged that our nursing practice is dependent on flexibility and adaptability. Practitioners far too often jealously guard what they perceive as their expertise and their knowledge. Indeed, it is not too Machiavellian to suggest that knowledge is power, and challenges to what we believe we know and do can be extremely uncomfortable. As discussed earlier, even an authoritarian 'put-down' can await the unwary student or junior colleague who questions our practice.

Yet, for quality learning and professional growth to become central to our practice, criticism is exactly the commodity we should be seeking rather than attempting to avoid. Where criticism is often vainly taken as being harmful, it is in reality usually a strength. We only grow, professionally speaking, when we can see the immense benefits of having our less than successful, or even desirable, practices exposed so that we can correct, enhance or update them.

Supervision can at first invoke suggestions of subordinate status or being under scrutiny by a superior, but it is in fact a thoroughly professional process of the facilitated self-scrutiny of one's beliefs and/or actions. The direct association with reflective practice is immediately apparent, and as Burns and Bulman (2000) state, clinical supervision is now being seen as a formal means of legitimising reflection by practitioners as a means of learning. Indeed, the creation of a culture that combines clinical practice and supervision is a long-established target for NHS Trusts (Johns and Freshwater, 1998).

For Fisher (1996), clinical supervision is a blend of education, support and management, although, as the UKCC (1996) cautions, clinical supervision and managerial supervision must be kept firmly separate. This demarcation is a critical condition for achieving success if, as Bond and Holland (1998) urge, the supervisee is to remain the central figure retaining overall control. For this to work, however, each individual supervisee must first have attained, or be working towards developing, in-depth reflective skills.

Although clinical supervision is now widely seen as a key tool in the pursuit of quality and excellence in practice, reflection is the toolbox. To maximise the very real benefits of supervision, reflection, be it personal, shared or guided, is an essential skill, to be developed early on in one's career. Unless we can learn to accept our own close scrutiny, even be our own worst critics, it will be impossible to accept the constructive scrutiny and criticism of others.

■ Chapter Summary

Reflective practice is for many still a rather nebulous concept with properties that are seen as abstract and vague, yet it can perhaps be seen that the basic principles of reflection are quite simple, even though their mastery will take some time. The time taken to achieve this will, however, be worthwhile.

It is hoped that, through this chapter, students will now be able to define the true structures of the process and will start to develop the mechanisms by which they can implement it in their own personal practice. These are skills worth developing as they hold the real promise of seeing what we do with greater clarity.

For the student, such skills acquisition offers a special imperative in that it holds the key to taking charge of our own professional development and more especially our learning. Nurse education programmes, even the most empathic and revolutionary, can go only part way towards equipping us with the skills and insight necessary to becoming an effective practitioner.

The best nursing practice is invisible and anticipatory, buried in the depths of the meaningful, interpersonal relationships we develop with our patients, clients and co-workers. Through reflection in and on our actions, processes such as the analysis of critical incidents and the true worth of experiential learning, best practice can be unearthed and used to refine our further development, not just during our period of training, but throughout our careers.

● **Test Yourself!**

1. In your own words, describe ritualistic actions and compare your response with that offered by Jarvis (1992).

2. An effective trigger for reflective potential has been described by Boyd and Fales (1983) as 'a sense of inner .... '.

3. Using the reflective framework offered by Atkins and Murphy (1994), what follows an analysis of feelings and knowledge relevant to the situation?

4. What does Schön (1983) call the two types of reflection?

5. The tacit comparison of an impending care situation against previous experience is described by Van Manen (1977) as .... reflection.

6. Write your own definition of a critical incident and compare it with those offered within the chapter.

7. What are the key features of Burnard's (1987) practice knowledge and experiential knowledge?

8. Name the four stages of Kolb's (1984) experiential learning cycle.

9. What growing professional initiative does Fisher (1996) describe as a blend of education, support and management?

10. When experiential learning is being facilitated by teachers or supervisors, what must they regard as a key condition?

References

Atkins, S. and Murphy, K. (1994) Reflective practice. *Nursing Standard* **8**(39): 49–56.

Benner, P. (1984) *From Novice to Expert: Excellence and Power in Clinical Nurse Practice.* Addison Wesley, Menlo Park, CA.

Berger, P. and Luckman, T. (1967) The social construction of reality. Cited in Jarvis, P. (1992) Reflective practice in nursing. *Nurse Education Today* **12**: 174–81.

Bond, M. and Holland, S. (1998) *Skills of Clinical Supervision for Nurses.* Open University Press, Buckingham.

Boud, D., Keogh, R. and Walker, D. (eds) (1985) Reflection: turning experience into learning. In Burnard P. (1991) Improving through reflection. *Journal of District Nursing* May, pp. 10–12.

Boyd, E. and Fales, A. (1983) Reflective learning – key to learning from experience. Cited in Powell, J. (1989) The reflective practitioner in nursing *Journal of Advanced Nursing.* **14**: 824–32.

Burnard, P. (1987) Towards an epistemological basis for experiential learning in nursing education. *Journal of Advanced Nursing* **12**: 189–93.

Burns, S. and Bulman, C. (2000) *Reflective Practice in Nursing,* 2nd edn. Blackwell Science, Oxford.

Cervero, R. (1988) Effective continuing education for professionals. In Jarvis, P. (1992) Reflective practice in nursing. *Nurse Education Today* **1**: 174–81.

Coutts-Jarman, J. (1993) Using reflection and experience in nurse education. *British Journal of Nursing* **2**(1): 77–80.

Crouch, S. (1991) Critical incident analysis. *Nursing* **4**: 30–1.

Darbyshire, P. (1993) In the hall of mirrors. *Nursing Times* **89**(49): 26–30.

Dewey, D. (1933) *How We Think*. DC Heath, Boston.

Dewing, J. (1990) Reflective practice. *Senior Nurse* **10**(10): 26–8.

Driscoll, J. (1994) Reflective practice in practice. *Senior Nurse* **13**(7): 47–50.

Fisher, M. (1996) Using reflective practice in clinical supervision. In Burns, S. and Bulman, C. (2000) *Reflective Practice in Nursing*, 2nd edn. Blackwell Science, Oxford.

Greenwood, J. (1993) Some considerations concerning practice and feedback in nursing education. *Journal of Advanced Nursing* **18**: 1999–2002.

Habermas, J. (1977) Knowledge and human interests. Cited in Atkins, S. and Murphy, K. (1994) Reflective practice. *Nursing Standard* **8**(39): 49–56.

Jarvis, P. (1992) Reflective practice in nursing. *Nurse Education Today* **12**: 174–81.

Jarvis, P. and Gibson, S. (1985) *The Teacher Practitioner in Nursing, Midwifery and Health Visiting*. Croom Helm, Beckenham.

Johns, C. and Freshwater, D. (eds) (1998) *Transforming Nursing Through Reflective Practice*. Blackwell Science, Oxford.

Kolb, D. (1984) *Experiential Learning*. Prentice Hall, Englewood Cliffs, NJ.

Melia, K. (1987) *Learning and Working: The Occupational Socialisation of Nurses*. Tavistock, London.

Menzies, I. (1960) A case study in the function of social systems as a defence against anxiety. Cited in Melia, K. (1987) *Learning and Working: The Occupational Socialisation of Nurses*. Tavistock, London.

Mezirow, J. (1981) A critical theory of adult learning and education. Cited in Jarvis, P. (1992) Reflective practice in nursing. *Nurse Education Today* **12**: 174–81.

Palmer, A., Burns, S. and Bulman, C. (1994) *Reflective Practice in Nursing*. Blackwell, London.

Parker, D., Webb, J. and D'Souza, B. (1995) The value of critical incident analysis as an educational tool and its relationship to experiential learning. *Nurse Education Today* **15**: 111–16.

Polanyi, M. (1967) The Tacit Dimension. Cited in Schön, D. (1983) *The Reflective Practitioner*. Avebury, New York.

Powell, J. (1989) The reflective practitioner in nursing. *Journal of Advanced Nursing* **14**: 824–32.

Powell, J. (1992) Reflection and the evaluation of experience: prerequisites for therapeutic practice. In Driscoll, J. (1994) Reflective practice in practice. *Senior Nurse* **13**(7): 47–50.

Schön, D. (1983) *The Reflective Practitioner*. Temple Smith, London.

Schön, D. (1987) *Educating the Reflective Practitioner*. Jossey Bass, London.

Stockwell, F. (1984) *The Unpopular Patient*. Croom Helm, Beckenham.

Street, A. (1991) From image to action – reflection in nursing practice. In Palmer, A., Burns, S. and Bulman, C. (1994) *Reflective Practice in Nursing*. Blackwell, London.

UKCC (United Kingdom Central Council for Nursing, Midwifery and Health Visiting) (1992) *Scope of Professional Practice.* UKCC, London.

UKCC (United Kingdom Central Council for Nursing, Midwifery and Health Visiting) (1996) *Position Statement on Clinical Supervision for Nursing and Health Visiting.* UKCC, London.

Van Manen, M. (1977) Linking ways of knowing with ways of being practical. In Atkins, S. and Murphy, K. (1994) Reflective practice. *Nursing Standard* **8**(39): 49–56.

Warner Weil, S. and McGill, I. (eds) (1989) Making sense of experiential learning: diversity in theory and practice. Cited in Parker, D., Webb, J. and D'Souza, B. (1995) The value of critical incident analysis as an educational tool and its relationship to experiential learning. *Nurse Education Today* **15**: 111–16.

Williams, M. (1996) Reflection, thinking and learning. *British Journal of Theatre Nursing* **6**(5): 26–9.

SUSAN MOORE

Chapter

The Politics of Health Care

14

Contents

Learning outcomes

This chapter explores the wider context of health care, looking at how health-care policy is made. The first section describes the British political system and the parts of the process that contribute to the formation of health policy. The second section examines some health policies and legislation that affect nursing and midwifery practice today. First, the whole structure of the NHS is described. Next, we turn to an outline of the legal structures that govern the professions of nursing, midwifery and health visiting. Finally, specific branches of practice are discussed in relation to the legislation that provides a framework for practice. After completing this chapter, you will be able to:

- Outline the key political institutions involved in the development of social policy

- Justify the need for nurses to have a knowledge of social policy

- Describe the key features of policy relating to midwifery, children's nursing and mental health and learning disability practice

- Discuss the development of the statutory regulation of nursing, midwifery and health visiting.

■ The Political Process

Why study politics?

This is surely a legitimate question to pose. Why do nurses need to know about political institutions and how social policy is devised, enacted and implemented? How will this affect the way in which they deliver effective care to their clients? What will it matter to a client who is in severe pain or hallucinating, how politically astute the nurse is who offers him help? The immediate answer is that, at this stage in an illness, a client will not be interested in any other skills that a nurse has but those which help to ease the pain or distract him from the hallucinations. Later on, however, a significant proportion of acute illnesses become chronic conditions that affect significant areas of a person's life. It is possible in this situation, where service users and nurses alike are motivated by a need, to influence and improve the service. They are facilitated in doing this if they understand the social and political systems that created it.

It can be argued then that several justifications can be put forward for nurses to understand the process of policy formation in health care. First of all, the nurse is a citizen, and it may be argued all citizens should have an understanding of the systems and processes by which decisions are made that affect their lives. Second, nurses who begin their career at 18 years old may work within the health-care system for 30 years or more, during which they will have the potential to effect care for a significant number of people. Nurses will be more effective if they understand the history, development, values and beliefs of the health-care delivery system and its institutions within which they operate. Third, when nurses are acting as advocates for clients or client groups, it may be helpful to assist them to understand the system and why care is delivered in the way it is. In addition, as care is increasingly delivered outside the hospital setting and in the community, care packages have to be put together with contributions from a range of agencies such as social services, housing and education. Nurses who aim to deliver effective care to clients need to have an understanding of these agencies and the legal frameworks within which they operate. Finally, having gained an understanding of the system, the nurse may seek, either individually or as part of a pressure group, to change or improve health-care policies. For example, the Royal Colleges of Nursing and Midwives and the Community Psychiatric Nurses Association are organisations that seek to influence health policy on behalf of their members.

Political values and beliefs

It is important, when considering health policy, to have an understanding of the values and beliefs that shape it. Ranade (1994) argues that the philosophy that

CONNECTIONS

Pain is discussed further in Chapters 1 and 6.

health policy

the principles that govern public actions to deliver health services

provided an impetus for the 1948 National Health Service was rooted in the principles of socialism. Before 1948, people were aware of the significant inequalities in health care. Beveridge, the author of the report that provided the blueprint for the NHS (Ministry of Health, 1942), was also concerned with the economic benefits that would result for society if health were improved. These values of shared social responsibility for welfare provision and extensive state economic intervention continued to dominate during the 1950s and 60s. They were based upon the optimistic view that resources invested in health and welfare would support economic growth by improving the quality of the work-force and contributing to full employment.

In the 1970s, academic writing challenged the view that public welfare services were an equalising force in society. It was suggested by the Black Report (DHSS, 1980) that, despite 30 years of a welfare state, there were still significant inequalities in health. The medical dominance of health care was also challenged (Illich, 1976; McKeown, 1976). It was argued that medicine focused too much on science and the promotion of the profession and not enough on meeting clients' needs.

The values and beliefs that underpinned the policies of the Conservative administrations from 1979 onwards have been summarised by the term 'New Right'. At that time, the welfare state seemed to be failing, and a 'crisis of welfare' was described in which the growth in the population of older people would coincide with a reduction in the population of wage-earners, combined with slow economic growth. This would result in economic disaster. The New Right solution to this problem was to reduce the level of state intervention in the economy. It was argued that market forces were distorted by too much economic planning and regulation. Furthermore, citizens had to fund welfare from taxation, and this resulted in a tax burden that stunted free enterprise. Last, economic decline resulted from having a large public sector that did not contribute to wealth creation.

The New Right believed that professionals tended to promote their own interests above those of the service, which resulted in inefficiency. In addition, they felt that because welfare was provided by state monopolies, the service was inefficient and wasteful, which would not be tolerated in organisations that were motivated by competition. It was argued from a moral stance that citizens were being coerced in two ways by the welfare state: first, by having to pay more tax because the service was wasteful; and second because, as a prospective consumer, the citizen was offered no choice.

In 1997, a new Labour government was elected, the values and beliefs that characterise its health policy having been termed the 'Third Way'. This approach calls for economic growth founded on free market policies. Emphasis is placed on shifting the balance from financing pensions and cash benefits towards the provision of better public services, particularly education and health. Those to

socialism
a political doctrine that seeks to organise society on the basis of fairness and equity

welfare state
a collective term to describe all the government provision, for example education, health or social security, that offers aid to those who need it

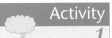

Activity
1

Compare the three approaches to policy – the 'Old Left', the 'New Right' and the 'Third Way'. Decide which you think is the most convincing and say why.

be targeted are disabled people, single parents and, by being offered retraining, unemployed people. Another characteristic of the Third Way is stakeholder involvement, the aim of the whole policy being for stakeholders to have a say in the development of services (Leathard, 2000).

There are significant differences between the 'Old Left', 'New Right' and 'Third Way' philosophies. These have been the driving force behind the development of social policy, and it is essential, when evaluating the effectiveness of policies, that the underpinning values and beliefs are understood.

How are political decisions made?

It is important to be aware that social policies start with governments. Social policies are the expression of that government's values and beliefs. In order for the nurse to understand, analyse and criticise social policies, he or she must first have some understanding of the political system that produces them and the process of government that enacts them.

British central government

the Cabinet

the executive decision-making body of government, made up of ministers of state, led by the prime minister

In Britain, there is a system of democratic representative government whereby approximately 650 representatives are elected every 5 years by a 'first past the post' or simple majority voting system. After a general election, the monarch formally requests the leader of the majority party to form a government. The majority party leader then becomes the prime minister. When forming a government, there are over 100 positions to be filled, which will be taken up by members of the winning party. The most important positions are those of members of **the Cabinet**, the executive body of government, which is made up of between 15 and 25 members. These are mainly ministers who lead government departments, but there may in addition be members without departmental responsibilities who have political or co-ordinating roles, for example the deputy prime minister.

The Cabinet is a key body in the decision-making process. Any new policy proposal or change to legislation is discussed, argued through and negotiated within the Cabinet forum. When such proposals need detailed work, Cabinet committees are set up to complete this. These then refer work back to the Cabinet for a final decision.

Within the UK, some powers have now been devolved to the Scottish Parliament and the Welsh and Northern Ireland Assemblies. These bodies have locally elected members and leaders who can make local decisions about a range of matters that includes health and social policy.

Government ministers

A **government minister** has the role of and responsibility for leading a government department, such as **the Treasury** or the Department of Health (DoH). A department consists of a large staff of permanent civil servants who administer it and put policy into effect. Ministers accept responsibility for work carried out in their name and are accountable to Parliament. A government minister can find himself in some considerable conflict as he has to contribute to both developing and co-ordinating central policy and strategy for the government. At the same time, he has a partisan commitment to his department to advance and protect its interests.

> **government minister**
>
> a person with responsibility for running a government department

> **the Treasury**
>
> the government department that has the responsibility of receiving the government's financial income, distributing it to other departments and setting the annual budget. Its chief minister is the Chancellor of the Exchequer

There are four main aspects to the role of government ministers. First, they put forward legislation. Second, they have to attend to a high workload of departmental administration, perhaps the development of policy that does not require legislation. Third, ministers have to respond to questions put to them in the House of Commons. These might be probing questions posed by opposition Members of Parliament (MPs), designed to embarrass or challenge the government. Equally, they may be questions asked by members of their own party that are designed to offer the opportunity to announce new policy or report favourable statistics. The final aspect of a minister's role is public relations. This will involve a programme of formal visits, speeches and meetings aimed to publicise the work of the department.

The House of Commons

In the UK, the seat of government is the Houses of Parliament. This is situated in Westminster in London and comprises two chambers.

The House of Commons is the chamber within which government policy is presented, debated, negotiated and finally voted upon by MPs. Policy starts as an Act of Parliament. Proposals for change are set out in the form of a 'Bill', which requires skilled presentation and wording, carried out by civil servants, who are permanent government employees. They are engaged in a wide variety of administrative roles within each of the government departments.

> **Bill**
>
> a draft of proposed legislation. It is work in progress until it becomes an Act of Parliament

Bills have to pass through four stages in both the House of Commons and the House of Lords. Stage one is the 'first reading', which occurs when the Bill is formally presented to the House. The 'second reading' is when the main principles of the Bill are debated by all parties within the House. The third stage, called the 'committee stage', involves an examination of the Bill in detail by a small standing committee. This is the stage during which changes or amendments can be made. The final stage is known as the 'third reading' or 'report stage': the revised Bill, having been examined by the committee, is referred back to the House, where it can yet again be amended.

The House of Lords

This is the second chamber of government, made up of non-elected representatives. The purpose of the House is to offer a second opinion on the Bills that appear before it. It works as a check and a balance to the House of Commons.

Bills go through the same four stages in the House of Lords. This second house can recommend amendments to Bills, but the House of Commons does not have to accept them. The final stage for a Bill to become an 'Act of Parliament' is for it to receive royal assent from the monarch.

The work performed by the ministry

The secretaries of states or ministers are the statutory heads of the departments. They have a number of junior ministers, themselves elected MPs, who support the secretary in his or her function. The junior ministers are appointed by the prime minister, and they are in turn supported in administering the work of the department by a staff of civil servants. It is important to note the differences between these two groups. The ministers may be at the department for a relatively short period of time, during which they may well wish to make their mark and achieve significant policy change. Civil servants, however, are likely to work in one department for the whole of their career. They tend, therefore, to see policy change in the longer term. This can cause some difficulties and disharmony in the promotion of policy change. The most significant civil service role in this context is that of the permanent secretary, the most senior civil servant within a department. This person is in daily contact with the minister and is the minister's source of communication and information about the department.

Financing policy

An important part of any policy relates to how it will be funded: Where will the money come from? How will it be distributed? How much money is there? The NHS provides a good example of how a budget is agreed and subsequently distributed. Money to finance the NHS derives from three sources: central government tax revenues, national insurance contributions and charges to service users. The largest proportion (81 per cent) comes from national taxation, national insurance representing 16 per cent and the remaining 3 per cent charges to service users. The allocation of funding for public services is regulated by the

Treasury and is dictated by the economic policy of the current government, which, for either economic or social reasons, may decide to restrict or develop spending on public services.

The DoH negotiates with the public services division of the Treasury, submitting to it revised annual plans for spending. The result of the joint work of these two government departments is to produce the Public Expenditure Survey Committee Report. This is subsequently presented to the Treasury ministers and is studied in the light of the current economic climate and the government's overall strategy. The allocation of funding between various departments is finally decided at Cabinet level, the eventual decisions being set out in the White Paper on Public Expenditure. The end result is that Parliament votes on the money for the year ahead for all public expenditure, including the NHS.

How is policy effected?

The previous sections have described how policy is made at governmental level and the political institutions that support that process. Equally important, however, is to understand how that policy is effected at the level of the workforce. Hill (1993) suggests that policy-making and policy implementation are not discrete operations but in fact merge: the implementation process influences policy design from an early stage and continues throughout it.

Policy implementation involves several sets of relationships. Initially, there is the relationship between central government agencies, in the case of health policy, for example, the DoH, and local agencies such as health authorities or NHS Trusts. The relationships underlying policy implementation become more complex when the effective realisation of the legislation involves the collaboration and co-operation of several organisations, each with its own discrete culture and operating system.

Policy implementation will also be influenced by the values and beliefs of the practitioners who put the policy into effect. Because there is such a distance between the central controlling agency and the individual who is delivering the service, there can be much room for discretion in how he or she acts. This can result in a considerable gap between the original principles and objectives of the policy and the actuality of the implementation.

Another important feature that influences policy implementation is finance. For change to take place, extra resources are sometimes required to make a change effective, perhaps to provide new environments or to train staff for new roles. Policy implementation is a complex, interactive process that shapes the nature of service delivery and also provides the feedback that ultimately results in policy change.

Activity 2

Are you a politically aware citizen? Which constituency do you live in? What is the name of its MP? Which political party does he or she represent? Does your MP hold a government office? Where and when does he or she hold constituency 'clinics' to obtain feedback and meet constituency residents?

■ Social Policy and Nursing Practice

In this second section, the structure and function of the NHS will be outlined before describing how nursing is regulated. The final part of the chapter examines specific legislation that governs mental health and children's nursing and midwifery.

The National Health Service

The NHS came into existence on 5 July 1948. It represented a significant social reform, the underpinning idea being that all members of society are entitled to health care, whatever their ability to pay. The service is paid for from the taxation of the whole population, and the organisation of the service is taken on by the government. Patients are able to receive treatment whenever they need it without having to negotiate payment. It is argued that this is the most cost-effective way of delivering health care to a population. Furthermore, it contributes to the overall health potential of that population and is fair and equitable. In 1948, hospitals and community services that had been run and financed by charities or on a commercial basis were all brought under the public umbrella of the NHS.

The NHS experienced funding difficulties almost from its inception. Delivery costs escalated, and successive governments have since struggled to deliver an effective service when faced by economic recession, an old and crumbling infrastructure and an ageing population. Both Conservative and Labour governments have struggled to make the NHS more effective by reorganising its structure. In 1974, an attempt was made to solve the problem by including more layers of bureaucracy to control its operations. Health service management had three layers of administration – regional, area and district – but this very quickly became untenable as decision-making had to fight its way through several layers of red tape.

In 1982, the Conservative Government attempted to control the NHS by introducing a new kind of management system called 'general management'. In this system, a new breed of manager was introduced who might or might not have a professional training. The important feature was that the manager had the skills to manage human and material resources.

A further attempt was made in 1990 to control the overwhelming public expenditure on health and social welfare by introducing systems based on the 'internal market'. In this approach, various parts of the health system competed for contracts in a similar way to that seen in commercial enterprise. Different parts of the system were termed 'purchasers' and 'providers', health authorities and some general practitioners purchasing health care from NHS

Trusts. Operation like a commercial business in a competitive internal market was designed to reduce costs and increase quality.

None of these reforms has, however, entirely worked. The NHS still struggles to fund the renewal of antiquated buildings, keep up with constant growth of technology and manage a huge workforce. In 1997, the country elected a new Labour government that made the reform of the NHS its foremost priority. This government has also reorganised and restructured the NHS with the objective of delivering an effective service.

Throughout all these changes, what has remained constant is the belief of the British people that the NHS is the best way to deliver health care to the whole population.

The new NHS: modern and dependable

In December 1997, the Labour government published a White Paper *The New NHS: Modern, Dependable* (DoH, 1997). This set out the government's strategy to reform the NHS using values and beliefs that can be summarised in the phrase 'the Third Way'. This Third Way lies between the central control approach of the 1970s NHS and the inequity of the internal market of the 1990s. Underlying this social policy are the principles of partnership and collaboration. The policy was further developed and presented as the *NHS Plan* (DoH, 2000a), which sets out 10 core principles:

> CONNECTIONS
>
> *Other relevant legislation is outlined in Chapter 15.*

1. The NHS will provide a universal service for all based on clinical need
2. The NHS will provide a comprehensive range of services
3. The NHS will shape its services around the needs and preferences of individual patients, their families and their carers
4. The NHS will respond to different needs of different populations
5. The NHS will work continuously to improve quality services and to minimise errors
6. The NHS will support and value its staff
7. Public funds for healthcare will be devoted solely to NHS patients
8. The NHS will work together with others to ensure a seamless service for patients
9. The NHS will keep people healthy and work to reduce health inequalities
10. The NHS will respect the confidentiality of individual patients and provide open access to information about services, treatment and performance.

These core principles embody Third Way thinking and are the principles that will guide NHS strategy over a period of 10 years.

The NHS structure for 2002

The current blueprint for the NHS aims to give local citizens and local health providers more power to decide upon and deliver health services locally. This is set out in the document *Shifting the Balance of Power within the NHS* (DoH, 2001b), which describes the structures that will be put in place in order to make this happen.

Department of Health

Ultimate management and control will rest, as it always has done, with the DoH, the government department led by the Secretary of State for Health, who is a full member of the Cabinet. The department has traditionally been highly directive in terms of how health care is organised and delivered. From April 2002, the department aims to facilitate rather than direct service delivery.

From 2003, the interface between the DoH and local services will occur via four Regional Directors of Health and Social Care, whose job will be to oversee the development of the NHS. There will be four regional directors for England, the country being divided into the South, the North, London and the Midlands.

England has approximately 30 strategic health authorities whose main role is to lead the strategic development of the local health service and manage the performance of primary care Trusts and NHS Trusts. This level of management relates to a geographical area that has a population of around 1.5 million people. It is the health authorities' job to focus upon the overall needs of the health economy. They are charged with the responsibility of ensuring that all the NHS organisations work together, managing performance by how they negotiate targets and ensure that these are achieved.

The local delivery of care is managed by primary care Trusts, which have two functions. First, they assess local health need and then negotiate and commission services for an improvement in health of the local population. Second, they manage and deliver primary and community service. Working through local strategic partnerships, primary care Trusts co-ordinate planning and community engagement and the influence of the wider government agenda. They also have a responsibility to work with local authorities to integrate health and social care. From April 2004, primary care Trusts will receive 75 per cent of NHS funds directly from the DoH. This will give them significant power as they will then determine how those funds will be distributed.

NHS Trusts differ in that they have only a responsibility to provide specialist health services, for example district general services, mental health services and ambulance services. The intention, expressed in the Third Way, is to ensure patient-centredness by devolving power to clinical teams able to make decisions about patient care.

Activity

3

To investigate structures in your locality, identify the members of your local NHS Trust or primary care Trust, whom they have contracts with and the Trust's annual income. A good source of information is the annual report available from the Trust's headquarters, copies of which may be available in clinical departments.

CONNECTIONS

More about clinical teams may be found in Chapters 1 and 15.

Regulating the profession

The profession of nursing itself is also subject to social policy and legislation. After a protracted campaign at the beginning of the twentieth century, nurses eventually persuaded the government to create a professional register. This was finally achieved in 1919, when the Nurses Registration Act was passed, creating registers for different parts of the profession. The aim of the register was to protect the public as only those who had trained as nurses would be admitted to it. Equally, those nurses who did not uphold the required standard of professional conduct would be removed from the register and would not be able to practise as registered practitioners.

The Act also created the General Nursing Council, a governing body for the profession whose role was to set the standards of education necessary to prepare nurses, examine nurses and maintain the register. Council members were appointed by the minister of health, and a similar council was created for midwives.

This system remained in place for 60 years. In 1979, the systems for regulating the profession were reorganised by the Nurses, Midwives and Health Visitors Act, creating a new body, the United Kingdom Central Council for Nursing, Midwifery and Health Visiting (UKCC). This brought together all the separate organisations and councils of the four kingdoms under one administration, so all the parts of the profession – nursing, midwifery and health visiting – were regulated by the same body. The principal functions of the UKCC were to establish and improve standards of training and professional conduct.

Since April 2002, the regulatory body has been the Nursing and Midwifery Council. It is composed of a smaller number of elected nurses, midwives and health visitors and appointed lay members and includes representation from all the four countries of the UK (DoH, 2001c). The Health Act 1999 defines its functions as:

- Keeping the register of members admitted to practice
- Determining standards of education and training for admission to practice
- Giving guidance about standards of conduct and performance
- Administering procedures (including making rules) relating to misconduct, lack of fitness to practise and similar matters.

Midwifery services

The practice of midwifery has always been considered to be distinct from that of nursing, and it developed its own set of policy provision over the twentieth century. There were several attempts to introduce legislation to regulate the profession of midwifery during the nineteenth century, the main driver behind this being the Matrons Aid Society, founded in 1881. The Society comprised a small group of educated midwives who wanted to improve standards of care and the professional status of midwives. In the late nineteenth century, eight Bills proposing a midwives register were introduced to Parliament, but all failed. As this had partly been because the government did not give it priority, the proposed legislation was then put forward by a Private Members Bill. The Bill was opposed by the medical profession because it trespassed upon their professional territory, but equally there was opposition from the developing nursing profession, led by Mrs Bedford Fenwick, who wished to see the professions united and regulated jointly.

A Midwives Act was eventually passed in 1902, its main provision being to establish a Central Midwives Board, initially for England and Wales, provision later also being made for Scotland and Ireland. The CMB was charged with maintaining a roll of certificated midwives, and it also set up local supervising authorities (LSAs) to supervise the practice of midwives. The Central Midwives Board set out rules governing midwifery practice, provided for the education of midwives and set up structures to maintain professional discipline.

In the first half of the twentieth century, the practice of midwifery took place largely in the client's home. Women had to pay a fee to the midwife, and to the GP if he was required. As many clients could not afford the doctor, the midwives would often pay the fee, so the Midwives Act 1918 provided for the LSA to pay the fees of doctors who were called to obstetric emergencies. The later Midwives Act of 1936 made it compulsory for the LSAs to provide a salaried domiciliary midwifery service; the fact that midwives could now receive a salary allowed them to provide a fuller service, which included antenatal care.

The Second World War had an effect upon the organisation of obstetric care. As a result of the war effort, there were fewer friends and family available to support a woman through a delivery, so women were drawn to having their babies delivered in hospital. The advent of the NHS in 1948 again changed the nature of obstetric care. As the service was now free, women took it up more readily and were more prepared to have their babies in hospital.

The 1979 Nurses, Midwives and Health Visitors Act created a statutory committee for midwives, important in the regulation of practice. The committee is required to make midwives' rules, which relate to the LSAs and to midwives' practice.

The recent reform of nursing regulation (DoH, 2001c) proposes to maintain this policy. The Nursing and Midwifery Council will still have a midwifery committee, and the council will make midwives' rules. Supervision of midwifery will continue under LSAs, which will still require midwives to attend educational courses to update their practice.

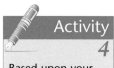

Activity

4

Based upon your reading of this section and your observations in obstetric practice, make a list of the ways in which the regulation of midwifery differs from that of nursing.

Mental health care

Care for people with mental health problems in the nineteenth and the first half of the twentieth century was based in large asylums, later to be termed psychiatric hospitals. More recently, however, there has been a movement to assist clients to live independently in the community, and policy and legislation have been developed to support this movement.

Caring for people who have mental health problems sometimes involves the use of powers that infringe civil liberties, so this area of client care is subject to significantly more legal involvement. In their daily practice, mental health nurses have to be knowledgeable about the law that regulates mental health practice.

Mental Health Act 1959

A significant change occurred in mental health care in the late 1950s. Before this, the delivery of care had occurred through the large psychiatric hospitals built in the nineteenth century. Admission to hospital was by a system of certification, all clients who were admitted being legally committed into the care of the hospital and detained against their will. During the 1950s, however, there was considerable social change, which created the climate for the development of legislation that was revolutionary in its approach.

The Mental Health Act of 1959 repealed all previous mental health legislation, introduced a single code for all types of mental disorder and set out new definitions of mental disorder. Clients could be admitted for treatment on a voluntary basis, as with any other hospital. Provision was made for compulsory admission to hospital only for those who were a danger to themselves or others because of mental illness. A new body, the Mental Health Review Tribunal, consisting of legal, medical and lay members, was created to safeguard clients' civil rights. This allowed clients who were detained to have a right of appeal. The Tribunal also has the power to discharge clients from hospital following a successful appeal. The effect of the Act was to reduce the number of clients who were compulsorily detained as clients could be admitted to hospital before they became severely ill. The stigma associated with mental illness was significantly reduced, discharging clients from hospital became much easier, and staff could contemplate the concept of the client living in the community.

Hospital closure

In 1961, Enoch Powell, then Minister of Health, announced a new policy – a programme of closure of the mental hospitals. He recognised that a huge proportion of the NHS budget was spent on maintaining mental hospitals and envisaged that this programme would lead to a reduction in spending on the NHS. Powell wanted to see the development of mental illness units within general hospitals, so a trend was started to decrease institutional care and increase community services, although this did not happen with anything like the speed that Powell had anticipated.

Better services for the mentally ill

The Department of Health and Social Security (DHSS) published a report (1975) showing that although the client population of mental hospitals had been reduced, not one hospital had been closed and the volume of work was in fact increasing (DHSS, 1975). The report drew a picture of how future services would be centred on general hospitals, provision also being made for hostels for recovering clients, outclient clinics and day care.

Mental Health Act 1983

As services developed in the community and more effective drug therapies were discovered, the nature of mental health care changed. Once again, the legal framework required amendment, a Mental Health Amendment Act being passed in 1983. The main tenets of the 1959 Act were upheld but new provisions were added. Clients who are detained under treatment orders may be treated without their consent for the first 3 months after admission, after which a second opinion has to be sought to continue treatment. This second opinion is supplied by a qualified psychiatrist appointed by the Mental Health Act Commission (MHAC). Treatment in this case is most often electroconvulsive therapy or drug therapy.

The MHAC, created by the 1983 Act, is a special health authority whose role is to be an independent inspectorate, its powers being limited to detained clients. MHAC members are charged with the duty of visiting and interviewing detained clients and investigating their complaints. In addition, the MHAC makes an annual report to Parliament.

The Act also makes provision for social care. Social services departments are required to appoint approved social workers, who have to be competent in the care of mentally ill people. The approved social worker has the duty to apply to the hospital for a client to be detained. Before doing this, however, he or she must interview the client and ensure that there is no means of providing care other than compulsory admission. Health and social services are charged with a duty to provide aftercare for clients who have been detained on a treatment order.

Care programme approach

In 1991, the government responded to several incidents that had caused public concern by developing a system for the organisation of mental health care for people with severe mental illness living in the community. The approach is to be followed by all health practitioners who deliver care to people with mental health problems. The first essential element of this **care programme approach** is a systematic assessment of health and social care needs, based on which the client possesses an agreed care plan. A key worker is appointed to co-ordinate the care plan and liaise with all the agencies that contribute to the package of care. The client's progress is subject to regular review, and he or she is involved in care decisions at every stage.

> **care programme approach**
> a systematic framework for mental health practice which ensures that the service user has an assessment, a care plan and a key worker, and ensures that the client is fully involved

The care programme approach is still the framework that is employed to structure the care of people with mental health problems, especially those who are seriously mentally ill.

Supervision register

Another measure was introduced in 1994, this being designed to address the problem of responding to and monitoring the care of people with complex needs who might be a risk to themselves or others. The supervision register is a list kept by each mental health-care provider unit of three types of client: those at risk of suicide, of serious violence to others and of severe self-neglect. The decision to include someone on the register is made in consultation with all members of the mental health team, and clients must have an opportunity to state their views. The final responsibility for inclusion lies with the consultant psychiatrist. The client must be informed of this decision both orally and in writing. The register constitutes a confidential health record, and computerised registers are subject to the provisions of the Data Protection Act.

Supervised discharge

The **supervised discharge** order came into effect in 1996. This is an arrangement by which a client who has been treated in hospital under the provisions of the Mental Health Act 1983 is subject to formal supervision when discharged. The aim of the order is to ensure that the client receives aftercare services. Clients who are placed on this order will have been assessed as being at substantial risk to themselves and others, and will normally also be included on the supervision register.

> **supervised discharge**
> provides for a patient to receive aftercare under supervision

Arrangements for aftercare under supervision are drawn up as part of a normal discharge planning process, following the principles of the care planning approach. The supervision order has the power to require the client to live in a particular place and attend a particular place at set times for medical treatment, occupation, education and training. The client may also be required to allow access to his place of residence to the supervisor or anyone else authorised by the supervisor. Despite having the power to require the client to attend for treatment, the order does not give the power to impose medication or any other treatment against the client's wishes. The Act specifies that a range of people must be consulted before the order is applied: the client, members of the team caring for the client in hospital, the community team and informal carers and relatives.

The client has a supervisor, a member of the community mental health team who is suitably experienced and qualified. This can be any professional but is often a community mental health nurse. The supervisor is responsible for monitoring the implementation of the care plan and liaising with other members of the community team, as well as for ensuring that the order and care plan are reviewed. Most importantly, the supervisor is responsible for ensuring that the client complies with the requirements of the order. The supervisor has the power to require entry to the client's place of residence and to convey the client to a place where he or she is required to live or attend. The order is applied for a period of 6 months, and the client has the right to appeal against it to the Mental Health Review Tribunal.

All these legal measures have been devised in order to meet the demands of caring for people who have severe mental illness but can live in the community with support rather than staying in a large institution.

Reform of the Mental Health Act

At the beginning of the twenty-first century, further reform has been proposed, the proposals being set out in a White Paper *Reforming the Mental Health Act* (DoH, 2000b). This legislation is designed to take account of recent social change. Mental health care is increasingly being delivered in community settings, individuals spending less time in mental hospitals. The Act is to be based on a common framework for compulsory care and treatment, set out in a single pathway based on three distinct stages.

- *Stage One: Decisions on the use of compulsory powers*
  This concerns decisions to begin assessment and initial treatment under compulsory powers. It has to be supported by objective evidence and based on a preliminary examination by appropriately qualified professionals
- *Stage Two: Formal assessment and initial treatment under compulsory powers*
  Patients will receive a full assessment of their health and social care needs

before receiving treatment based on a preliminary care plan. This will be limited to a maximum of 28 days. There will be a fast-track procedure for patients to refer their cases to the Tribunal for review. After 28 days, the continuation of compulsory powers must be authorised by an independent decision-making body – the new Mental Health Tribunal

- *Stage Three: Care and treatment order*
  The Tribunal will be empowered to make a first care and treatment order for up to 6 months. The next order may be for a further 6 months, after which the orders will be for 12 months. The care and treatment order will authorise the care and treatment specified in a care plan that has been designed by the clinical team.

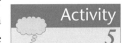

Activity 5

Mental health legislation has to achieve a balance between protecting the rights of the individual with a mental health problem and those of society. To what extent is this balance likely to be achieved by the changes outlined in the White Paper *Reforming the Mental Health Act* (DoH, 2000)?

The Act proposes the role of 'clinical supervisor'; this will normally be the appropriately qualified consultant psychiatrist in charge of the case, but it can also be a consultant clinical psychologist. This person has the power to discharge a patient from compulsory care and treatment. The patient may also appeal to the Mental Health Tribunal.

An order for care and treatment under compulsory powers can be applied if the patient is living in a community setting. Against each requirement set out for the patient, the order will outline what action the clinical supervisor is empowered to take if the patient fails to comply. Any patient who is actively resisting treatment will be given medication only in hospital.

Learning disability nursing

The legal framework that supports learning disability practice is the Mental Health Act 1983. Practitioners use this legal framework to detain clients, give compulsory treatment and offer protection of rights.

In 2001, the government published the White Paper *Valuing People: A New Strategy for Learning Disability for the 21st Century* (DoH, 2001a). This document offers a blueprint for the way in which services are to be planned and delivered for people with a learning disability. It is presented as an action plan that will be rolled out over the 5 years from 2001 to 2006. The paper outlines a considerable amount of funding that is to be allocated to learning disability services, specifically to be spent on supporting people with a learning disability in a move from long-stay hospital facilities to more appropriate supported accommodation, modernising day centres and improving services for children. A key feature of the development is effective advocacy services, which will be carried out in conjunction with voluntary agencies. Significant funding, partly financial support to be offered through increased social security benefits, is allocated to increasing the support offered to carers. Support is also offered via a national information centre and helpline developed in partnership with the charity MENCAP.

A key deficiency in learning disability services has been that clients have found it difficult to gain equal access to the health services, so the White Paper proposes to develop systems able to cater for complex health needs. Equally, it sets out to enable people with a learning disability to have the same right of access to mainstream health services as any other citizen.

Significant factors in providing a high quality of life are the comfort of and the facilities available in one's housing accommodation. People with a learning disability are to be offered a greater choice and control over where and how they live. Similarly, services will be developed to enable a greater choice of employment and to design services that meet the needs of people from a wide range of cultural and ethnic backgrounds. This policy is supported by the four principles of rights, independence, choice and inclusion.

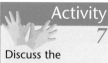

Activity 7

Discuss the argument that the principles of *Valuing People* (DoH, 2001a) arise from the values and beliefs of the 'Third Way'.

Working with children and young people

Children and young people are a group who are vulnerable, especially when in need of health and social care. As with mental health care, there is a legal framework that supports and guides practitioners in their work with children.

The Children Act

The legal framework that currently supports practice is the Children Act 1989, which took effect from 1991. It is addressed mainly to the court and to local authority social services, but parts of it are important for nurses to understand.

The main principles of the Act are child and family focused: the welfare of the child is paramount, and the overall aim is that children should be brought up and cared for within their own family. If children are in danger, they should be protected by effective intervention. An important tenet is that children should be kept informed about what happens to them and be involved in the decision-making process. Care should also be designed to support parents, ensuring that **parental responsibility** is maintained and that effective support is provided.

parental responsibility
a set of rights and duties against which parents can be assessed

The Act requires health practitioners to work with parents to enable them to care for their children to the best of their ability by enhancing their knowledge and understanding of child care and development. Working in the spirit of the Act means listening to the child, providing appropriate information and taking account of his or her feelings and wishes. Health-care professionals are also required to co-operate with the social service and education departments to meet the health needs of the child. Most important is the identification of children in need and their referral to social services if that is appropriate.

Section 17(10) of the Act specifically defines a 'child in need' as one who:

> is unlikely to achieve or maintain, or to have the opportunity of achieving or maintaining, a reasonable standard of health or development without the provision for him of services by a local authority [or whose] health or development is likely to be significantly impaired, or further impaired, without the provision for him of such services [or who] is disabled.

The Act recognises the role of midwives, health visitors and school nurses in having contact with the child from birth. They are likely to be the first to recognise a child in need and are expected to refer the child to social services using agreed health authority protocols. They are also expected to co-operate with social workers to provide the health care needed to promote the child's welfare.

The Act outlines a new concept of 'parental responsibility', which has replaced the phrase 'parental rights', emphasis being placed on the ongoing obligations of the parents' role. This includes the duties, rights, powers, responsibilities and authority that a parent has in respect of a child and his or her property. Parental responsibility is not affected by parental separation or divorce.

The nurse may be involved in a case in which a court order may be applied, so it is important to be aware of of the different types of order that might be granted. A *care order* is made if a court decides that a child is suffering or is likely to suffer significant harm through a lack of adequate parental care or control. The child is placed in the care of the local authority, which then has parental responsibility for the child that is shared with the parents. It does not take parental responsibility from the parents, but the local authority may decide how the parents exercise it.

A *supervision* order is made if the court decides that the local authority should observe a child closely and give guidance, the child then being under the supervision of a local authority or probation officer. Under this order, the local authority or the supervisor has parental responsibility.

A *child assessment order* is for use in situations in which there are reasonable grounds to suspect that the child is suffering significant harm but is not at immediate risk. The applicant may form the opinion that an assessment is needed but that the parents are unwilling to co-operate. Either the local authority or the National Society for the Prevention of Cruelty to Children may apply for this order. It has a maximum duration of 7 days, and the court decides on the nature of the assessment.

An *emergency protection order* is reserved for extremely urgent cases in which the child's safety is immediately threatened. This order can be applied for 8 days, with a additional 7 if necessary, but the order may be challenged by the parents after the first 72 hours of the order have elapsed. Parental responsibility is given to the applicant but only insofar as it is necessary to safeguard the child and promote his or her welfare. All these orders can be made by the court under public law.

In addition, there are a number of orders that are at the disposal of the courts but which are under private law proceedings relating to cases of divorce, domestic violence or adoption.

A *residence order* states with whom the child will live. This order may be made while the child is in the care of the local authority. It can thus end any care order and give parental responsibility to the person with the benefit of the order.

A *contact order* requires the person with whom the child lives to permit the child to have contact with those named in the order.

A *prohibited steps order* prevents the child's parents or any other person taking steps as outlined in the order without first obtaining the permission of the court.

Nurses may be required to attend a child protection conference before an application is made for a court order; the conference has to be clear and certain about the evidence before applying for an order. Nurses must also be prepared to write reports for court proceedings. In a child protection case, the nurse is required to provide documentation describing the nature of the significant harm that the child has already suffered. In addition, a statement of the child's future risk is required.

Almost any nurse, midwife or health visitor may, at some time in his or her practice, encounter a child who is at risk, so having a working knowledge of the principles and powers of the Children Act is important for all practitioners.

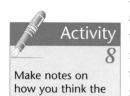

Activity

8

Make notes on how you think the Children Act protects and supports the rights of children.

▪ Chapter Summary

This chapter has described the main institutions of government and the processes that are undertaken in order to enact social policy. It has outlined how the NHS came into being and its subsequent development, and has discussed the statutory regulation of the profession and the development of education. In addition, social policy relating specifically to midwifery, children's nursing and mental health practice has been described in some detail. Finally, it should be emphasised that nurses can sometimes be a support and help to service users as much because of their knowledge of the wider social context of care as because of their clinical skill.

● **Test Yourself!**

1. How many stages must a Bill pass through in the House of Commons?

2. In which year did the NHS begin?

3. What are the main functions of a primary care Trust?

4. In which year did midwives gain the power to establish a Central Midwives Board?

5. What is the name of the inspectorate created by the Mental Health Act 1983?

6. What is the name of the order of the Children Act in which the court decides that the local authority should observe a child closely and give guidance?

| *Further Reading* | Dimond, B.C. and Barker, F.H. (1997) *Mental Health Law for Nurses.* Blackwell, Oxford. | Hanson, A.H. and Walles, M. (1990) *Governing Britain*, 5th edn. Fontana, London. |

References

DHSS (Department of Health and Social Security) (1975) *Better Services for the Mentally Ill.* HMSO, London.

DHSS (Department of Health and Social Security) (1980) *Inequalities in Health* (Black Report). HMSO, London.

DHSS (Department of Health and Social Security) (1983) *NHS Management Inquiry* (Griffiths Report). HMSO, London.

DoH (Department of Health) (1992) *The Children Act 1989: An Introductory Guide for the NHS.* HMSO, London.

DoH (Department of Health) (1997) *The New NHS: Modern, Dependable.* HMSO, London.

DoH (Department of Health) (2000) *Reforming the Mental Health Act.* HMSO, London.

DoH (Department of Health) (2000a) *The NHS Plan.* HMSO, London.

DoH (Department of Health) (2001a) *Valuing People: A New Strategy for Learning Disability for the 21st Century.* HMSO, London.

DoH (Department of Health) (2001b) *Shifting the Balance of Power within the NHS.* HMSO, London.

DoH (Department of Health) (2001c) *Shaping the Future.* HMSO, London.

Hill, M. (1993) *Understanding Social Policy*, 4th edn. Blackwell, Oxford.

Illich, I. (1976) *Limits to Medicine: Medical Nemesis*, 2nd edn. Marion Boyars, London.

Leathard, A. (2000) *Health Care Provision: Past Present and into the 21st Century*, 2nd edn. Stanley Thornes, Cheltenham.

McKeown, T. (1976) *The Modern Rise of Population and the Role of Medicine: Dream, Mirage or Nemesis?* Rock Carling Monograph. Nuffield Provincial Hospitals Trust, London.

Ministry of Health (1942) *Report of Committee on Social Insurance and Allied Services* (Beveridge Report). HMSO, London.

Ranade, W. (1994) *A Future for the NHS?: Health Care in the 1990s.* Longman, London.

Chapter

Nursing Practice in an Interprofessional Context

15

Contents

Learning outcomes

At the end of this chapter, the reader will be able to:

- Define the term 'interprofessional practice'

- Identify elements of good and bad practice in teamwork settings

- Highlight different professionals' contributions to teamwork

- Describe the role of the primary health-care team

- Discuss the challenges that the primary health-care team presents to different professionals

- Plan methods of working in practice that will support effective interprofessional teamwork

- Consider the ethical issues that interprofessional practice may create.

■ What is Interprofessionalism?

interprofessional

involves a group of different professionals working to achieve mutually agreed goals

'Interprofessional' is the term most recently used to describe professionals from different disciplines working together. The definition suggests that these professionals are working in collaboration to achieve the same goals for the client, patient or service user. Interprofessional practice can occur in a range of settings, from that of the acute medical ward to community support for elderly people.

multidisciplinary

often used to describe interprofessional teamwork in an academic context

Other terms are also used in place of and in preference to 'interprofessional': Leathard (1994) notes that, in health care, 'multidisciplinary' and 'interdisciplinary' have commonly been used to describe practice. Marshall et al. (1979) define multidisciplinary practice as the work of a group of individuals with different training backgrounds, for example nursing, medicine, occupational therapy, health visiting and social work, who share common objectives but make a different but complementary contribution. 'Interdisciplinary' has been described by Payne (2000) as work 'where professional groups make adaptations to their role, to take account of and interact with the roles of others'. The term 'multi-agency' is also used to describe the involvement of a range of services and professionals in the delivery of health and social care to an individual. To help the reader, the term 'interprofessional' will be used when describing teamwork that involves working towards the same goal for patients or clients.

transdisciplinary

working across ordinary professional boundaries to meet the needs of the client, patient or service user

Transdisciplinary teamwork (Garner and Orelove, 1994) may be a more radical form of practice. It can include working across ordinary professional boundaries to meet the needs of the client or service user. A nurse in the field of learning disability may, for example, give advice on housing or welfare benefits to a young man, although, in day-to-day practice, this would usually be the role of the social worker.

Two key features of interprofessional practice are teamwork and collaboration. Thus, the concept of interprofessional practice may be interpreted in a range of ways, which will be explored in this chapter.

■ Moves Towards Interprofessional Practice

CONNECTIONS

Chapter 14 reviews how government policy is enacted.

Over the past 30 years, changes in the delivery of health and social care have placed a different emphasis on the role and work of professionals. These changes have been created by government policy and concerns about the cost and focus of health and welfare provision. In addition, the developing role of some professional groups and the need to respond in order not to undermine the provision of services has required a new look at practice. Advances in technology that have reduced the time spent in hospital, in addition to the deinstitutionalisation movement, have placed an emphasis on care in the community. This has had an impact on more vocal and questioning consumers and service user groups seeking an understanding of, or participation in, decisions about the treatment and services offered, together with welfare rights. These changes have not occurred in isolation: all can be attributed to one or more of the factors identified. Because this chapter explores interprofessional work, it may be worth reviewing each of these elements separately.

Government policy and the focus of health and welfare provision

Moves to introduce general management structures created by the Griffiths Report (DoH, 1983) refocused the activity and roles of professionals within the NHS, one of the greatest changes being the movement of nurses and clinicians into general management. A second change was the division of the functions of delivering and purchasing care, Owens and Petch (1995) explaining this move as an attempt by the government to control budgets and resources. These changes also occurred in social care and formed part of the NHS and Community Care Act 1990. The separation of the functions of purchasing and providing health and social care was also to influence general practice and the role of the GP. In addition, it offered social workers and nurses new opportunities to support other groups with long-term needs, for example people with learning disability.

CONNECTIONS

Chapter 14 considers how government policy is enacted.

Following the election of a new Labour government in 1997, the ongoing implementation of the White Paper *The New NHS: Modern, Dependable* (DoH, 1997) and the *NHS Plan* (DoH, 2000), together with *Primary Care, General Practice and the NHS Plan* (DoH, 2001a), has confirmed the emphasis on primary health care, with the creation of **primary care groups** and Trusts. These groups are responsible for consulting with local communities on health-care needs as well as commissioning the health care needed from a range of services, for example acute health care. Such changes will continue to affect the way in which professionals work together and will create different partnerships and relationships for practice. The government sees these groups as being pivotal in achieving changes in public health as set out in the document *From Vision to Reality* (DoH, 2001b).

primary care groups

groups of GP practices set within a specific locality

In practice, this means new roles for some professionals. In primary care groups, for example, practice nurses may take on the responsibility for managing specific elements. Equally, some of the roles traditionally undertaken by the GP, for example caring for people who have a terminal illness in their own homes, may now be undertaken by community or practice nurses.

In other sectors of health care, multiprofessional working continues to be an essential part of the NHS's agenda modernisation, as is seen with cancer services, where patient outcomes may be more positive if support is offered in a multiprofessional context (Audit Commission/Commission for Health Improvement, 2001).

Role expansion

The Greenhalgh Report (Greenhalgh and Company, 1994) reviewed the role of junior doctors and recommended the reduction of their weekly working hours. One response to this initiative has been that of a broader role for nurses. The document *The Scope of Professional Practice* (UKCC, 1992) identifies several areas in which nurses could take on broader and more autonomous roles, for example nurse prescribing and nurse practitioner roles within community hospitals and nurse-led clinics.

The National Health Service and Community Care Act 1990 has also created alterations in the provision of long-term care, which has resulted in a closer working relationship between nurses and social workers. This is most common in care for elderly people and in developing services for those with a learning disability.

Finally, there has been a blurring of the boundaries between health visitors, district nurses and community nurses. All of this means a greater emphasis on teamwork and multiprofessional co-operation as clinical work that lay in the domain of the GP or hospital-based doctor is now being transferred to other professionals.

Changes in service provision

CONNECTIONS

Chapter 14 expands upon the issue of deinstitutionalisation.

As technology and approaches to treatment have changed, some patients and clients are spending less time in acute hospital settings. Many people are discharged and supported by community or district nurses in their own homes, the majority of care being provided by family members. Running parallel to these developments has been the deinstitutionalisation movement for those who are elderly or have a learning disability or mental health need.

The transition from institution to community care has seen a change in role for the professional groups of nurses, occupational therapists, psychologists and speech therapists, which has been compounded by an increasing emphasis on voluntary and independent sector provision in the community. Work that might once have been undertaken by qualified professionals may now be carried out by support workers or vocationally trained employees. Professional roles have in contrast become more specific because of the different types of support required in community settings.

At the same time, the cost of some roles has been questioned and the need for a professionally qualified individual challenged. Interwoven throughout these changes has been an increased demand for interprofessional collaboration in order to co-ordinate service delivery in the community.

The rights of service users, clients and patients

The recognition of the changing position of service users with regard to the services offered has gained momentum. An acknowledgement of fragmented services and a need to create a seamless service has built the foundation for change. Responses from service user groups have ranged from the formal voice of the Community Health Council and other representative bodies, to the radical position of others, notably those involved in the Council for Disabled People. Such activity has challenged the power of the professional and set the scene for a partnership between the service user and professional, as well as a greater input into decision-making on the use of resources. This change in position of the service user or client has meant that the involvement of a large number of professionals in their specific care group is no longer accepted; and greater collaboration within and across professional teams will be needed in order to minimise this and ensure access to the appropriate services.

Why is interprofessionalism important to nurses?

For nurses practising in a range of health-care and social care settings, the need for collaboration to meet service user needs will be a priority, and working together with other professionals will be part of everyday practice. In order to make sense of interprofessional working, and to enhance its success, it is necessary to have a clear picture of how nursing practice in the interprofessional team has evolved over time and what factors have impinged upon its success. A greater understanding of the role of other professional groups may be gained by thinking about interprofessional practice, which may give nurses greater confidence in collaboration.

> **Activity**
> *1*
> From your recent practice experience, identify all the different professionals you have come into contact with. What is their role and how does it link with yours?

■ Teamwork

When interprofessional or multidisciplinary work is described, it is usually a function of **teamwork**. The World Health Organization (1984) describes a team as:

> **teamwork**
> a group of identified professionals working together to achieve a specific outcome or set of outcomes

> A group who share a common health goal and common objectives determined by community needs, to the achievement of which each member of the team contributes, in accordance with his or her competence and skill and in coordination with the function of others.

Similarly, Rubin and Beckhard (1972) and Gilmour et al. (1974) describe it thus: 'a team is a group of people who make different contributions towards the achievement of a common goal.' Others would offer a three-strand definition:

belonging and being part of something successful and synergy, a common objective or purpose, and being able to achieve more collectively than as individuals outside the teamwork setting.

Collaboration

collaboration
a term to describe working together. The use of the term 'collaboration' often suggests that there may be conflict present and that the work may at times be difficult

Collaboration can be defined as 'work across boundaries, work with difference' (Loxley, 1997), successful collaboration depending on team members having clear ideas about what they hope to achieve. These ideas should be clear not just to the individual team members, but also to all those contributing to the team activity. Equally, team members should be working to meet the same goals or objectives for service users, patients or clients.

Effective collaboration requires mutual support and space for disagreement or the exploration of different views to take place. Part of the process of collaboration is deciding when it is needed and when individual team members can make autonomous decisions. In emergency situations, for example, there may be limited time for collaboration, but this does not stop collaboration occurring in emergency or crisis intervention work. Instead, team members may need to develop protocols or guidelines that take into account the decision-making process so that these guidelines can be followed in difficult situations or circumstances.

CONNECTIONS

For an example of emergency working, see cardiac arrest in Chapter 6.

Factors affecting teamwork

Although, from the definition, the route to teamwork may seem straightforward, it is in reality a more complicated process. Many factors can influence the ability of a team to practise effective co-operation, all of these occurring in the changing context of health and social care practice.

Financial

When budgets and resources are constrained, the issues of cost and who will foot the bill for intervention can create tension within teams. Practitioners at ground level often wish to work collaboratively to solve problems with service users, but the managers who hold the budgets may be constrained and be less able to be facilitative, perhaps placing restrictions on the amount of collaboration that takes place.

Team support

A key factor in team development is that of co-ordination, and resources may once again influence the level of support. Teams need accountable individuals to help the problem-solving process and take practice-focused solutions forward. These individuals may be identified as leaders or co-ordinators. Those teams lacking leadership or co-ordination are not as likely to achieve effective outcomes for clients. As a result, the cost in terms of an individual leader's time has to be met. Equally, teams require a physical environment in which to meet, as well as scheduled time to discuss problems, evaluate progress and plan future developments. All of these have both obvious and hidden cost implications.

Endorsing teamwork

Team members need to be able to see the benefits of a team-based model of care. When professionals are under pressure to maintain their current workload, finding time for additional means of collaborating and reviewing their current practice may seem yet another, and somewhat onerous, task.

The lynchpin of good practice may be evaluation as this enables team members to consider the effectiveness of their intervention and whether it has achieved the outcome that was anticipated. Balancing the results of intervention against the time and cost involved may help team members to decide on the relevance of the team activity that they have undertaken. Team members may need to consider the best use of their time together and set priorities, all of which may change following review. As teams work together over a longer period of time, they may be able to make decisions more swiftly, but ongoing evaluation may help them to decide whether such teamwork processes ensure the best outcomes for service users or patients.

Activity
2

Think again about your recent practice experience. What sort of formal and informal methods of evaluation have you seen? How effective have they been? Consider, for example, reading case notes or care plans, or review meetings within social care agencies.

◼ Professional Boundaries

For teamwork to be centred on clear outcomes for service users, clients and patients, team members need to be clear about the nature of their role within the team and what the boundaries of that role are. In other words, they need to ask what their professional role is, and where it ends and becomes the responsibility of a different professional. Hudson (1999) notes the significance of professional boundaries and the need for clarity with regard to professional roles and models of care. What practice activity, for example, is defined as core and to be taken on by all members, and what is seen as specific and thus the role of one discipline? Do differing approaches to practice, for example the medical versus the social model of care, impact on collaboration? Without clarifying the roles, team members may drift towards a common ground, which means that some areas of practice can be neglected.

This is illustrated by McGrath's (1993) study of community teams in the field of learning difficulties in the late 1980s, her research reviewing the practice of 27 teams in Wales. Team members were nurses, social workers, psychologists, physiotherapists or speech therapists, and one of the main aims of the team was to establish individual care plans for each person with a learning difficulty requiring a service intervention. McGrath's research indicates that, during the period of the study, a number of benefits were perceived by individual team members, but these did not result in the establishment of a higher level of individual programme or care plans. In contrast, collective responses to such developments as advocacy schemes increased, and individual team members felt that their knowledge of learning difficulty was heightened. However, the key aim of creating formal care plans made little progress.

All of the above are significant barriers to good practice that need to be overcome or acknowledged by both those working in teams and those co-ordinating them. Other elements can also inhibit or sustain good working practices.

■ Professional Socialisation

Individuals' socialisation into and integration within a specific professional group may impact upon their ability to work within an interprofessional team. When a person enters a career pathway with the intention of registering as a professional nurse, for example, a key element of the process is that of **professional socialisation** into the role. This may include guidelines on what clothing to wear in practice, the particular skills and competencies learnt in the common foundation programme and the way in which the client or patient is described, all manifesting themselves in how the learner develops the role or identity of a nurse. Similar processes will occur in all professional groups, a consequence being that when teamwork is practised, such factors may impinge on team integration. Some specific elements of professional socialisation are language, values and professional status.

professional socialisation

the process of taking on a set of values and an identity that are associated with and underpin a particular profession

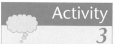

Activity 3

Think about your first weeks of nurse education. What activities formed part of the socialisation process? Were you aware of this process at the time?

Language

A vocabulary of terminology and abbreviations is used continuously within each professional group to communicate information, and the language involved may be unique to that profession. When teamwork is undertaken, the meaning of particular words and expressions will need clarification. If clarity is not sought, assumptions may be made about the meaning of specific language and actions, one result being conflict or conflicting views when language is interpreted in different ways by those who do not belong to that particular professional group.

Personal values

A **value** is something that individuals hold at the centre of their being. Values are developed over time and from experience, and personal values may reflect an individual's culture, moral stance or lifestyle. Values may be a product of age or historical tradition. Such values may be translated into action through the development of specific views or attitudes, either positive or negative. Values held may suggest that all individuals have the right to the same opportunities, for example that all people with learning disability should be part of ordinary community life. In this case, attitudes, shown in terms of behaviour, might involve becoming an independent advocate for an individual when the person needs help with communicating his wishes. In contrast, attitudes may remain observable only in terms of how positively or negatively an individual views a person or situation.

value
something that an individual holds at the centre of his or her being, developed over time and from experience

Professional values

In addition to personal values, individuals who participate in professional education may also develop a further set of values, and there may be assumptions made within teams about the values of the different professional groups. All are working towards similar goals for the client or service user, ideally in partnership with that person, but values may in reality be different. Social work may, for example, be concerned with interprofessional practice and achieving outcomes for service users based on a recognition of oppression and inequality in society, and the care plan or care management assessment set in place might reflect this. Equally, physiotherapists may be focused on physiological factors that inhibit good health for service users. In working towards collaborative practice, discussion based on values and what they mean to individual professions may work towards an understanding of professional action. If values are ignored, however, this may lead to greater tension in teams (Braye and Preston-Shoot, 1994).

Activity 4

What do you think the values of the nurse are? What are these values based on? Do they differ from your own?

Interprofessional values

Loxley (1997) describes the core values of interprofessional work as trust and sharing. She uses the word '**utilitarian**', that is, being or having practical worth, to endorse their validity in teamwork. Essential components of trust and sharing are that they must remain two way. This means not only relying on people's commitment to the team's purpose or task, but also taking on the team members' belief in oneself as being able to deliver the goods or take on the role, and meeting these expectations. Achieving the ability to trust others and to share

utilitarian
a solution that aims for the greater good, one which has a practical outcome

practice with them will require confidence and a clear understanding of one's own professional role, which may become more complex when individuals are of a different status.

Ethics

Interprofessional practice may bring to the fore ethical dilemmas in the practice setting. Sheppard (1996), for example, describes potential areas of conflict between professions. GPs will have as their highest priority respect for the life of the patient, whereas a social worker's major concern will be the wishes of the clients themselves. This could lead to conflict over issues regarding the clinical treatment of individuals, particularly if they are already unwell or have a mental illness or learning disability. Child protection work can also create ethical dilemmas if the needs of the child conflict with those of other family members at home. Nurses too can be involved in a range of complex situations, for example when planning discharge for older people. There may be a difference between the wishes of the older person in question and the family members. The elderly person may wish to go home, whereas the hospital consultant may think a nursing home more appropriate. As a nurse, whose wishes do you act upon?

Status

For teams to work effectively, mutual trust and a respect for all members' contributions to the team are required. Part of the means of achieving this trust is by holding a greater understanding of the key role of other professional groups and acknowledging the differences and similarities in language, values and models of practice used by other professions. The team co-ordinator or leader should facilitate this process as a model for teamwork is developed.

Nurses have traditionally been seen as semi-autonomous practitioners working to guidelines drawn up by medical staff; doctors themselves have been seen as making autonomous clinical decisions and advising other members of the health-care and social care teams on practice. Speech therapists and physiotherapists, although autonomous practitioners, work largely on an individual basis with clients, advising on very specific areas of intervention. Because of these differences, power and status may become an issue when teamwork is undertaken. Doctors, for example, may have difficulty taking advice from other health-care professionals, whereas nurses may lack the confidence to advise or provide information related to a specific area of practice. Social workers' views of good practice in mental health services may clash with a more medically orientated response from a consultant psychiatrist. All this can influence the way in which teams function and create future stress for team members.

■ Good Practice in Teamwork

At this point, nursing practice in an interprofessional context may seem complex and to be avoided at all costs! Nevertheless, having realistic expectations of teamwork may help the nurse to prepare for practice with greater confidence and maintain a focus on what is significant to the outcomes for the client or service user. Some reasons for this are as follows.

Knowledge

Knowledge that identifies some probable causes of friction within the teamwork setting can help to make sense of difficulties and begin to shape the problem-solving process, in other words to help the practitioner to find a workable solution to the situation. Because of the knowledge held, an acceptance of team members' differences and different contributions to teamwork can lead to a gradual mutual trust. This will in turn contribute towards a working environment in which it is safe to air conflict or state different opinions. A further spin-off will be the prevention of isolation and an increased willingness to share information.

Methods of practice intervention

The responses to a client's or service user's needs may differ across a range of different professionals. A medical model approach may favour giving information and a course of treatment to individuals; this model may be used by doctors. Some nurses may also adopt an information-giving role. In contrast, other professionals may seek a more partnership-based model of practice, seen for example, as Oliver (1996) suggests, where the professional is viewed as a resource to be used by the particular service user. In other words, the client or individual service user will direct the professional's approach, personally requesting specific information, action and responses. This approach is developing within social work and care management-type roles. The different models of practice of different professional groups can lead to an inconsistency of information for the client or service user and cause greater confusion. The teamwork process should, however, provide a framework within which issues such as what information should be given and the level of commitment required by each professional are clearly stated and agreed.

Pritchard (1995) adopts Bruce's (1980) 'teamwork for presentation' matrix to identify stages of team co-operation (Table 15.1). Pritchard's matrix illustrates the steps toward the committed team by describing co-operation in a range of teamwork activities. The main use of this tool has been in the assessment or diagnosis of a team's current position. Here it is used to give an example

Table 15.1 Stages of team co-operation

Co-operation in:	'Nominal'	'Convenient'	'Committed'
Team goal-setting	No explicit goals	Follow doctors' goals	Shared explicit goals
Role perceptions	Stereotypes common	Some understanding	Roles clearly understood
Professional status	Wide differences	Differences inhibit co-operation	Differences ignored
Referral of patients	To agency rather than individual professionals	Referral by delegation	Easy two-way referral and open access
Interaction within team	Very little and irregular interaction	Some interaction	Close regular interaction, formal and informal
Mutual trust	Lacking	Guarded	Strong and developing
Communication failure	Often	Sometimes	Exceptional
Confidentiality	A problem	Problems partly solved	Not a problem
Advice to patients	Inconsistent	Poor co-ordination	Consistent
Preventative care	Not possible	Possible	Optimum conditions

Source: Modified from Bruce (1980).

of what could be achieved within the teamwork setting. Moreover, as Pritchard (1995) notes, there is a need to link teamwork performance to outcomes for service users and, as such, to begin to meet need.

Meeting need

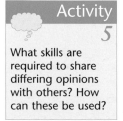

Activity 5

What skills are required to share differing opinions with others? How can these be used?

CONNECTIONS

Chapter 11 provides more information on teamworking.

In a team where conflict is aired and individual members feel safe to share differing views, steps can be taken towards clear mutual goals. These can help the teamwork forward, preventing obstruction and avoiding difficult issues. Rubin and Beckhard (1972) suggest that, in order to meet need, the team must be able to identify agreed objectives and be able to articulate and resolve differences. Finally, the team must be able to manage interpersonal issues – how the team feel about each other – and make a commitment to teamwork. In learning to manage all of these factors, the needs of service users or clients can remain central to the team's purpose.

■ Working in Teams

The first section of this chapter has reviewed some of the factors that can affect teamwork, these being generic in setting and content. In this section, the role of the primary health-care team will be explored to provide a specific example of teamwork and multiprofessional practice.

What is the primary health-care team?

In the foreword to the summary of the early White Paper *Primary Care: Delivering the Future* (DoH, 1996), primary health care was described as 'the NHS most people see – the NHS of the family doctor and their team, community nurses, therapists as well as pharmacists, dentists and optometrists'. It will also include midwives, district nurses and health visitors. Since the implementation of the White Paper *The New NHS: Modern, Dependable* (DoH, 1997), the role of the primary care team has continued to develop and grow: traditional teams based around health centres may now include counsellors and mental health nurses, and social workers will be involved in areas such as child protection and provision for elderly people. Plans set in place by the 1996 White Paper will review and expand the role of the nurse in learning further skills, such as prescribing medication. Equally, the role of the practice nurse has expanded to take on referrals from people who would ordinarily have seen their GP. In addition, the new strategy for people with learning disabilities, *Valuing People* (DoH, 2001c), highlights the relationship between the primary health-care team and other services in meeting the ongoing health-care needs of this group of people as one means of preventing social exclusion.

primary health care
the continuing health and social welfare care offered appropriately to individuals in need living in private households

CONNECTIONS
Chapter 14 outlines other relevant legislation.

How has it evolved?

Jeffereys (1995) wrote that, as a result of the Family Doctor's Charter (BMA, 1965) in 1966, arrangements were set in place for positive community-based practice. This charter established a positive role for non-hospital-based medicine, a structure for interprofessional work being instigated. Jeffereys identified the elements of this structure as allowances for GPs who worked together on one site, and promoting the employment of receptionists and practice nurses, by providing reimbursement for their services, and offering interest-free loans for more modern premises. The Health Services and Public Health Act 1968 endorsed a health-promotion role for general practice that involved the prevention of ill-health and support for families. Thus, the role of the primary health-care team gradually emerged.

Further changes were to occur in the 1980s as the Conservative government set about cutting the increasing public expenditure. Pietroni (1994) reported that the White Paper *Priorities for Health and Social Services in England* (DHSS, 1976) and the *NHS Management Inquiry* (DoH, 1983) were to culminate in the

NHS and Community Care Act 1990 (DoH, 1990). These placed further responsibilities for care within the primary care team, making it the first point of call for all referrals. Alongside this, budgets have devolved to GPs, with practices taking on GP fundholding responsibilities. These moves have enabled GPs to decide on purchasing priorities for primary and secondary care across the spectrum of demographic needs. These developments have placed GPs at the centre of decision-making within the primary health-care team despite suggestions that other professionals, such as nurses, might take on the initial assessment role. Chart 15.1 highlights the key developments within primary health-care nursing practice.

Quality services in the community

As part of the NHS modernisation agenda, the primary health-care team is continuing to face the challenge of effective teamwork and the need to develop further professional roles. The government's aim to achieve a seamless service remains, in order that clients and patients are not seen by a vast number of different professionals and to prevent their continual assessment and attendance at different clinics. An emphasis on developing primary health care remains a top priority, the principles of good primary care, shown in Figure 15.1 below, being highlighted with regard to quality. In addition, one of the key functions of primary care groups will be that of **clinical governance**, ensuring that effective, high-quality care is offered to a specific population.

clinical governance

a comprehensive method of determining the quality of provision of service, focusing on professional accountability, audit, patient or client perception of the service and value for money

CONNECTIONS

Chapter 16 reviews clinical governance.

Role of the professional within the primary health-care team

There are still decisions to be made about the extended roles of nurses and how these will contribute to the primary health-care team. Equally, the need to use resources effectively remains an issue. Also unanswered is why there is still an ongoing need to re-emphasise interprofessional teamwork when primary health-care teams have been in existence for more than 25 years. Teamwork should be seen as an essential part of working together, yet some gaps still exist. Some broad reasons for the difficulties encountered in teamwork were raised earlier in the chapter. If we look specifically at primary health-care teams, all the factors identified may inhibit good practice, but it is worth looking at this point at some further constraints on teamwork within primary care teams.

Location

It is probable that the core members of the primary health-care team are situated on one site within a local health centre. Other professionals, such as social

Chart 15.1 ● Key developments in primary health-care nursing

District nursing

1970s	Introduction of attachment schemes
	District nurses based at GP practices. Established primary health-care teams
1972	Report of the Committee on Nursing made recommendations for formal post-basic education, which became law in 1979
1974	Royal College of General Practitioners published *Nursing in General Practice in the Reorganised NHS* (RCGP, 1974)
1990s	Extended role of the district nurse may include the prescribing of medication, previously the task of the GP
	Review of educational requirements of the role as part of the English National Board specialist pathway curricula

Practice nursing

1970s	Nurses attached to GP practice
1986	Cumberlege Report, *Neighbourhood Nursing: A Focus for Care* (DHSS, 1986)
	Recommended development of the nurse practitioner role – taking on direct referrals to ease the pressure on GPs
1987	Government rejected these plans
1990s	Role of practice nurses under review
1996	White Paper *Primary Care: Delivering the Future* (DoH, 1996) advocates major changes to practice nurse education and role within the primary health-care team
1998	Configuration of primary care groups may mean changes in the practice nurse role

Health visiting

1976	Court Report identified the health visitor as a major agent of prevention in family work (Orr, 1975)
1970s and 80s	Central Council for the Education and Training of Health Visitors continued to assess the role of the health visitor, especially when the focus on child protection and children at risk increased
1980	Standing conference on health visitor education, *A Time to Learn*, looked at the changing role of health visiting
1990s	Role still unclear. Purchaser concern with cost of health visitor intervention
1998	Configuration of primary care groups may mean changes in the role of the health visitor

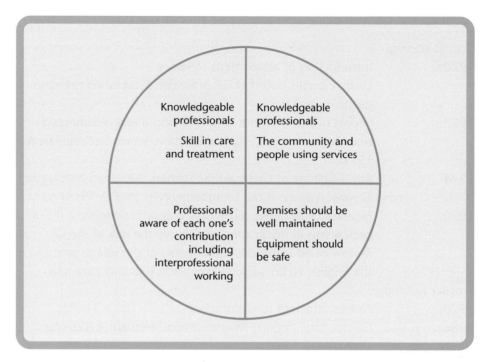

Figure 15.1 ● Principles of good primary care (adapted from DoH, 1996)

workers, who provide an input to the team may, however, be based at different locations. As a consequence, they may miss out on informal contact and lines of communication.

Team size

Within the primary health-care team, a range of individual professionals may be involved in providing services, and the size and extent of this may impact on team development. Too large a team may prevent clear and focused discussion and inhibit the decision-making process. Examples of this may be seen in the child protection and mental health services.

Payment

Individual professionals working as part of the primary health-care team will be employed on different rates of pay and conditions of service. This could lead to a feeling of resentment among some team members.

Resource management

Within the primary health-care team, responsibility for practice and performance may not be clearly identified. In some teams, GPs may be the decision-makers when funding for services is allocated. In contrast, practice nurses and other nurse practitioners may have limited financial or budgetary control. Although individual practitioners may see themselves as autonomous, issues such as payment and access to resources can lead to an inequality of status, and individual contributors to teamwork may as a consequence be seen as being of more or less value.

In the changing climate of primary care, in which GPs may have greater financial autonomy, the position of other professionals may be under greater scrutiny, for example when making decisions about the effectiveness of the input of various professionals and, in doing so, questioning roles and performance. Part of this process may lead to a narrowing down of certain roles and a limited input of some professionals to primary health-care teams. Such activities may restrict good teamwork.

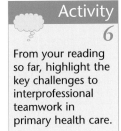

Activity

6

From your reading so far, highlight the key challenges to interprofessional teamwork in primary health care.

■ Moving Towards Co-operation

The place of interprofessional work currently remains uncertain. Pockets of good practice are observable, but mutual co-operation and the desires of service users can be in conflict with government policy, the way in which funding mechanisms operate and the struggle for power of some professional groups (Figure 15.2).

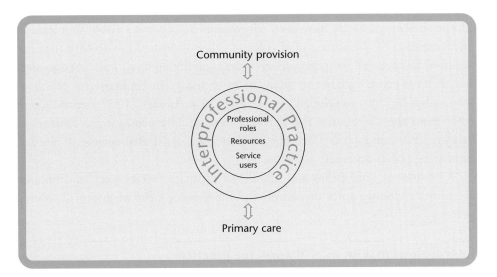

Figure 15.2 ● Factors affecting interprofessional work

◾ Responses to Teamworking

Research and reports

A considerable amount of research and evaluation has been undertaken in the area of teamwork in primary and community care. Many of the findings of earlier studies in the 1980s focusing on primary health-care settings were negative, and the reluctance to collaborate of some specific professional groups, such as doctors, is well documented. More recently, however, the value of interprofessional work has become the focus of research and evaluation. Most of the work published emphasises the positive responses to collaboration across different professional groups, although it is too early to review the impact of this research on practice development. As the body of research grows, along with an increasing amount of research funding for such projects, it is, however, likely that effective mechanisms for change will be identified and implemented. At the time of writing, several key reports have been published that focus on the value of collaboration, including:

- the Sainsbury Foundation for Mental Health report (Sainsbury Foundation, 1997)
- the Standing Medical, Nursing and Midwifery Advisory Committee (1996) report
- the Standing Committee on Postgraduate Medical and Dental Education (SCOPME, 1997) Working Paper.

Educational developments

Education has been one response to the interprofessional agenda. Providers of educational programmes have seen educational activity as a route to a greater understanding of the professional roles of others. Most of the activity that has occurred has been at postregistration or post-qualifying level. Individual professionals have come together to share units of study, an emphasis on problem-solving having been developed during the 1990s. Loxley (1997) reproduces a table from the Centre for the Advancement of Interprofessional Education, Primary and Community Care (1996) that gives a detailed review of the co-ordinating bodies and their activities.

A number of universities and schools of medicine, social work and nursing are also developing units or forums for the development of interprofessional practice initiatives.

Interprofessionalism as a 'theory' for practice

Many of the elements that form interprofessional practice have been brought together in this chapter. Much of this has centred upon teamwork and collaboration, and a review of roles and professional boundaries. We have seen how the developments in community care have created many of these changes. In reality, interprofessionalism has been seen as a set of skills or competencies rather than a whole new way of informing practice, with a theoretical underpinning. For example, from what knowledge base does interprofessional work come? Loxley (1997) suggests that assumptions are made about what knowledge from a certain discipline might be helpful but that this has not been investigated or studied in a coherent way. It is largely driven by what services need, and because of this, a sound theoretical framework has not yet developed.

A number of academics and practitioners are beginning to study and build a theory for interprofessional practice. As this develops, it is possible that those professionals who have been reluctant to make interprofessional practice a priority may begin to participate.

Personal responses

The moves forward outlined above tackle complex issues at a societal service and organisational level. An individual in practice can still, however, begin to create change. For a nurse practising in a multiprofessional setting, thinking about individual responses to teamwork and reflecting on their cause or foundation may be helpful. Observing professionals who hold effective team member skills may also provide ideas for the development of personal knowledge and skills.

> **CONNECTIONS**
>
> *Chapter 13 describes an approach to thinking about this in a structured and useful way.*

From this perspective, individual methods of working that can help effective teamwork can be shaped. Part of this exercise should include an active consideration of the role of service users in the process.

■ Chapter Summary

The route to interprofessional practice is a complex one. At times, the agendas of government, service managers, professionals and service users seem to be in conflict, but positive examples can nevertheless be seen in practice. As practitioners, educationalists and service managers design the organisational structures needed to develop further multiprofessional work, professionals can build on their skills in collaboration. The interface of health and social care delivery can then become a positive one.

● **Test Yourself!**

1. What does the term 'interprofessional practice' mean?

2. Provide examples from your own experience of good and bad teamwork.

3. How do different professionals contribute to teamworking?

4. What challenges does working in a primary health-care team create for the nurse?

References

Audit Commission/Commission for Health Improvement (2001) *NHS Cancer Care in England and Wales*. Audit Commission, London.

BMA (British Medical Association) (1965) *Family Doctors Charter: A Charter for the Family Doctor Service*, BMA, London.

Braye, S. and Preston-Shoot, M. (1994) *Empowering Practice in Social Care*. Open University Press, Buckingham.

Bruce, N. (1980) *Teamwork for Preventative Care*. Research Studies Press/John Wiley & Sons, Chichester.

Centre for the Advancement of Interprofessional Education, Primary and Community Care (1996) *National Coordinating Bodies and their Interests*. CAIPE, London.

DHSS (Department of Health and Social Security) (1976) *Priorities for Health and Personal Social Services in England*. HMSO, London.

DHSS (Department of Health and Social Security) (1986) *Community Nursing Review. Neighborhood Nursing – A Focus for Care*. Cumberlege Report. HMSO, London.

DoH (Department of Health) (1983) *NHS Management Inquiry* (Griffiths Report). HMSO, London.

DoH (Department of Health) (1990) *Caring for People. Community Care in the Next Decade and Beyond*. HMSO, London.

DoH (Department of Health) (1996) *Primary Care: Delivering the Future*. HMSO, London.

DoH (Department of Health) (1997) *The New NHS: Modern, Dependable*. Stationery Office, Norwich.

DoH (Department of Health) (2000) *The NHS Plan*. Stationery Office, Norwich.

DoH (Department of Health) (2001a) *Primary Care, General Practice and the NHS Plan*. Stationery Office, Norwich.

DoH (Department of Health) (2001b) *From Vision to Reality*. Stationery Office, Norwich.

DoH (Department of Health) (2001c) *Valuing People. A New Strategy for Learning Disability in the 21st Century*. Stationery Office, Norwich.

Garner, H.G. and Orelove, F.P. (1994) *Teamwork in Human Services. Models and Application across the Life Span*. Butterworth Heinemann , Boston.

Gilmour, M., Bruce, N. and Hunt, M. (1974) *The Work of the Nursing Team in General Practice*. Council for the Education and Training of Health Visitors, London.

Greenhalgh and Company (1994) *The Interface Between Junior Doctors and Nurses: A Research Study for the Department of Health*. HMSO, London.

Hudson, B. (1999) Primary health care and social care: working across professional boundaries. *Managing Community Care* **7**(1): 15–22.

Jeffereys, M. (1995) Primary health care. In Owens, P., Carrier, C. and Horder, J. (eds) *Interprofessional Issues in Community and Primary Health Care*. Macmillan – now Palgrave Macmillan, Basingstoke.

Leathard, A. (1994) *Going Inter-professional. Working Together for Health and Welfare*. Routledge, London.

Loxley, A. (1997) *Collaboration in Health and Welfare*. Jessica Kingsley, London.

McGrath, M. (1993) *Multidisciplinary Teamwork*. Avebury, Aldershot.

Marshall, M., Preston, M., Scott, E. and Wincott, P. (eds) (1979) *Teamwork For and Against: An Appraisal of Multidisciplinary Practice*. British Association of Social Workers, London.

Oliver, M. (1996) *Social Work. Disabled People and Disabling Environments*. Jessica Kingsley, London.

Orr, J. (1975) Health visiting in the UK. In Hockey, L. (ed.) *Primary Care Nursing*. Churchill Livingstone, London.

Owens, P. and Petch, H. (1995) Professionals and management. In Owens, P., Carrier, J. and Horder, J. (eds) *Interprofessional Issues in Community and Primary Health Care*. Macmillan – now Palgrave Macmillan, Basingstoke.

Payne, M. (2000) *Teamwork and Multiprofessional Care*. Macmillan – now Palgrave Macmillan, Basingstoke.

Pietroni, P. (1994) Interprofessional teamwork. In Leatherhead, A. (ed.) *Going Inter-professional*. London, Routledge.

Pritchard, P. (1995) Learning to work effectively in teams. In Owens, P., Carrier, J. and Horder, J. (eds) *Interprofessional Issues in Community and Primary Health Care*. Macmillan – now Palgrave Macmillan, Basingstoke.

RCGP (Royal College of General Practitioners) (1974) *Nursing in General Practice in the Re-organised NHS*. RCGP, London.

Rubin, I.R. and Beckhard, R. (1972) Factors influencing the effectiveness of health teams. *Millbank Memorial Fund Quarterly* **50**(3): 317–37.

Sainsbury Foundation for Mental Health (1997) *Pulling Together*. Sainsbury Foundation for Mental Health, London.

Standing Committee on Postgraduate Medical and Dental Education (SCOPME) (1997) *Multiprofessional Working and Learning. Sharing the Educational Challenge*. SCOPME, London.

Sheppard, M. (1996) Primary care roles and relationships. In Watkins, M. et al. (eds) *Collaborative Community Mental Health Care*. Arnold, London.

Standing Medical, Nursing and Midwifery Advisory Committee (1996) *In the Patient's Interest: Multiprofessional Working Across Organisational Boundaries*. HMSO, London.

UKCC (United Kingdom Central Council for Nursing, Midwifery and Health Visiting) (1992) *The Scope of Professional Practice*. UKCC, London.

World Health Organization (1984) *Glossary of Terms Used in the 'Health for All' Series*. WHO, Geneva.

16 Challenges to Professional Practice

Contents

- Defining Professional Practice
- Philosophies and Ideologies
- Clinical Governance
- Models and Frameworks of Care
- Where to Next?
- Test Yourself!
- References

Learning outcomes

The aim of this chapter is to start you thinking about some of the issues that influence the ways in which nurses operate as registered practitioners to manage and deliver nursing care. At the end of the chapter, you should be able to:

- Define professional practice and discuss the responsibilities involved

- Understand the *Code of Professional Conduct* in relation to your own roles and responsibilities as a student, with particular relationship to accountability and informed consent

- Describe the role that personal, organisational and professional beliefs and values play in underpinning practice

- Identify the influence of models and frameworks of care in nursing practice

- Discuss the significance of quality assessment, standards and the role of clinical governance in evaluating nursing care

- Identify your own responsibilities for evidence-based practice and lifelong learning.

By the time you reach the end of the common foundation programme, you will have gained some confidence in clinical skills, experienced a range of placements aimed at broadening your perceptions of nursing and your clients, and developed a theoretical foundation on which to build the more specialised theory of your chosen branch of nursing. The issues raised in this chapter can be seen as challenges that nurses have addressed in an effort to move from an occupation dominated and directed by medical practitioners, to one with a developing knowledge and skill base of its own, which has a direct influence on client care. All of these subjects will be addressed in more detail in your branch studies and are merely touched upon here in terms of raising your awareness of what the responsibilities of being a **registered practitioner** are.

The issues to be considered are:

registered practitioner

a nurse, midwife or health visitor who is registered on the professional register with the NMC

- Defining professional practice
- The responsibilities of professional practice
  - The Nursing and Midwifery Council *Code of Professional Conduct*
  - accountability
  - informed consent
  - credibility
  - lifelong learning
- Evidence-based practice
- Philosophies and ideologies (beliefs and values)
- A knowledge base for nursing – frameworks of care, models and the nursing process
- Quality, standards and clinical governance.

Before addressing the theoretical issues, however, it is worth taking time to consider just what we mean by 'professional practice'.

■ Defining Professional Practice

The debate over whether or not nursing is a profession has been raging for over a decade, and each of us has our own views on it (for an overview of this, see Rafferty, 1996). The whole issue is largely a sterile one that has little impact on the way in which nurses practise nursing; what is far more important for nursing students is how we choose for ourselves what constitutes 'professional' behaviour and how we enact that in our practice. So perhaps the best place to start this chapter is by identifying what we mean by professional practice. Try Activity 1.

Some of the issues that you identified probably relate to such things as:

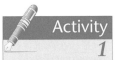

Activity

1

Take a few minutes to think back over your experience to date and note down the expectations you would have of any person whom you consulted as a professional, for example a lawyer, a doctor or an architect.

- The knowledge that people have
- Their professional qualifications or evidence of belonging to a professional body or organisation that licenses or registers them to practise
- The skill that they exhibit in their practice
- Their conduct – for example, the way in which they dress, their manner, how they treat you, the respect they show you and the confidence they have in their ability to help you
- A recommendation from other people or the fact that they are recognised for their particular expertise.

Hence we all carry with us a personal view of what professional practice is.

Superimposed on this will be external definitions that arise from the professional bodies governing the people whom they license to practise, for example codes of practice, and criteria established by government policies. Similarly, there may be expectations of professional practice that derive from employers and contracts of employment.

Moloney (1992) suggests that the set of attributes displayed by people in professional practice can be seen as 'professionalism' and that they relate essentially to the attitudes and attributes that they display. The first of these is that a profession is indeed 'practised' or engaged in rather than being a theoretical activity. Other attitudes may be a commitment to work and an orientation towards service rather than personal profit. Similarly, there may be a requirement for accountable practice that is based on evidence and an inherent motivation for learning and the development of a knowledge base. These arise, as we have seen, from a multitude of sources.

The responsibilities of professional practice

CONNECTIONS

Chapter 14 describes in greater detail the regulation of the professions.

The UKCC and four National Boards were established in the 1979 Nurses, Midwives and Health Visitors Act as the regulatory bodies for the professions. These were superseded by the Nursing and Midwifery Council (NMC) in 2002. Although the UKCC was intended to be an elected body, it functioned in its first years, from 1980 to 1983, as an appointed body as responsibilities were transferred from the previous authorities such as the General Nursing Council, the Central Midwives Council and the Council for the Education and Training of Health Visitors. Similar transitional arrangements enabled the NMC to shadow the UKCC for a year prior to taking over its full powers.

One of the main functions of the UKCC was the maintenance of a 'live' register of qualified nurses, midwives and health visitors. According, however, to Section 2(1) of the 1979 Act:

The principal function of the Central Council shall be to establish and improve standards of training and professional conduct for nurses, midwives and health visitors.

In order to carry this out, four key objectives and priorities were been identified (UKCC, 1988).

Objective one

To determine an education and training policy and programme to ensure that nurses, midwives and health visitors who are trained and registered meet the needs of society in the 1990s and beyond.

In order to achieve this objective, the UKCC established a set of training rules and for the first time included a statement of the outcomes of training. While clarifying and developing initial training for registration, the Council also developed a policy for the standards of post-qualifying education under the heading 'Post-registration Education and Practice' (PREP). The UKCC provided practitioners with *The PREP Handbook* (UKCC, 2001), which consolidated all the previous guidance, provided details of the continuing professional development (CPD) standard that was to be achieved and clarified the definitions used.

There are two separate standards that affect a practitioner's registration, one relating to practice and one to CPD. When completing your notification to practise for triennial registration, you are signing to confirm that you:

- have worked in some capacity by virtue of your registration for a minimum of 100 days (750 hours) during the previous 5 years or undertaken a return to practice course (practice standard)
- undertake a minimum of 5 days (35 hours) CPD over the 3 year period and record this in your personal portfolio.

Objective two

To promote a heightened awareness among nurses, midwives and health visitors of:

- professional standards and responsibilities
- the opportunities of being members of a profession.

These two issues have resulted in several publications that provide professional advice and guidelines for nurses, midwives and health visitors. The most significant of these for student nurses are probably the *Code of Professional Conduct*

(NMC, 2002), *Exercising Accountability* (UKCC, 1989), *Confidentiality* (UKCC, 1987) and *Guidelines for Professional Practice* (UKCC, 1996).

The purpose of the *Code of Professional Conduct* (2002) is to:

- inform the professions of the standard of professional conduct required of them in the exercise of their professional accountability and practice
- inform the public, other professions and employers of the standard of professional conduct that they can expect of a registered practitioner.

The Code states that, as a registered nurse or midwife, you must:

- protect and support the health of individual patients and clients
- protect and support the health of the wider community
- act in such a way that justifies the trust and confidence the public have in you
- uphold and enhance the good reputation of the professions.

Chart 16.1 shows the responsibilities placed on practitioners by the Code of Conduct.

Objective three

To develop professional conduct work positively and in dealing with matters of professional misconduct to ensure a consistency of approach throughout the UK.

The NMC offers professional advice about standards of conduct and ensures that practitioners have access to any current information available. **Professional**

Chart 16.1 ● *Code of Professional Conduct*

As a professional nurse or midwife, you are personally accountable for your practice. In caring for patients and clients, you must:

- respect the patient or client as an individual
- obtain consent before you give any treatment or care
- protect confidential information
- co-operate with others in the team
- maintain your professional knowledge and competence
- be trustworthy
- act to identify and minimize risk to patients and clients.

Source: NMC (2002). Available at www.nmc-uk.org.

CONNECTIONS

Chapter 15 explores teamworking.

Conduct Committees hear cases of alleged misconduct against any registered practitioner; they sit in different regional venues and are open to members of the profession. In addition, two panels – the Panel of Professional Screeners and the Health Committee – meet to consider other issues relating to practitioners' fitness to practise, such as alcohol or drug abuse.

Professional Conduct Committees

committees of the NMC whose purpose it is to hear cases of alleged professional misconduct

Objective four

To make the Central Council financially viable and a cost-effective and efficient organisation.

The Nursing and Midwifery Council (NMC) became effective on 1 April 2002. As well as taking on the professional regulatory role of the UKCC in terms of accountability in practice and determining standards for practice, the NMC will be responsible for two significant aspects of quality assurance in the education of nurses, midwives and health visitors (UKCC, 2002):

Activity 2

Access and review the contents of the new NMC website (www.nmc-uk.org). Note any information about the revised Code of Conduct.

Discuss your findings with your practice-based mentor or study group.

- Setting standards for preregistration education and also for those education programmes leading to a recordable qualification (that is, one that is entered on the register of practice)
- Monitoring the quality of all education programmes leading to registerable or recordable qualifications.

The NMC quality assurance framework will incorporate elements of institutional approval, approval in principle, validation, annual monitoring, periodic review and subject review. To achieve this, the NMC will work in partnership with:

- education purchasers – strategic health boards and workforce confederations
- quality assurance organisations such as the CHI (England and Wales), Clinical Standards Board (Scotland), Northern Ireland Practice and Education Council and EC
- Quality Assurance Agency
- Service providers, both NHS and independent
- Higher Education Institutes
- Multiprofessional regulatory bodies such as the General Medical Council, Health Professions Council and General Social Care Council.

One of the most significant issues to have been highlighted by the UKCC, and which has transferred to the NMC, in terms of standards of professional practice is that of accountability.

What is accountability?

Although we tend to talk in terms of *professional* responsibility, there are in fact four different types of accountability that can be identified for registered nurses:

1. Accountability to society under criminal and civil law.
2. Accountability to the employer under a contract of employment.
3. Accountability to the patient under existing law provision.
4. Accountability to the profession under the Nurses, Midwives and Health Visitors Act 1979.

Thus, although we usually focus on the latter in terms of professional issues, it is important to remember that nurses, as individual members of society, need to be accountable in terms of the expectations of any other member of society; that is, they cannot commit a criminal act and expect to be defended by a professional code.

Features of professional accountability

Professional accountability means using one's professional judgement and being answerable for it. We can therefore identify two features of it – decision-making and an obligation to explain and justify any actions taken.

As a nurse, you are privileged to be allowed to make decisions about areas of care based on your knowledge, skills and experience. These will quite often be life-saving decisions or decisions that have a huge potential impact on your clients: think, for example, of the responsibility underlying a health visitor's decision to refer a suspected case of child abuse to the social services department. Practitioners are imbued with the power to make decisions because they are recognised as being competent in their area of practice and their clients trust them to act in their best interests. On the other side of the coin, however, lies the expectation that all practitioners will, if asked, be able to justify the basis on which they made their decisions. This implies that there is both a right and a duty attached to professional accountability. In recognising the nurse's autonomy, there is a concomitant responsibility to act in the best interests of the client.

Student nurses and accountability

Students clearly cannot be professionally accountable because they are not entered on the professional register, but they are accountable in the other three ways. A registered nurse may, for example, delegate the task of giving an intramuscular injection to a student. The student is accountable for not causing harm

---

accountability

being answerable for one's actions

CONNECTIONS

Chapter 10 discusses accountability in the context of wound care.

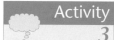

Activity

3

Try to identify examples from your own life that would fit under each type of accountability listed in the text.

professional accountability

being answerable to the NMC for decisions made and actions taken in the course of practice

CONNECTIONS

Chapter 3 outlines the technique of intramuscular injection.

to the patient and should therefore not give the injection if he or she does not feel competent to do so. The registered nurse, however, retains the professional accountability in terms of ensuring that the correct drug and dosage are administered and for ensuring that the student is, in the registered nurse's opinion, competent to administer the drug. Thus, students may be given responsibility by qualified nurses who themselves retain accountability.

The nurse's role in obtaining informed consent

The nurse's role in informed consent has for a long time been vague and confused both in legal terms and in practice, but it was clarified in 2001 with the publication of the *Reference Guide to Consent for Examination or Treatment* (DoH, 2001). This is summarised in Chart 16.2. The 12 key points clarify the need to obtain consent for *anything* that is done to patients, the issues surrounding obtaining consent for children, who is responsible for obtaining consent, the notions of competence to give consent and rights to refusal of treatment.

The public are becoming more informed about their rights within health care and also more litigious in pursuing infringements of those rights through the

Chart 16.2 ● Twelve key points on consent: the law in England

1. Before you examine, treat or care for competent adult patients you must obtain their consent.

2. Adults are always assumed to be competent unless demonstrated otherwise. If you have doubts about their competence the question to ask is 'can this patient understand and weigh up the information needed to make this decision?' Unexpected decisions do not prove the patient is incompetent, but may indicate a need for further information or explanation.

3. Patients may be competent to make some health care decisions, even if they are not competent to make others.

4. Giving and obtaining consent is usually a process, not a one-off event. Patients can change their minds and withdraw consent at any time. If there is any doubt, you should always check that the patient still consents to your caring for or treating them.

5. Before examining, treating or caring for a child, you must also seek consent. Young people aged 16 and 17 are presumed to have the competence to give consent for themselves. Younger children who understand fully what is involved in the proposed procedure can also give consent (although their parents will ideally be involved). In other

cases, someone with parental responsibility must give consent on the child's behalf, unless they cannot be reached in an emergency. If a competent child consents to treatment, a parent cannot over-ride that consent. Legally, a parent can consent if a competent child refuses, but it is likely that taking such a serious step will be rare.

6. It is always best for the person actually treating the patient to seek the patient's consent. However, you may seek consent on behalf of colleagues if you are capable of performing the procedure in question, or if you have been specially trained to seek consent for that procedure.

7. Patients need sufficient information before they can decide whether to give their consent: for example information about the benefits and risks of proposed treatment, and alternative treatments. If the patient is not offered as much information as they reasonably need to make their decision, and in a form they can understand, their consent may not be valid.

8. Consent must be given voluntarily: not under any form of duress or undue influence from health professionals, family or friends.

9. Consent can be written, oral or non-verbal. A signature on a consent form does not itself prove the consent is valid – the point of the form is to record the patient's decision, and also increasingly the discussions that have taken place. Your Trust or organisation may have a policy setting out when you need to obtain written consent.

10. Competent adults are entitled to refuse treatment, even where it would clearly benefit their health. The only exception to this rule is where the treatment is for a mental disorder and the patient is detained under the Mental Health Act 1983. A competent pregnant woman may refuse any treatment, even if this would be detrimental to the fetus.

11. No-one can give consent on behalf of an incompetent adult. However, you may still treat such a patient if the treatment would be in their best interests. 'Best interests' go wider than best medical interests, to include factors such as the wishes and beliefs of the patient when competent, their current wishes, their general well-being and their spiritual and religious welfare. People close to the patient may be able to give you information on some of these factors. Where the patient has never been competent, relatives, carers and friends may be best placed to advise on the patient's needs and preferences.

12. If an incompetent patient has clearly indicated in the past, whilst competent, that they would refuse treatment in certain circumstances (an 'advance refusal'), and those circumstances arise, you must abide by that refusal.

Source: Reference Guide to Consent for Examination or Treatment (www.doh.gov.uk/consent)

legal justice system. Nurses are in a vulnerable position with regard to their accountability to both the patient and those who may be directing the patient's care; this is often the case when nurses are carrying out treatments and procedures under the instruction of others. It is easy to assume that consent has been obtained by others, but the guidelines suggest that it is the responsibility of the person giving the treatment to obtain that consent.

The Nursing and Midwifery Council

The registered nurse is accountable for his or her actions as a professional at all times, whether or not engaged in current practice, and whether on or off duty. Ultimately, the nurse is accountable to the NMC for any failure to satisfy the requirements of the introductory paragraph of the *Code of Professional Conduct*. The interests of the public and client must predominate over those of the practitioner and profession, and, as such, practitioners are accountable for both their actions and their omissions.

Essential parts of accountability are making contemporaneous and accurate records of nursing care, and the consequences for clients if they have not been given the care they require. Health-care records are increasingly being written and stored on computers, so it is worth spending some time considering the implications of computer-held records for nurses.

The use of computers

Using computer facilities in record maintenance and care-planning can be a definite advantage to the profession providing that clear guidelines for practice are established. Issues that need to be considered before implementing any system on a large scale are:

- The acquisition and storage of client-related data
- The compilation of a database of nursing care practices, including the generation of alternatives
- Accountability for individualised care plans
- The maintenance of records
- Confidentiality, security and access.

Data Protection Act 1998

The first Data Protection Act, passed in 1984, was designed to offer UK citizens protection in terms of information held about them on computer. This Act was updated in 1998, the eight data protection principles being retained but modified in the light of advances in both technology and our use of it over the past decade.

All users of computerised records need to be registered under this Act, employers having block registration that covers all employees using their facilities. Chart 16.3 shows the eight principles to be observed with reference to storing information about people.

The eight principles of the Data Protection Act 1998

First principle

Personal data shall be processed fairly and lawfully and, in particular, shall not be processed unless:

- At least one of the conditions in Schedule 2 is met and
- In the case of sensitive personal data, at least one of the conditions in Schedule 3 is also met.

The principles are set out in Part I of Schedule 1 of the Act. Part II of Schedule 1 consists of interpretation provisions applicable to the first, second, fourth, sixth, seventh and eighth principles.

- Schedule 2 of the Act provides conditions for the processing of any personal data in compliance with the first principle, while schedule 3 provides conditions for the processing of sensitive personal data in compliance with the first principle over and above those set out in Schedule 2
- Schedule 4 of the Act consists of cases in which the eighth principle (prohibiting the transfer of personal data outside the European Economic Area) does not apply.

Conditions of processing

This changes the requirements of the previous Act by ensuring that personal data *may not* be processed unless at least one of the following conditions are met:

1. The data subject has given their consent to the processing.
2. The processing is necessary:
   - for the performance of a contract to which the data subject is party or
   - for the taking of steps at the request of the data subject to entering into a contract.
3. The processing is necessary to comply with any legal obligation to which the data controller is subject, other than an obligation imposed by contract.

Chart 16.3 ● The principles of the Data Protection Act 1984

1. The information to be contained in personal data shall be obtained, and personal data shall be processed, fairly and lawfully.
2. Personal data shall be held only for one or more specified and lawful purposes.
3. Personal data held for any purpose or purposes shall not be used or disclosed in any manner incompatible with that purpose or those purposes.
4. Personal data held for any purpose or purposes shall be adequate, relevant and not excessive in relation to that purpose or those purposes.
5. Personal data shall be accurate and, where necessary, kept up to date.
6. Personal data held for any purpose or purposes shall not be kept for longer than is necessary for that purpose or purposes.
7. An individual shall be entitled:
   a) at reasonable intervals and without undue delay or expense:
      i) to be informed by any data user whether he holds personal data of which that individual is the subject
      ii) to access any such data held by a data user
   b) where appropriate, to have such data corrected or erased.
8. Appropriate security measures shall be taken against unauthorised access to, or alteration, disclosure or destruction of, personal data and against accidental loss or destruction of personal data.

4. The processing is necessary in order to protect the vital interests of the data subject.
5. The processing is necessary:
   ● For the administration of justice
   ● For the exercise of any functions conferred by or under enactment
   ● For the exercise of any functions of the Crown, a Minister of the Crown or a government department, or
   ● For the exercise of any other functions of a public nature exercised in the public interest.
6. The processing is necessary for the purpose of legitimate interests pursued by the data controller or by the third party or parties to whom the data are disclosed, except where processing is unwarranted in any particular case because of prejudice to the rights and freedoms or legitimate interests of the data subject.

Sensitive personal data

The Act expands the previous four categories of sensitive data to eight:

1. The racial or ethnic origin of the data subjects.
2. Their political opinions.
3. Their religious beliefs or other beliefs of a similar nature.
4. Whether they are members of a trade union.
5. Their physical or mental health or condition.
6. Their sexual life.
7. The commission or alleged commission by them of any offence.
8. Any proceedings for any offence committed or alleged to have been committed by them, the disposal of such proceedings or the sentence of any court in such proceedings.

Conditions are laid out in the Act for processing these sensitive data. As many of these categories are involved when nurses record patients' details, it is important for practitioners to be aware of any infringements of patients' rights that they may make. Your employer, as the data controller, is ultimately responsible for ensuring that the systems used comply with the Act and that you as an individual are not compromised in carrying out your duties. The conditions can be read at www.dataprotection.gov.uk/chpt3.htm.

Second principle

Personal data shall be obtained only for one or more specified and lawful purposes, and shall not be further processed in any manner incompatible with that purpose or those purposes.

On the whole, data collected by nurses are used explicitly to inform patient care, and the patient's consent is given with that as implicit. Problems can occur however, where data are used for a purpose different from which they were originally recorded, such as for retrospective use in research studies or even auditing procedures.

Third principle

Personal data shall be adequate, relevant and not excessive in relation to the purpose or purposes for which they are processed.

Nurses record many personal details from patients, some of which may never be used. It is important, when reviewing nursing assessment processes and the data

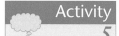

Activity

5

Consider the last time you made a patient assessment and think about the types of information you recorded. Review these against principles 1,2 and 3. Are you satisfied that you are working within the spirit of the Act?

recorded on patients, to ensure that information that is irrelevant or unnecessary for the patient's care is not recorded.

Fourth principle

Personal data shall be accurate and, where necessary, kept up to date.

Problems of accuracy may occur when nurses are recording information about a patient from a third party, such as a relative or another health-care professional or interested party. There is no longer any defence in saying that the information was supplied by someone else: steps have to be taken to ensure that the information is accurate.

Fifth principle

Personal data processed for any purpose or purposes shall not be kept for longer than is necessary for that purpose or those purposes.

Sixth principle

Personal data shall be processed in accordance with the rights of data subjects under this Act.

Seventh principle

Appropriate technical and organisational measures shall be taken against unauthorised or unlawful processing of personal data and against accidental loss or destruction of, or damage to, personal data.

Eighth principle

Personal data shall not be transferred to a country or territory outside the European Economic Area, unless that country or territory ensures an adequate level of protection for the rights and freedoms of data subjects in relation to the processing of personal data.

More details regarding all of these principles are available from the website (www.dataprotection.gov.uk/chpt3.htm).

These principles derive from society's beliefs about people's rights and responsibilities when living within it, arising from a concern to promote fairness and equality. Each profession in society is, similarly, founded on a set of beliefs and principles that underpin how it relates to society and how its members practise. These principles can be seen as **philosophies** and **ideologies**.

philosophies
sets of beliefs and values that guide the way in which we operate in the world

ideologies
sets of ideas, assumptions and images that help people to make sense of society and provide individuals with distinctive social identities

■ Philosophies and Ideologies

Personal beliefs and values

We all practise from a belief and value system that has arisen from our own personal experiences of life and what we have encountered. Jasper (1996) suggests that personal beliefs and values arise from the following sources:

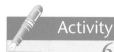

Activity

6

Take a few minutes to list the beliefs and values that you hold that made you want to become a nurse. Can you attribute any of these to Jasper's sources?

CONNECTIONS

Chapter 15 investigates values.

CONNECTIONS

Chapter 13 contains details of reflective practice.

- Our religious beliefs and moral upbringing
- Our ethnic origins
- Our educational opportunities
- Our social class
- The environment in which we grew up
- Our life experiences.

In addition to these personal life experiences, we accumulate various other beliefs and values that are accommodated into the way we practise as nurses.

You will already have encountered different ways of looking at the world from your nursing education, from the practitioners and educationalists with whom you work, and from your reading. You will have developed particular ways of looking at things that direct the way in which you give care. Think, for example, about concepts that you have met, such as 'holistic care', 'individualised care' or 'reflective practice'. Or even about the difference between your ideas of what nursing is now compared with what you thought it would be when you started your nursing education.

In addition to these beliefs and values, you will also have been exposed to professional ones as defined by the NMC in the *Code of Professional Conduct* (2002) and illustrated in Chart 16.1 above. Such professional codes of conduct clearly identify the standards of practice that are expected from practitioners and provide them with a baseline of values and beliefs deemed appropriate at that particular time. Indeed, the NMC possesses the power to sanction any practitioners who contravene the code, even in their personal lives. The beliefs and values of the professional codes are absorbed into the individual belief and value system of the practitioner. Thus, anyone calling themselves a nurse, midwife or health visitor is assumed to behave in the way expected of a registered practitioner, as set out in the *Code of Professional Conduct*.

The final sources of influence on your personal beliefs and values are those arising from your employing organisation and from wider societal issues such as government policy relating to health and social care. These sources of beliefs are likely to change, or be modified, at an even more rapid rate than those arising from educational or professional philosophies because they will be subject to political influences and trends, for example the impact that the introduction of the internal market has had on the provision of infertility treatment by the NHS or the decisions taken in some health authorities to restrict access to health care depending on the age of the client.

Wright (1986) suggests that the combination of these sources of values and beliefs can be regarded as a personal philosophy that is used to shape our practice and education, provide motivation, prompt research and set our management style.

CONNECTIONS

Chapter 14 contains more information on the internal market.

Nursing philosophies

As nurses, we tend to work in teams to provide nursing care. The care delivered by a team of nurses working together will be directed by our beliefs and values in the same way that our own style of nursing is.

CONNECTIONS

Chapter 15 explores teamworking.

The word 'philosophy' in nursing tends to refer to a way of doing things that is underpinned by a written statement of beliefs and values. Mawdsley (1991) sees a nursing philosophy as:

> an invaluable tool which directs and influences patient care. It is a series of beliefs, values and outlooks that can be developed in any area concerned with patient care, with the purpose of demonstrating what nurses feel their particular specialty should be achieving both for patients and nursing staff.

For a philosophy to be a true representation of the care delivered by a team, there are two key elements that must be contained in it. First, it must be an agreed statement that reflects the shared perceptions, beliefs and values of all those concerned. Second, it must be related to their own practice and have practical applications. Johns (1989, cited in Johns, 1991) identifies the value of a philosophy when he says:

> Staff who share a common positive belief about nursing, within the context of their workplace, are more likely to give consistent and congruent care for the benefit of their patients.

A nursing philosophy is therefore:

- A statement of intent and belief
- An explanation of how and why things are done
- A statement of the purpose of the organisation and individuals
- A statement of the ideas behind our behaviour and actions
- A reflection of members' ideals and ideas for nursing, which should be endorsed by their peers
- An outlook that should include the future, expectations and reflection
- A consideration of the role of nursing.

Activity 7

All clinical areas providing placements are required to have a nursing philosophy. Think back to your last placement. Were you introduced to the philosophy? How was its relationship to care explained?

Look again at the six components of a written philosophy. How successful is your example in covering these? To what extent are the characteristics of a philosophy present? Does your example really reflect the nursing care given in that clinical area?

A written philosophy includes:

- What you do
- Why you do it
- What you value and why
- What is important and why
- The uniqueness of your practice or ward and so on
- The qualities offered.

The success of a philosophy as a working document for a clinical area will often depend on the way in which it was devised in the first place. If it is meant to reflect the combined values of the area or team to which it relates, it is essential that those people were involved in developing it. Described below are two approaches to philosophy development.

The top-down approach

In this case, the philosophy tends to be imposed by the managerial system and is a reflection of organisational beliefs, which are not necessarily applicable to the nursing care. As a result, the philosophy may become a paper exercise, the components not being shared by the nurses, who lack any ownership or motivation to use it within their practice. This, however, may not necessarily be the case because organisations adopt change and responsibility and accountability are delegated downwards. Many nurses are using broad policy statements created within an organisation and developing their own philosophies from them, incorporating the beliefs and values of their own nursing environment. These are fine as broad statements, but they do not necessarily relate to the specific environment of nursing in which teams of nurses are working and, although helpful as value statements, are not necessarily useful as operational policies.

The bottom-up approach

In this case, it is the people who will have to use the philosophy who are involved in writing it. Philosophies developed in this way tend to include the 'how, what, when, why, who and where' of practice, which can then be used as a way of directing and delivering care within a specific environment. An excellent example of the creation of a philosophy in which all the team members were involved is described by Johns (1991) in relation to the Burford Nursing Development Unit.

Purposes of a philosophy

Practical application

It can now be seen that a nursing philosophy must, if it is to be effective, have

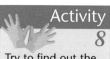
Activity 8
Try to find out the origins of the philosophy you used in Activity 7. Ask your supervisor how it was developed, for example who wrote it, where the underpinning beliefs and values came from, and how these were identified. What part did the members of the ward team play in its development?

practical application to the area for which it has been written and must reflect the practices that currently occur. It will therefore serve the purpose of stimulating nurses to reflect on their practice in terms of being able to justify the nursing care delivered and learning from their experiences. The philosophy can also be used to teach nursing care to students or other types of worker, and can form the basis of the development of nursing care in that area.

Facilitating teamwork

Similarly, a philosophy as a working document will facilitate teamwork as all members of the team will share common values and beliefs that have been made explicit and open. A published philosophy may even be used to recruit new members of the clinical team as it can be used to advertise the beliefs and values underpinning care to potential applicants and form the basis of exploring whether a person will fit into the ward team. A philosophy will also encourage continuity of care while the client is being looked after in that clinical area and enable a smooth transfer to other areas or upon discharge.

> **CONNECTIONS**
>
> *Chapter 15 looks further at values and beliefs in teamworking.*

Setting a baseline for the development of quality and standards in practice

It seems logical to assume that if a philosophy for a clinical area has been agreed by the team working in it, it will serve as a starting point for setting the **standards of care** and assessing the **quality of care** delivered. If the philosophy identifies your beliefs and values, and these are translated into the way in which you work and what you intend to provide, you have already set some *standards* to be achieved. The *quality* of your care can be measured by finding ways of evaluating the outcome of care against your original intentions.

standards of care

these usually identify the minimum standard to which an aspect of care is expected to conform and provide the criteria against which the quality of care can be measured

quality of care

the measure of the standard of care that is used to evaluate the services being delivered. The term 'quality' needs to be accompanied by an adjective describing the standard to be achieved, for example 'high'-quality care

Quality

On the surface, this aspect is very simple, but let us take some time to think about what we mean by quality. Quality is a nebulous term that means different things to different people. One problem lies in the necessity to qualify the term with a value word such as 'high' or 'low' in order to give it some meaning. It is, for example, clearly meaningless to talk about 'quality' care without defining the standard of quality that you are aiming for – 'quality' could refer to anything.

Another problem relates to who defines the quality. Think, for example, of the values that you might attribute to high-quality care in giving a blanket bath. You might identify privacy, time, skilled staff and other issues relating to assessing the condition of your client and completing the task in a certain length of time. Your client may well, however, look for different measures of quality – what might these be? Your ward manager may well, on the other hand, think of good-quality procedures as relating to completing the work schedule, meeting the client's needs as identified in the care plan and complying with the treatment schedule.

It is therefore important, where any measurement or assessment of quality is attempted, to ask several overarching questions about what it is that is being attempted.

What is being assessed?

This evolves from the definition of quality that is in operation, from organisational needs, from externally imposed criteria such as government targets, and from the beliefs and values that underpin the model of quality being used. Koch (1994) suggests that there have previously been three generations of quality evaluation: measurement orientated, objective orientated and judgement orientated.

In a *measurement-orientated approach*, boundaries or quality criteria are selected by the health-care professionals and data are collected in statistical terms. Examples of this are the waiting times of clients attending a particular outpatient department and the wound infection rate following a specific surgical procedure.

Objective-orientated approaches use observational techniques to assess the strengths and weaknesses of care against stated objectives. Many of the well-known quality audit tools, such as Phaneuf's audit of documentary records (Phaneuf, 1976), use this approach.

Judgement-orientated techniques involve the evaluation of care against standards set by 'experts', usually in the form of quality assurance committees. Approaches within this category often have a dual purpose in terms of quantifiable standards of practice and the marketing of services as labels such as 'excellent' or 'poor' are awarded. QUALPACs (Wandelt and Ager, 1974) can be seen as falling into this category of approaches as value assessments are made of the care given. Another recent initiative of this type is the assessment of nursing outcomes (Higgins et al., 1992; Griffiths, 1995), which relates the outcome achieved to the process used to achieve it.

These three categories of approach share the characteristics of the standards being set by health-care experts, thus ignoring client-generated concerns, and of being of a quantifiable nature, data being collected by a disinterested observer (Koch, 1994). They might not, however, suit the purposes of nurses wanting to evaluate the quality of their own work, especially as few of these approaches involve client-generated issues relating to the everyday care received. Koch (1994) suggests that this can be achieved by using a fourth-generation approach to the evaluation of quality that is negotiation orientated, involving a skilled negotiator who acts as facilitator in setting the agenda for quality among all the stakeholders.

Another approach to involving clients in assessing the quality of care has been the development of client satisfaction schedules (Bond and Thomas, 1992; Avis et al., 1995; Simpson et al., 1995). These have the advantage of enabling the clients' perspectives to be drawn into the quality debate and often use **qualitative approaches** to data-gathering, which generate material relating to clients' experiences, rather than **quantitative approaches**, which rely on objective statistics yet do not describe subjective experiences. Thus, when exploring quality assessment in your own area of practice, it is important to be able to identify exactly what you are assessing. This leads to the next question of *what purpose you are assessing it for*.

Although you have probably not yet had to think very much about the quality of care that you deliver because you have been closely supervised in clinical practice, you will, as you move into your branch studies, need to make such decisions and clarify the purpose of evaluating that quality for your own personal and professional development. This is where the skills of reflective practice that you met in Chapter 13 will be useful to you. Now refer to Activity 9.

This activity highlights one purpose of quality assessment – meeting individual practitioners' needs to ensure their own high-quality care. Many other purposes can, however, be identified if you refer back to the beginning of this section. These are listed briefly below and can be a stimulus to further reading as you go through your branch studies. Quality may be assessed in order to:

- Ensure value for money
- Attract funding for a service
- Demonstrate target achievements
- Audit a service
- Award training status to a clinical area
- Verify that standards of practice are being achieved
- Publicise a service
- Provide new business or services.

The next question that needs to be addressed is *what structure will the approach take*? This is not the place to outline the strategies available for assessing quality; suffice it to say that there is a whole range of approaches depending on what it is you want to assess and the purpose of your assessment. Examples of nursing assessment tools are the Phaneuf audit (Phaneuf, 1976), QUALPACs (Wandelt and Ager, 1974) and DYSSSY (RCN, 1990).

qualitative reseach approaches

research approaches that use in-depth and holistic methods through the collection of narrative data and a flexible design

quantitative research approaches

approaches to investigating phenomena that lend themselves to precise measurement and quantification, often involving a rigorous and controlled design

CONNECTIONS

Chapter 13 outlines a way of performing a structured and thoughtful review of your care activities.

■ Clinical Governance

The NHS has been subject to numerous reviews since its inception, many of which have attempted, either implicitly or explicitly, to address concerns relating to the quality of the service provided. Experienced health service personnel may, somewhat cynically, find themselves asking: clinical governance – why now? (been there, done that, got the T-shirt!). 'Clinical governance' certainly seems to be the current 'buzz phrase' within certain NHS and government circles.

Approaches such as total quality management, quality circles, continuous quality improvement, the King's Fund initiative, Investors in People, re-engineering, the dynamic standard-setting system and medical/clinical audit, to name but a few, have been among the quality intitatives employed in the past. But this begs the question, 'If we have been down this road before, why do we appear to be making a return journey?'

Recent key concerns emerging appear to be *responsibility* and *accountability* for *quality of performance*. The introduction of the clinical governance framework can be described as a direct response to these concerns.

What is clinical governance?

The New Labour government was elected to power, with a significant majority, in May 1997, producing in the autumn of that year the first of a series of key documents setting out the agenda for health care into the next century. The notion of clinical governance (DoH, 1997; emphasis added) was thus introduced:

> The Government will require every NHS trust to embrace the concept of Clinical Governance, so that *quality* is at the core, both of their *responsibilities* as *organisations*, and of each of their staff as *individual professionals*.

The challenge was laid down but the rules remained unclear, further illumination (DoH, 1998) being provided several months later:

> Clinical Governance is a *framework* through which NHS *organisations* are *accountable* for *continuously improving* the quality of their services and *safeguarding high standards* of care by creating an environment in which excellence in clinical care will flourish.

Key deadlines were set although the details remained 'fuzzy' and those looking for a 'blueprint' for clinical governance were disappointed. Scally and Donaldson (1998) describe, however, how:

> For the first time, all health organisations will have a statutory duty to seek quality improvement through clinical governance.

The message became clear and a line of accountability was drawn, identifying individual responsibility for ensuring organisational performance, in terms of not only sound financial management, but also the integration of existing quality assurance and performance monitoring systems into a framework for continuous quality improvement. The chief executive or chair of the governing body was to be 'the accountable officer' and NHS Trusts were required to produce their first clinical governance reports in spring 2000, with annual monitoring. These documents will come into the public domain, encouraging openness and emphasising accountability.

In addition to this a statutory body, the Commission for Health Improvement (CHI), has been set up with powers to scrutinise, support, investigate, police and inquire, backed by the legal duty of quality imposed on every organisation. Quality assurance and improvement are no longer 'optional extras' but a statutory obligation.

The stated aim of clinical governance (DoH, 1998) is seductive and deceptively simple:

Safeguarding high standards of care by creating an environment in which excellence in clinical care will flourish.

The reality is, however, rather more complex, requiring a change in culture that could in some cases almost be described as a 'paradigm shift'. Organisations, and the individuals who comprise them, will face a number of developmental challenges.

The following could be described as prerequisites for clinical governance:

- A supportive culture, nurturing integrity and honesty
- A consensus regarding the meaning of the concepts underpinning clinical governance
- Time to do 'it'
- Clearly defined lines of accountability within the organisation – who is responsible for what and when? Who holds the decision-making authority and is therefore accountable for discharging a responsibility?
- Leadership across all professional groups
- Robust communication and record-keeping systems
- Mechanisms to support clinical supervision/peer review and critical reflection for all professional (and, increasingly, non-professional) groups.

Elements of clinical governance

It is increasingly apparent that clinical governance is a framework within which a number of existing systems and processes are integrated. The key elements of the clinical governance framework can be summarised as:

- Education
- Continuing professional development
- Clinical audit (multiprofessional)
- Evidence-based practice
- Clinical effectiveness
- Clinical risk assessment, management and reduction
- Improving practice
- Defining outcomes of care, treatment or therapy
- Collecting good-quality clinical data
- Monitoring clinical practice
- The systematic dissemination of 'best practice', both within *and* outside the organisation
- Professional self-regulation
- Service user involvement.

These key elements can also be described in a series of logical (albeit overlapping) groupings (Figure. 16.1).

Many, if not all, of these systems and processes already exist in one form or other. In some areas, they are well defined; in others, they operate in an ineffective, piecemeal fashion. The challenge posed by clinical governance is to develop these systems to an uncommonly sophisticated level of integration. This will be

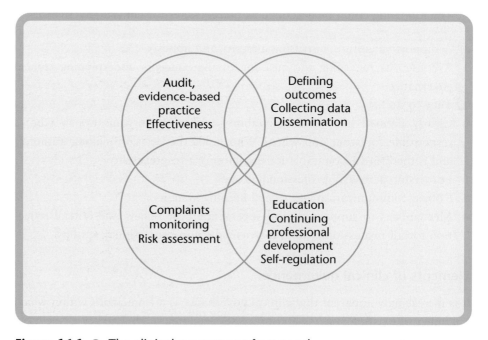

Figure 16.1 ● The clinical governance framework

characterised by moving away from a culture of self-protection and blame to one of self-regulation and learning through experience. It will include progress from a position of isolation and professional tribalism to one of collaboration and multiprofessional teamworking. The challenge will incorporate moving from practice based upon tradition, ritual, folklore and personal preference to practice that is centred around expert professional judgement that is itself informed by sound, appropriate evidence, critical analytical and reflective skills.

Organisational systems and processes will need to transform from being isolated 'pockets' of activity to being an integrated, coherent framework with the service user firmly located at the centre. The design of service provision will be the vehicle for achieving excellence in care, whether this is operationalising health improvement plans within specific, nationally agreed performance frameworks or enhancing individual quality of life and well-being in chronic, life-limiting or terminal conditions. Exemplars in practice will be recognised and systematically disseminated. Complaints and risk management systems will be used to identify and analyse problems so that they too can become part of the 'flow of information' feeding into the quality improvement cycle that lies at the heart of clinical governance (Figure 16.2). Unlike other cycles, the clinical governance cycle can be broken into at any point. The challenge is to ensure that, no matter where the cycle is entered, all the components are engaged (Severs, 1998).

> **CONNECTIONS**
>
> *Chapter 15 contains explanations of multiprofessional teamworking.*

> 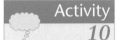 **Activity**
> **10**
>
> Look again at Figures 16.1 and 16.2. Which elements of the clinical governance framework do you think have the greatest impact on each part of the clinical governance cycle and why?

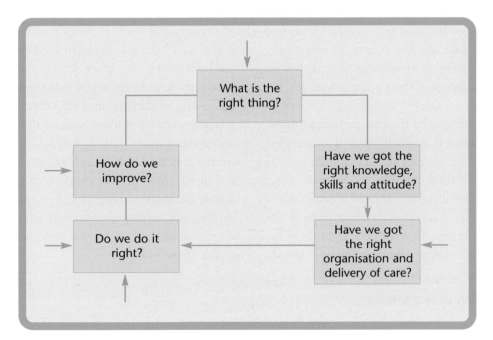

Figure 16.2 ● The clinical governance cycle

All of these issues have a direct link to the philosophy of care that has been created for the clinical area. This philosophy sets the baseline for determining the focus that quality assessment will take and relates directly to the standards of care to be achieved.

The development of nursing

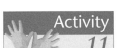

Activity 11

Gather together from your clinical area as many examples as you can in an attempt to assess the quality of care being provided.

Consider such aspects as a tracking form for client care, the presence of written standards for procedures, the evaluation of care against the written philosophy and the collection of statistics relating to bed occupancy.

Although written philosophies tend to be the end result of values clarification and teamwork, they mark just one stage in the overall process of developing nursing knowledge, a process that begins when nurses start to think about what they are doing and why. Creating a philosophy of care for a clinical area, or being able to articulate your own philosophy, sets the baseline for thinking about and making connections between our knowledge base, our skills and our experience, and for considering how these can be taken forward.

■ Models and Frameworks of Care

Another purpose of a nursing philosophy is to underpin the model of nursing that is used to direct care in the clinical area.

One of the major challenges that nurses have faced in the quest for professional practice is the development of a knowledge base that can be seen to relate specifically to nursing. Prior to the 1950s, there was very little theory that could be seen to be exclusively concerned with the ways in which nurses practised in a specific capacity. Since that time, and related in particular to the move of nursing education into American universities, nurse theorists have attempted to identify a nursing knowledge base that is separate or built eclectically from other foundations of theory. Some authors, usually from outside nursing, argue that there is no specific knowledge that can be seen to belong to nursing, and they therefore justify the designation of nursing as a semiprofession. Others suggest that there is no such thing as a knowledge base belonging to any particular profession; instead, it is the special combination of the way in which knowledge from different sources is collected together and used to underpin practice that provides the focus of a profession. In addition, although nursing is still in the infant stages of creating nursing knowledge, this has developed effectively over the past 40 years. The creation of models of nursing was one of the first attempts at creating a knowledge base specific to nursing in this way.

What is a model?

Wright (1990) defines a nursing model as:

a collection of ideas, knowledge and values about nursing which determines the way nurses, as individuals and groups, work with their patients or clients.

Models therefore:

help nurses to organise their thinking about nursing and then set about their practice in an orderly and logical way.

Hence the primary purpose of a model is to help nurses to understand nursing from a particular viewpoint and use that to direct their care. But what do we mean by a model? In everyday life, a model is often seen in a physical way, as with a model house, boat or aeroplane. Although it does not contain all the elements or components of the real thing, it acts as a representation of that thing. So how does this help us with models of nursing? Models of nursing also act as a representation of reality but from a particular viewpoint: nursing models describe, or represent, nursing from the viewpoint of the writer and present different ways of looking at or understanding nursing. Nursing models are thus abstract models that help us to make sense of the way in which nursing happens.

These models do not have to be published, formal models written by theorists: each one of us has our own informal model that we carry around in our head. These comprise individual collections of ideas about nursing, socialised behaviour and experience from both nursing and life, and determine a great deal of nursing care as they form the basis of the way in which each nurse practises. Although these informal models are obviously important to the individual, there are certain problems associated with individuals practising their own model rather than one that is shared by others in the team. Informal models are usually value laden and are not necessarily based on commonly held values. In a way, they are 'secret' models, but at the same time we seem to make the assumption that everyone else shares our values.

Formal models occur, however, when the values, beliefs and ways of working are made explicit and shared by the team of nurses in the clinical area. They enable groups of nurses to think about, and carry out, nursing in a fairly similar way, with clear objectives for the delivery of care because the model purports to represent the nursing care to be achieved by that team.

Over the past 60 years, many models have been created that claim to represent the reality of nursing. Although most of these originate in the USA, the most commonly used model in practice in the UK, the activities of daily living (ADL) model, was devised by Roper et al. in Edinburgh in the 1980s; this will be used as an illustration for the rest of this section. The ADL model developed from Virginia Henderson's description of what nursing does in helping clients with 14 activities of living (Henderson, 1966). These were refined by Roper et al. (1980) as an educational model to help students learn about nursing.

Components of models

Philosophies and beliefs

The basic starting point for a model is a statement of the beliefs and values that underpin it, usually referred to as the philosophy of the model. Roper et al. (1980) use Henderson's (1966) definition of nursing as a starting point. This suggests that:

> The unique function of the nurse is to assist the individual, sick or well, in the performance of those activities contributing to health or its recovery (or to a peaceful death) that he [sic] would perform unaided if he had the necessary strength, will or knowledge, and to do this in such a way as to help him to gain independence as rapidly as possible.

Thus, the underpinning beliefs here relate to nursing as a 'helping' activity by which the nurse, using the framework of the ADLs (Chart 16.4), aids a client to gain independence or die peacefully. There is a focus on the individual as an active part of the nursing process because it identifies the notion of partnership, in which nurses will only do things for clients that they are unable to do themselves. There is also a notion of **holism** running through this definition, in that although the activities are identified as separate elements, there is no attempt to address each one without the presence of the individual client. The definition implies that all individuals can grow in some way, whether by direct nursing interaction, by the provision of information or by the support necessary to gain independence. There is also the underpinning assumption that the ADLs are indeed the activities that enable people to live and grow.

From this brief discussion, it can be seen that a philosophy is composed of many different ideas that together set the scene for each particular model. Each model has a different set, or combination, of these ideas that underpin it and will therefore see nursing, and the delivery of nursing care, in a different way. The ideas within the philosophy and that make up the model are usually referred to as 'concepts'.

holism

a philosophy addressing the person as an irreducible whole

Chart 16.4 ● Roper et al.'s activities of daily living

1. Maintaining a safe environment
2. Communicating
3. Breathing
4. Eating and drinking
5. Eliminating
6. Personal cleansing and dressing
7. Controlling body temperature
8. Working and playing
9. Mobilising
10. Sleeping
11. Expressing sexuality
12. Dying

CONNECTIONS

More information on these activities of daily living (activity numbers in brackets) can be found in Chapters 3(1), 6(3), 4(4), 5(5), 8(9), 7(11) and 9(12).

Concepts

Concepts can be viewed not only as ideas, but also as a mental picture of these that is made up of a collection of ideas and constructed within the mind (Walker and Avant, 1996). We can see immediately that concepts are therefore open to individual interpretation depending upon experience. To illustrate this, try Activity 12.

The words you have written are likely to have arisen from your own experiences of marriage. Single readers may, for example, rely on memories from childhood, whether or not their parents were married, the socio-economic stability of marriage, religious beliefs and any experiences of a 'married' partnership. Students may well have experienced happy or traumatic marriages themselves and may indeed be divorced or separated, with experience of abuse or economic problems. So although we all have an understanding of the concept of 'marriage', the word and its meaning are likely to possess different components for each individual.

This immediately poses a problem for nurse theorists in constructing the philosophy of a model and its component parts. It is therefore extremely important for concepts to be defined within each model so that the reader can understand what the basis of the model is.

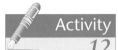

Activity 12

To illustrate what is meant by the fluid nature of concepts, write down the images, ideas or words that come into your head when you hear or read the word 'marriage'.

The metaparadigm of nursing

There are four major concepts that are found in nursing models or frameworks, which are collectively known as the **metaparadigm** or grand framework of nursing. These concepts (constructs) are: man or the person, the environment, health and nursing. All nursing models describe and define these concepts, the way in which they are combined determining how the client will be approached and how the nurse will serve the client. Chart 16.5 summarises the metaparadigm concepts as defined by Roper et al. (1980).

Other concepts may be included in the model and give it a particular and specific focus. In Peplau's (1952) model, for example, the concept of 'interpersonal relations' is central, in Orem's (1980) model we find the concept of 'self-care', and in Roy's (1984) model there is 'adaptation'. The concepts central to Roper et al.'s model are summarised in Chart 16.6 below.

Hence we can see that each model of nursing will define and develop concepts in a way that 'fits' the overall nature of the model. Although it is important to understand a model for concepts to be clearly defined and unambiguous, the concepts do not exist in isolation – the model itself needs in some way to explain the *relationship* between them.

metaparadigm of nursing

the defining combination of concepts that are seen to make up nursing: man, the environment, health and nursing

CONNECTIONS

Chapter 11 explores interpersonal relations.

Chart 16.5 ● Roper et al.'s metaparadigm concepts

The person – the model focuses on the client as an individual engaged in living throughout his or her life span, and moving from dependence to independence according to age, circumstances and environment. The important ideas relating to the person are:

- the progression of a person along a life span
- a dependence–independence continuum
- the activities of daily living and factors influencing these
- individuality

CONNECTIONS

Chapter 2 develops concepts of health and reviews environmental factors influencing health.

Health – Roper et al. (1990) develop this concept in the third edition of their model and draw attention to the notion that the concept of health changes, as does society and current thought. They see health as a dynamic process with many facets

Environment – this is defined as anything external to the person and is deemed to be an essential component of 'living activities' as it is one of the influential factors that impinge upon all activities of daily living

Nursing – this is involved when an individual is unable to be independent in any of the activities of daily living and cannot draw on the support of family or social group to meet them. Nursing aims at:

1. The individual acquiring, maintaining or restoring maximum independence in the activities of living, or enabling him or her to cope with dependence on others if circumstances make this necessary

2. Enabling the individual to carry out preventative activities independently to avoid ill-health

3. Providing comforting strategies to promote recovery and eventual independence

4. Providing medically prescribed treatment to overcome illness or its symptoms, leading to recovery and eventual independence

Source: Adapted from Pearson et al. (1996).

Statements

Statements are used to link two or more concepts together and, according to Walker and Avant (1996), must be present before explanations or predictions can be made. Statements may occur in two forms:

Chart 16.6 ● Other concepts in Roper et al.'s model

Life span – an individual begins living at conception and ends it at death. As people engage in the process of living, their position along the life span influences their capacity for independence. Progress on the life span is, of course, unidirectional

Dependence–independence continuum – this continuum is moved along dynamically and is affected by a whole range of factors

Activities of daily living – 12 of these are defined in the model; the individual is seen as engaging in them in different capacities as he or she moves through the life span. The activities of daily living are listed in Chart 16.4. Each activity has five components:

● Physical
● Psychological
● Socio-cultural
● Environmental
● Politico-economic

Preventative activities – these are adopted in order to prevent those things which will impair living, such as accidents and illness. They include, for example, eating a balanced diet to maximise health and restricting alcohol intake to prevent car accidents

CONNECTIONS
Chapter 4 discusses the current concept of a balanced diet.

Comforting activities – these are performed to give physical, psychological and social comfort; an example is doing stretching exercises to relieve muscle tension

Seeking activities – these are activities carried out in the pursuit of knowledge, new experiences and answers to new problems

The latter three activities tend to be interrelated and overlapping, and may occur simultaneously in actions taken by the individual

Individuality in living – each person will be affected by a unique range of influential factors, the result being that they will manifest differences in the way in which they live.

Source: Adapted from Pearson et al. (1996).

1. *Relational statements* declare a relationship of some kind between two or more concepts, for example 'A water temperature above X°C will cause skin damage'. Thus, relational statements assert either an association between concepts or causality – the effect of one concept on the other.

2. *Non-relational statements* either assert the existence of a concept or define a concept, and act as adjuncts to relational statements. They give meaning to concepts in a theory. An example is Roper et al.'s statement that:

> Basically, people are envisaged as carrying out various activities during a lifespan, from conception to death.

Once statements have linked concepts together, they can be built into theories.

Theories

Theories 'represent a scientist's best effort to describe and explain phenomena' (Polit et al., 2001). They help us to make sense of what we observe and perceive by suggesting relationships between concepts and propositions. Walker and Avant (1996, p. 22) suggest that a theory is:

> an internally consistent group of relational statements (concepts, definitions and propositions) that presents a systematic view about a phenomenon and that is useful for description, explanation, prediction and control. A theory, by virtue of its predictive potential, is the primary means of meeting the goals of the nursing profession concerned with a clearly defined body of knowledge.

The key words in this definition are the ones that identify the dynamic qualities of theories in terms of description, explanation, prediction and control. These move us from the notion that knowledge is fixed and given to the idea that knowledge is always in the process of being created or discovered. Dickoff et al. (1968) suggest that there are four levels of theory development to be seen through nursing history (Chart 16.7) and that these can be linked to Walker and Avant's key words. These clearly show how theory is inextricably bound to clinical practice; that is, theories have to have practical application or they are merely rhetoric or someone's ideas.

CONNECTIONS

Chapter 1 explains the nursing process.

You are, however, likely to have experienced the frustration of learning theory related to a particular aspect of practice (for example the ideas underlying the nursing process and nursing assessment) and then finding that this is not at all how it operates in practice. This is often referred to as the theory–practice gap and has perplexed many nurses over the past 20 years. Rolfe (1996) identifies this problem as originating with the notion of the separation between theory and practice in the first place. He suggests that 'nursing praxis' is a more realistic way of looking at the way in which nurses develop theories that originate and work in practice and proposes that:

Chart 16.7 ● Levels of theory development in nursing

1st level – factor isolating – identification of factors and their variables, and their subsequent definition. Walker and Avant's 'description'

2nd level – factor relating – explains by identifying possible relationships between factors. Walker and Avant's 'explanation'

3rd level – situation relating – predicts what may occur if factors are varied and manipulated. Walker and Avant's 'prediction'

4th level – situation producing – control of the situation can be achieved where the nursing intervention is highly likely to accomplish the desired goals. Walker and Avant's 'control'

nursing praxis begins with reflection-on-action, which except with very experienced practitioners, involves thinking about and analysing practice situations after the event and away from the clinical area. The outcome of reflection-on-action is personal knowledge about specific situations, which can be stored away for later use as paradigm cases, or which can be employed immediately in the construction of informal theory.

Rolfe goes on to describe a reflective, theory-proposing and testing model of the way in which nurses operate in everyday practice. Although this model incorporates many of the previous ideas about the relationship between theory and practice, Rolfe provides a way of looking at the creation of nursing knowledge that acknowledges their interdependency, the nurse being the catalyst for creating reality. There is a logical corollary to this approach – that theory without practice is of little use to the practitioner, and practice without theory is dangerous. We must thus explore the uses of theory and how the individual nurse can practise from an evidence basis that incorporates personal knowledge.

But why does nursing need to have theory at all? If nursing is just a conglomeration of facts and ideas generated within other disciplines, there does not appear to be a need for *nursing* theory. If, however, nursing has something special that delineates it from other disciplines, we need to develop a nursing knowledge base.

Now that you are probably at the end of your common foundation programme, it is important to identify just what nursing is to you as you will, from now on, increasingly be called on to defend your own practice as a nurse. Work your way down the questions in Activity 13 in an attempt to clarify your views at this time.

CONNECTIONS

Compare reflection-on-action with reflective practice, as described in Chapter 13.

nursing praxis

a model that integrates reflection-on-action, reflection-in-action and formal and informal theory

paradigm

in this context, a 'prime example' or model case

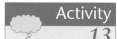

Activity

13

What knowledge base does nursing share with other disciplines? Think here about both the practical and theoretical components of your course and try to identify the disciplinary base that informs each one.

What makes nursing different from other disciplines; that is, what is special about nursing? Where does the knowledge come from that informs the 'special' nursing components? Where does nursing theory come from?

What is the purpose of nursing theory?

Having studied these questions, you are likely to have made the link between nursing being a special discipline in its own right, having a specific knowledge base, and the role that theory generation will play in that. We need to have evidence on which to base our practice, and there is little purpose for theory if it does not relate in some way to practice. We need to know what to do and why we do it, one of the purposes of theory being to enable us to practise from an informed basis. After all, that is why you are undertaking an educational programme in preparation for registered practice rather than working as an unqualified member of staff. But what are the other purposes of theory?

Purposes of theories

There are many purposes to which theories are put, one overall reason being to make scientific findings meaningful and generalisable. In nursing, the main purpose must be to enhance nursing practice. Subsidiary purposes include:

- The provision of knowledge
- Enhancing nursing's power by developing the knowledge base
- Explaining and predicting previously unexplained events
- The stimulation of new discoveries
- Aiding decision-making
- The support of professional autonomy in practice, education and research.

Finally, it is worth thinking about your own personal development in relation to being able to select the appropriate nursing action. Although much of the theoretical work that you have undertaken so far is based on learning facts and skills, you must remember that your critical powers are also being developed. It is very important to see theory in a developmental light, in terms of how being able to discuss and differentiate, evaluate and justify, helps your critical thinking.

Classification of nursing theories

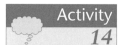

Activity

14

Work your way through Chart 16.8 and try to identify examples from your own experience to illustrate each level.

Nursing's knowledge base has now developed to such an extent that, instead of nurses being able to say with certainty, 'This is how you do it', there are a multitude of alternatives to consider. Although you may still find this confusing (especially when what you meet in practice bears little relationship to what you have learnt academically), you will, as you progress in your career, come to see that this points to the move by nursing from an occupation dependent on others to a fledgling discipline in its own right. Chart 16.8 considers the types or levels of theory development that you may come across.

As you can see, nursing models fit into the category of *grand theory*. It is worth taking some time to consider this as it helps to explain the problems that nurses have with trying to enact a model in a clinical area. Grand theory is

Chart 16.8 ● Levels of theory development

Meta-theories – these comprise the philosophical and methodological aspects of theory-building, for example philosophical issues about relationships between nursing theory, the philosophy of science and nursing knowledge or methodology (see, for example, Dickoff et al., 1968)

Grand theories – these define nursing broadly and abstractly from a global perspective, describing the 'whole of nursing's concern' (Chinn and Kramer, 1991). Theories at this level include nursing models that tend to provide a conceptual framework or overview of nursing. Because of the scope of nursing models, they tend not to provide testable theories but instead offer a direction for practice

Middle-range theories – although these are still abstract, they contain elements of grand theories but have less scope and fewer variables, thus making them more appropriate for testing. These include, for example, Watson's (1979) theory of caring and Peplau's (1952) theory of interpersonal relations

Practice theory – this is the situation-relating theory of Dickoff et al. (1968) that relates to the way in which nurses practise. Examples are techniques such as the Waterlow scale to assess the degree of risk of pressure sores and the management of incontinence

Source: Adapted from Walker and Avant (1996) and Manley (1991).

abstract – it is made up of concepts related to each other in some sort of framework that enables us to gain an overview of what is happening. Thus, nursing models are created by their author as a personal perspective on nursing; there is nothing fixed or 'true' about any one nursing model. If you take time to consider the plethora of models that we have (see, for example, Fawcett, 1984; Meleis, 1996), it becomes obvious that a model is an exposition of ideas that will help us to guide our practice. These ideas need to be operationalised and tested through middle-range and practice theories in order for them to be of practical use. Thus models are there to *guide* practice rather than tell nurses *how* to practise.

Many clinical areas have attempted to import models written by theorists in order to give a more theoretical foundation to their practice. The problem with this approach is that models of nursing are rarely founded on evidence. If, for example, we go back to Roper et al.'s model, the central concepts (apart from the life span continuum) are based on assumptions. Can we 'prove' that the 12 ADLs are in fact inclusive of all activities of daily living? Many nurses would argue that the concept of nursing contained within the model is too limited and does not cover many aspects of work carried out by community-based nurses. What the model does give us, however, is a way of looking at and directing our nursing practice.

The most common example of the use of the ADL model involves the way in which the assessment and planning of nursing care are enacted. The concept of the ADL has been used to develop comprehensive assessment strategies that enable nurses to gather data relating to the client's health status. This, in turn, informs nursing diagnosis, care-planning and much of the documentation that we see in nursing practice today. To what extent, however, does this interpretation of the ADL model represent the original model itself?

There have been numerous criticisms of the ADL model since its publication. These include the problem of mismatch between the concept of holism and the reductionist approach taken in the ADLs, and the largely physical focus of the model. As with any theory, however, it is up to readers to evaluate its usefulness for their own area of practice. It is extremely easy to engage in academic debate about the consistency that exists between the concepts and the lack of proven theory within the model, yet Roper et al. achieved a great deal in creating a model that appeared to reflect nursing in Britain when previous models had originated in America, with the associated problems of a culturally different conceptual understanding and a totally different health-care system. At the time of writing, nursing care delivered using the ADL model is alive and well in Britain despite attempts by other practitioners to create models in their own place of work.

There is of course a fundamental danger inherent in the notion of being able to adopt a model wholesale for a clinical area. Consider the fundamental principles underlying models, and nursing: by importing a ready-made model to guide practice, there is little likelihood that the nursing team will share the underpinning philosophy. Look back at the section concerning philosophies and the importance of joint ownership, and the two models of change. Imposed models are likely to be poorly received by staff who have no part in their creation. If staff do not give their commitment to the model as the way in which they practise, it is unlikely that the model itself will be implemented in its entirety. As a test, when you next visit your clinical area, ask the trained staff whether they have actually read the ADL model or whether they merely put into practice what they were told to do.

Finally, there is a fundamental problem with the idea of using a published model to guide all practice in one clinical area. Nursing today claims to provide holistic care and recognise clients as individuals with differing needs. How then can we assume that the same model can be applied to all the clients in one clinical area? The type of care that a client receives should be devised on an individual basis but it may vary depending on the model used in that particular area. If we can say that clients should receive care appropriate to their needs no matter which model is used, there is perhaps no need for different models, yet there are many models used to drive practice, all with differing starting points and a complicated conceptual development – despite the fact that there is little contemporary evidence published to show that the use of a model in practice affects client outcomes. What then is the purpose of using models in practice?

Effects on practice of using a model

Although there is scant evidence to support the direct effect of a model on client outcomes, there are documented benefits to using a model.

Teamwork

Many nurses draw attention to the benefits of choosing or creating a formal model of care that the whole team can share. By identifying, or even merely talking about, beliefs and values, and highlighting what is important to them in their practice, teams of nurses have found that their commitment to work and motivation have risen and that they feel valued as part of a team. In addition, the overt use of a model leads to a reduction in conflict between team members and is more likely to facilitate both continuity and consistency of care for clients.

Directing nursing care

Using a model can direct nursing care by providing a consistent focus for the way in which care is assessed, planned, implemented and evaluated. The use of Roper et al.'s model, for example, provides a comprehensive way of determining needs by using the idea of ADLs. Whether a nurse personally believes in such an approach is irrelevant if it is the model used in that area; it will lead the way in which care is given.

> **CONNECTIONS**
>
> *Chapter 1 explains the stages of the nursing process.*

Similarly, new ways of working or new policies for nursing care may arise from implementing a model as deficiencies can easily be identified through the application of the concepts.

Facilitating communication

The use of a model of care is usually accompanied by specific documentation or nursing records that comprehensively trace the client's progress through the system. These provide important data for charting progress and for enabling nurses to continue the chosen treatment regimen. They also force nurses to be accountable for their practice in a way unknown prior to the 1970s as detailed records have to be made and be signed by the supervising nurse. This has led to a vast improvement in the quality of nursing documentation as nurses learn to record their decision-making in client care as provision of the evidence on which their practice is based.

Selection of team members

CONNECTIONS

Chapter 15 looks at values and beliefs in teamworking.

There can be a more effective and appropriate selection of new team members if there is an active selection of people who share the same beliefs and values as the team. An active acknowledgement of the model to attract staff, and deliberate selection policies, will make it more probable that the right sort of people are selected.

Publicising good work

CONNECTIONS

Chapter 15 discusses values and beliefs in teamworking.

Models may also be used as the vehicle for demonstrating good practice. Some quality audit systems, such as that of Phaneuf, make the assumption that good documentation is a valid measure of the standard or quality of nursing care delivered. (Space precludes a debate on this here, but you might like to consider whether you believe that this is necessarily so.) The overt use of models, with public displays of the team philosophy, client and relative information booklets and active partnership in care, is likely to be seen by others as good practice. Similarly, other health professionals are likely to develop a greater understanding of the focus and direction of nursing care, and may well share it on a multidisciplinary basis, if a model is made public.

Aggleton and Chalmers (1990) suggest that models enable us to value what is effective in current practice, and encourage the search for new ways of improving care. There is thus an acknowledgement of the importance of nursing in health-care systems in its own right rather than just as the enactor of others' directions. In addition, models and theories may indicate the area of practice that distinguishes nursing from other health professions by defining a specific body of knowledge and describing nursing practice. This is particularly so when nurses have the courage to reject the use of published models and take the long, difficult road of creating one that suits their own nursing team.

Finally, this section ends with an analogy coined by Visintainer (1986), who likens the idea of models to different kinds of map. Maps are chosen for a specific purpose. If you wanted to drive from Portsmouth to Edinburgh, you would probably use a road map that showed motorways and main roads. However, that would not be much use if you wanted to go rambling on the Isle of Wight: for that, you would need a large-scale Ordnance Survey map. The same principle applies to models – they will work only if they are selected for a specific purpose. Models are clearly a positive tool for nursing but must be appropriate to the use to which it is intended to put them. Visintainer (1986) wisely says:

> The goodness of fit becomes the responsibility of the map-user not the map-maker, and the task can be a difficult one.

Nursing models and nursing process – the relationship

The nursing process has been fully covered in Chapter 1 so this ground will not be revisited here, but it is important to explore briefly the relationship between models and the nursing process.

Models tend to provide us with a representation of what nursing is and how it can be approached. They define the type of care and the concepts behind it. To use another analogy, models delineate the parcels and packages of care that can be expected. The nursing process is, however, a system of delivery – the vehicle for delivering the 'parcels', and in no way can the process be seen as a nursing model. The process says nothing about the content of care and is not specific to nursing; it is a sequence of steps passed through in order to achieve an end. The process can therefore operate effectively only within the beliefs and philosophies established by the model of care being used. Without the framework of the model, the process becomes just another form of work allocation.

■ Where to Next?

Congratulations – if you have read this chapter, you are probably about to embark on your chosen branch studies. This chapter has introduced many of the issues that you will meet in greater depth in the final 2 years of your course. What ties all of these issues together is the need for you to adopt the mantle of being a professional, registered nurse, with the accompanying privileges and responsibilities that this entails. On emerging fully qualified, from the branch programme, you will be expected to have adopted a professional ethos, to be competent and accountable for your practice, and to have acquired the necessary knowledge, skills and experience to give you professional authority.

Learning, however, does not, and cannot, stop on qualification. Quite apart from the UKCC's requirements for triennial registration, you will, as a qualified practitioner, need to be able to provide evidence-based practice (UKCC, 1995). In order to do this, you will continue to practise academic skills and will direct your own learning so that you can deliver care of the quality that you want to achieve. Courses for registration are only the beginning of a long and exciting journey but you will have acquired throughout the course the skills needed for lifelong learning. The next 2 years will consolidate those skills and enable you to take more responsibility for your own personal and professional development.

● **Test Yourself!**

1. (a) What is meant by professional practice?

    (b) What are the responsibilities associated with professional practice?

2. (a) What is meant by the *Code of Professional Conduct*?

    (b) What are your roles and responsibility, as a student, under the *Code of Professional Conduct*?

    (c) What is your accountability as a student nurse?

    (d) How does this differ from the accountability of a registered practitioner?

    (e) What does 'informed consent' mean? When is it needed, who can give it and who can obtain it?

3. How do beliefs and values influence nursing care?

4. How do models of care influence the care that a client receives?

5. (a) Why is quality assessment important in professional care?
    (b) What impact will the introduction of clinical governance have on nursing care?

6. Why is it necessary for registered practitioners to practise from a contemporaneous knowledge base?

■ **References**

Aggleton, P. and Chalmers, H. (1990) *Nursing Models and the Nursing Process*, 2nd edn. Macmillan – now Palgrave Macmillan, London.

Avis, M., Bond, M. and Arthur, A. (1995) Satisfying solutions? A review of some unresolved issues in the measurement of patient satisfaction. *Journal of Advanced Nursing* **22**(2): 316–22.

Bond, S. and Thomas, L.H. (1992) Measuring patients' satisfaction with nursing care. *Journal of Advanced Nursing* **17**(1): 52–63.

Chinn, P.L. and Kramer, M. (1991) *Theory and Nursing: A Systematic Approach*, 3rd edn. C.V. Mosby, St Louis.

Dickoff, J., Weidenbach, E. and James, P. (1968) Theory in practice discipline. *Nursing Research* **17**(5): 415–35.

DoH (Department of Health) (1997) *The New NHS: Modern, Dependable*. Stationery Office, London.

DoH (Department of Health) (1998) *A First Class Service. Quality in the NHS*. Stationery Office, London.

DoH (Department of Health) (2001) *Reference Guide to Consent for Examination or Treatment*. HMSO, London.

Fawcett, J. (1984) *Analysis and Evaluation of Conceptual Models of Nursing*. F.A. Davis, Philadelphia.

Griffiths, P. (1995) Progress in measuring nursing outcomes. *Journal of Advanced Nursing* **21**(6): 1092–100.

Henderson, V. (1966) *The Nature of Nursing*. Collier Macmillan, London.

Higgins, M., McCaughan, D., Griffiths, M. and Carr-Hill, R. (1992) Assessing the outcomes of nursing care. *Journal of Advanced Nursing* **17**(5): 561–8.

Jasper, M. (1996) *Evaluating Care and Effecting Change*. Unit Study Guide. Distance Learning Centre, South Bank University, London.

Johns, C. (1991) The Burford Nursing Development Unit holistic model of nursing practice. *Journal of Advanced Nursing* **16**: 1090–8.

Koch, T. (1994) Beyond measurement: fourth-generation evaluation in nursing. *Journal of Advanced Nursing* **20**(6): 1148–55.

Manley, K. (1991) Knowledge for nursing practice. In Perry, A. and Jolley, M. (eds) *Nursing: A Knowledge Base for Practice*. Edward Arnold, London.

Mawdsley, D. (1991) Who needs nursing philosophies? *Professional Nurse* **7**(2): 78–82.

Meleis, A. (1996) *Theoretical Nursing: Development and Progress*, 3rd edn. J.B. Lippincott, Philadelphia.

Moloney, M.M. (1992) *Professionalization of Nursing – Current Issues and Trends*. J.B. Lippincott, Philadelphia.

NMC (Nursing and Midwifery Council) (2002) *Code of Professional Conduct*. NMC, London.

Orem, D.E. (1980) *Concepts of Practice*, 2nd edn. McGraw-Hill, New York.

Pearson, A., Vaughan, B. and Fitzgerald, M. (1996) *Nursing Models for Practice*, 2nd edn. Heinnemann, Oxford.

Peplau, H. (1952) *Interpersonal Relations in Nursing*. G.P. Putnam, New York.

Phaneuf, M.C. (1976) *The Nursing Audit: Self-regulation in Nursing Practice*. Appleton-Century-Crofts, New York.

Polit, D.F., Beck, C.T. and Hungler, B.T. (2001) *Essentials of Nursing Research: Methods, Appraisal and Utilisation*, 5th edn. Lippincott, Philadelphia.

Rafferty, A.M. (1996) *The Politics of Nursing Knowledge*. Routledge, London.

RCN (Royal College of Nursing) (1990) *Quality Patient Care: The Dynamic Standard Setting System*. RCN, London.

Rolfe, G. (1996) *Closing the Theory–Practice Gap – a New Paradigm for Nursing*. Butterworth-Heinemann, Oxford.

Roper, N., Logan, W. and Tierney, A. (1980) *The Elements of Nursing*. Churchill Living-stone, Edinburgh.

Roper, N., Logan, W. and Tierney, A. (1990) *The Elements of Nursing*, 3rd edn. Churchill Livingstone, Edinburgh.

Roy, C. (1984) *Introduction to Nursing: An Adaptation Model*, 2nd edn. Prentice-Hall, Englewood Cliffs, NJ.

Scally, G. and Donaldson, L. (1998) Clinical governance and the drive for quality improvement in the new NHS in England. *British Medical Journal* **317**: 61–5.

Severs, M. (1998) The Clinical Governance Cycle. Lecture series, PG Cert Clinical Governance, Unit 1. University of Portsmouth, Portsmouth.

Simpson, R.G., Scothern, G. and Vincent, M. (1995) Survey of carer satisfaction with the quality of care delivered to in-patients suffering from dementia. *Journal of Advanced Nursing* **22**(3): 517–27.

UKCC (United Kingdom Central Council for Nursing, Midwifery and Health Visiting) (1987) *Confidentiality*. UKCC, London.

UKCC (United Kingdom Central Council for Nursing, Midwifery and Health Visiting) (1988) *UKCC – The First Five Years 1983–1988*. UKCC, London.

UKCC (United Kingdom Central Council for Nursing, Midwifery and Health Visiting) (1989) *Exercising Accountability*. UKCC, London.

UKCC (United Kingdom Central Council for Nursing, Midwifery and Health Visiting) (1995) *PREP and You*. UKCC, London.

UKCC (United Kingdom Central Council for Nursing, Midwifery and Health Visiting) (1996) *Guidelines for Professional Practice*. UKCC, London.

UKCC (United Kingdom Central Council for Nursing, Midwifery and Health Visiting) (2001) *The PREP Handbook*. UKCC, London.

UKCC (United Kingdom Central Council for Nursing, Midwifery and Health Visiting) (2002) The future of professional regulation. *Register* (Winter).

Visintainer, M. (1986) The nature of knowledge and theory in nursing. *Image* **18**(2): 32–8.

Walker, L.O. and Avant, K.C. (1996) *Strategies for Theory Construction in Nursing*, 3rd edn. Appleton & Lange, Norwalk, CT.

Wandelt, M. and Ager, J. (1974) *Quality Patient Care Scale*. Appleton-Century-Crofts, New York.

Watson, J. (1979) *Nursing: The Philosophy and Science of Caring*. Little, Brown, Boston.

Wright, S. (1986) *Building and Using a Model of Nursing*. Edward Arnold, London.

Wright, S. (1990) *My Patient – My Nurse*. Scutari Press, London.

Acknowledgement

With thanks to Nadia Chambers for the section on clinical governance.

Answers to Test Yourself! Questions and Activities

● Test Yourself!

Chapter 1

1. ● Assessment
   ● Diagnosis
   ● Planning
   ● Implementation
   ● Evaluation.

2. It enables the nurse to plan care for a client on an individual basis and to solve problems.

3. ● Physical health information
   ● Psychological information
   ● Social health information
   ● The activities of living.

4. Two: actual and potential.

5. ● Setting goals
   ● Identifying actions.

6. The MACROS criteria:
   ● Measurable and observable
   ● Achievable and time limited
   ● Client centred
   ● Realistic
   ● Outcome written
   ● Short.

7. ● Nursing handover
   ● Reflection
   ● Patient satisfaction or complaint
   ● Reviewing the nursing care plan.

Chapter 3

1. These data are available from the infection control department of your hospital Trust. The national average for hospital-acquired infection in the UK is about 9 per cent, so the number of patients affected will vary depending on the number of beds in the hospital.

2. The infection control department usually produces guidelines for infection control as well as the names of the infection control team. You are advised to consult the infection control manager/sister.

3. The following criteria should be used to evaluate the quality of hand-washing:
   ● The use of soap/detergent
   ● The use of continuously running water
   ● Positioning the hands to avoid contaminating the surface areas
   ● Rubbing the hands together vigorously
   ● Rinsing and drying the hands thoroughly.

4. Refer to the 10-point code outlined in Chapter 3.

5. Diarrhoea, vomiting, abdominal pain and pyrexia.

6. The source should be isolated. Spread must be prevented by following the infection control guidelines, for example employing a good hand-washing technique and protective clothing. Any further spread to staff/patients must be reported. The number of visitors should be restricted.

7. A general guide to ensure the patient's safety in the administration of medications is to check yourself against the five 'R's:
   ● The right medication
   ● The right amount
   ● The right time
   ● The right patient
   ● The right route.

8. The ventrogluteal muscle, the deltoid muscle and the dorsogluteal muscle.

9. Special precautions when giving injections to children:
   ● Take into account whether the infant has been walking for a year.
   ● Sites for intramuscular injection in infants who have not been walking for a year are:
     – the vastus lateralis muscle

  – the ventrogluteal muscle
  – the mid-anterior thigh muscle.
- Sites for intramusclar injections in older children who have been walking for more than a year are:
  – the vastus lateralis muscle
  – the dorsogluteal muscle
  – the deltoid muscle.

Chapter 4

1. - Fat: 37 kJ/g (9 kcal/g)
   - Alcohol: 29 kJ/g (7 kcal/g)
   - Carbohydrate: 17 kJ/g (3.75 kcal/g)
   - Protein: 16 kJ/g (4 kcal/g).

2. Fibre slows the release of glucose into the bloodstream (soluble fibre) and forms bulk to aid the passage of faeces (insoluble fibre).

3. Fruit, vegetables, whole grains, wholemeal bread, cereals, beans and pulses.

4. The fluid requirement is 30–35 ml/kg per day for adults with normal renal and cardiac function.

5. An antioxidant neutralises free radicals, the potentially damaging molecules within the body produced by normal processes such as digestion.

6. Vitamin A and beta-carotene, vitamin C, vitamin E and selenium.

7. Take your weight in kilograms divided by the square of your height in metres to estimate your body mass index.

Chapter 5

1. - The client's normal bowel habit
   - The frequency/time of faecal/urinary elimination
   - The presence of pain/discomfort when eliminating
   - The amount eliminated
   - Odour
   - Diet/fluid intake
   - Disease
   - Mobility.

2. - Drugs, resulting in reduced motility of the intestine
   - Laxative abuse, resulting in a diminished normal reflex
   - Pregnancy, due to reduced abdominal space and progesterone slowing peristalsis
   - Disease processes, altering the time of passage of the faeces
   - Pain, causing the client to be reluctant to defaecate

- Psychiatric problems, causing a lack of interest in the surroundings and diet, or an altered dietary intake
- A diet low in fibre, or an inadequate intake
- Fluids not sufficient for the patient's needs
- Immobility, reducing intestinal motility
- Ignoring the call to defaecate, allowing more fluid to be absorbed from the faeces, which therefore become harder and more difficult to eliminate
- Psychological factors caused by unfavourable conditions, the client delaying the defaecation process until more favourable conditions exist.

3. - Stress incontinence
    - Urge incontinence
    - Reflex incontinence
    - Overflow incontinence.

4. - Ileostomy: an opening from the ileum; faecal material liquid
    - Colostomy: an opening from the colon; faecal material ranges from semisolid to more formed stools
    - Urostomy: the bladder is removed and urinary excretion is diverted via a stoma formed on the abdominal wall.

5. - Embarrassment (the most common factor)
    - Depression
    - Anorexia nervosa
    - Chronic psychoses.

6. Calculated on a 30–35 ml/kg body weight, this equals 1950–2275 ml per 24 hours.

Chapter 6

1. 25 per minute.

2. Respiratory cycles of gradually decreasing rate and depth, followed by cycles of increasing rate and depth. Cheyne–Stokes respiration frequently indicates impending death.

3. - Mucoid: raw egg appearance, due to chronic bronchitis
    - Purulent: slimy and green, due to bronchopneumonial infection
    - Haemoptysis: red and frothy, due to bleeding in the lungs
    - Frothy: pink and bubbly, due to pulmonary oedema.

4. The jaw thrust is a method of opening the airway that maintains in-line stabilisation of the neck and is used if cervical injury is suspected.

5. - Decreased urinary output
    - Muscle weakness

- Peripheral cyanosis
- Cool extremities
- Grey, mottled skin in infants
- Tachycardia.

6. Using the brachial pulse in the infant and the carotid pulse for all other age groups.

7. 1. Sharp and clear
   2. Blowing and swishing
   3. Sharp but softer than 1
   4. Muffled but fading
   5. No sound.

8. By pressing one's thumb on a client's skin, causing it to blanch, and timing the return of the blood flow.

9. - Verbal descriptor
   - Visual analogue
   - Pain behaviour
   - Combined tool.

10. - Circulatory overload
    - Allergic reaction
    - Disease transmission
    - Pyrogenic reaction
    - Haemolytic mismatch.

Chapter 7

1. Read the section on body image and pick out the main words used to form a couple of sentences.

2. Circumcision, caesarean section, oopherectomy, lumpectomy, termination.

3. Body reality, body presentation and body ideal.

4. - A high incidence of sexually abusive experiences
   - Multiple experiences of bereavement and loss
   - Difficulties in talking about emotions
   - Limited sex education
   - Limited expectations and low self-esteem
   - A lack of assertiveness about sex and relationships
   - A lack of privacy.

5. Ancient Egyptian.

6. Intimacy; antidiscriminatory practice; empowerment and partnership.

Chapter 8

1. See below.

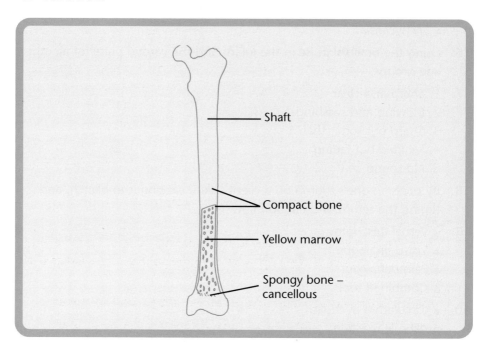

2. Collagen, calcium and phosphate, and bone cells.
3. The outer area of all the bones, in the shafts of the long bones and in the outer and inner parts of the flat bones.
4. Haversian systems.
5. To allow movement and aid the production of body heat.
6. The resistance offered to a passive stretch of the muscle. This is determined by the nerve supply to the muscle and its control, as well as by the contractile and elastic properties of the muscle.
7. Twenty per cent.
8. To facilitate movement, to ensure that movements are stable and to help to maintain the posture.
9. The elbow joint.
10. The shoulder girdle, hand, foot and vertebral column.
11. Flexion, extension, abduction, adduction, external and internal rotation, and circumduction.
12. Exercise slows osteoporosis, interrupts bone loss and encourages new bone mass. It may lessen dependency in individuals.

13. The development of deep vein thrombosis and pulmonary embolism, chest infections, constipation, urinary tract infections and renal calculi, muscle weakness and atrophy pressure sores and the demineralisation of bones.

14. A skin ulceration occurring as a result of unrelieved pressure and a combination of other variables. Nursing care involves the relief of pressure, encouraging mobility, a nutritious diet and adequate fluid intake. If the client is incontinent, incontinence aids should be used.

Chapter 9

1. Cessation of breathing, no palpable heart beat and fixed dilated pupils.

2. Valuing, preserving integrity, connecting, doing for, empowering and finding meaning.

3. The experience of pain influenced by physical, emotional, social and spiritual factors.

4. This a progressive stepwise approach to pain relief by giving increasing amounts of analgesics and adjuvants until the pain is controlled as fully as possible.

5. Pain, weakness, constipation, nausea and vomiting, and dyspnoea.

6. A term that describes the final aspects of caring following a patient's death. It involves preparing the body for removal but also helps to prepare relatives and staff in saying their goodbyes to the deceased.

7. Loss-orientated involves grief work, the intrusion of grief, breaking bonds and the denial/avoidance of restoration changes.

   Restoration-orientated involves attending to life changes, doing new things, distraction from grief, denial avoidance of grief and new roles/identities/relationships.

8. Any of the items listed below:
   - By being there
   - By listening in an accepting and non-judgemental way
   - By showing that you are listening and understand something of what they are going through
   - By encouraging them to talk about the deceased
   - By tolerating silence
   - By being familiar with your own feelings about loss and grief
   - By offering reassurance about the normality of grief
   - By not taking anger personally
   - By recognising that your feelings may reflect how they feel
   - By accepting that you cannot make them feel better.

9. Spiritual, situational and moral and biographical.

Chapter 10

1. The accountability relationships within which professional practitioners are required to discharge their duty of care to the client include:
   - Legal
   - Managerial
   - Organisational
   - Professional
   - Governmental
   - Moral and ethical.

2. Any kind of breach in the integrity of the skin or underlying tissues can be described as a 'wound'.

3. - According to causal factor(s)
   - According to depth
   - As 'open' or 'closed'
   - By the anticipated method of healing.

4. - Pressure area damage
   - Diabetic foot ulcer risk
   - Nutritional compromise
   - Manual handling.

5. - Epidermis
   - Dermis
   - Subcutaneous tissue
   - Hair and hair follicles
   - Nails
   - Sweat glands
   - Sebaceous glands
   - Sensory nerve receptors
   - Capillary network
   - Specialist cells, for example melanocytes.

6. The four main phases of wound healing are haemostasis, inflammation, proliferation and maturation.

7. The factors of the personal aspect that affect wound healing include:
   - Age
   - Mental state
   - Ability to communicate
   - Nutritional status
   - Cardiovascular status
   - Respiratory status
   - Mobility

- Continence
- Underlying pathophysiology
- Pain
- Type of wound
- Location of wound
- Condition of skin.

Those of the contextual aspect include:
- Socio-economic status
- Housing
- Access to the multidisciplinary team
- Access to voluntary organisations
- Method of care delivery
- Social network
- Exposure to environmental contaminants
- Ambient temperature
- Education
- Medication.

8.
- Moisture
- Protection from bacterial contamination
- Protection from particulate and toxic contamination
- Thermal insulation
- Removal of excess exudate
- Good blood supply
- Protection from mechanical damage
- Minimal disturbance.

9.
- General physical condition
- Mental state
- Mobility
- Nutritional status
- Continence
- Concurrent disease
- Cardiovascular status
- Pain
- Skin
- Risk assessment.

10. The purpose of a nursing care plan in wound management is to provide a systematic, rational documentary review, using a problem-solving approach, of the prescribed care required to meet nursing care needs and achieve specified nursing care objectives. The nursing care plan also provides documentary evidence of evaluations of nursing care,

providing a 'decision trail' for the rationale underpinning any modifications to the prescribed nursing care.

11. The term 'aseptic technique' refers to the method of carrying out procedures in an environment that is rendered as free as possible of micro-organisms and contaminants.

12. The evaluation of nursing care in wound management is concerned with the effectiveness of nursing interventions. The key considerations should be:
- Current versus previous wound status
- To what extent specified objectives have been achieved
- What factors have facilitated or impaired the achievement of these objectives
- Further assessment
- Revisions to planned care.

Chapter 11

1.
- Empathic understanding
- Genuineness
- Unconditional acceptance.

2.
- Prescriptive
- Informative
- Confronting
- Catalytic
- Supportive
- Cathartic.

3. Any of the interventions listed below could be used:
- Open questions
- Closed questions
- Checking for understanding
- Simple reflection
- Paraphrasing
- Logical building
- Empathic building.

5. A primary group is a close intimate group that usually has face-to-face contact. A secondary group is usually a large group in which members have less direct contact.

6.
- Task needs
- Team maintenance needs
- Individiual needs.

7.
   - Forming
   - Storming
   - Norming
   - Performing.

8.
   - Assertive
   - Aggressive
   - Submissive/passive.

9.
   - Listening carefully
   - Saying what you think and feel
   - Saying what you want to happen
   - Being persistent
   - Being prepared to compromise.

10. For valid criticism, accept the criticism. If the criticism is invalid, reject it. If it is partially valid, accept the valid aspects and reject the invalid aspects of the criticism.

Chapter 12

1. Self concept is the knowledge people have about themselves. It is an organised set of beliefs and feelings that are self-referent.

2. Self-awareness is a constructive appreciation of the self. Self-consciousness is a concern for others' perception of the self.

3. Stress occurs when the demands of the situation exceed the personal resources of the individual.

4.
   - Personality
   - Social support
   - Emotion.

5. Attitudes are the sum of one's beliefs and opinions. They have three components: behavioural, cognitive and affective.

6. It is people's attitudes to health behaviours that influence whether they will modify risky health behaviours such as smoking or a poor diet.

7.
   - Trust
   - Like/dislike
   - Credibility
   - Perceived attractiveness
   - Individual beliefs
   - Self-esteem.

Chapter 13

1. Ritualism – in which participants mindlessly go through the motions.

2. Boyd and Fales (1983) speak of this as 'a sense of inner discomfort'. Any deviation from that which is confidently known may generate feelings of insecurity, our actions no longer being guided by what is implicitly known through teaching or experience. Outcomes may seem risky, uncontrollable and unpredictable, and a sense of uncertainty results.

3. Evaluate the relevance of the knowledge.

4. Reflection-in-action and reflection-on-action.

5. Anticipatory reflection. This relates to the manner in which the care situation is approached, making a tacit comparison with previous experience to ensure that we are not already equipped in some way to deal with what is being met.

6. Crouch (1991) sees the critical incident as 'an observation or activity which was sufficiently complete in itself so as to permit inferences and predictions to be drawn from it'.

7. Practice knowledge is that achieved through a 'hands-on', skills acquisition mode. Of equal and possibly greater value, however, is experiential knowledge, gained through a direct, personal encounter with a subject, person or event.

8. ● An experience
   ● Observation and reflection
   ● The formulation of abstract concepts and generalisations out of that reflection
   ● Testing implications of concepts learned on new situations.

9. For Fisher (1996), clinical supervision is a blend of education, support and management.

10. Although experiential learning may be facilitated by a teacher or supervisor, it may equally well be an everyday event or a spontaneous or vicarious learning opportunity. It is essential that, when such methods are used, the pace must be set *by the learners* as it is their experience and their learning.

Chapter 14

1. Four.

2. 1948.

3. ● Block contracts
   ● Cost and volume
   ● Cost per case.

4. 1902.

5. Mental Health Act Commission.

6. A supervision order.

Chapter 15

1. 'Interprofessional practice' is one of the terms used to describe a group of professionals working together to achieve mutually agreed goals. These goals should involve the service user and the carer. Other terms are often used in place of interprofessional, for example interdisciplinary, multiprofessional and multidisciplinary. Interprofessional practice has been most common in primary care and community care settings, and more recently it has become an element of acute care practice.

3. With the establishment of primary care groups, the role of many professionals may change. Practice nurses, district nurses and health visitors, for example, may be involved in the management of primary care groups, bringing together the work of GPs and other professions. Social workers may also be represented, especially in child protection and mental health issues. In the hospital setting, nurses will be involved in the care-planning process for discharge in elderly care, as well as in working alongside physiotherapists and occupational therapists in the field of stroke rehabilitation. Ensuring that the client's or patient's needs are met by the person with the appropriate skill and knowledge is the most significant role that all professionals bring to teamwork. Equally, the ongoing evaluation and review of practice intervention will mean that the most effective use of resources is being made.

4. Ensuring that the specific skills and knowledge held by the nurse are recognised by others in the team. If the nurse is employed by the GP, he or she may have limited involvement in the allocation of resources for the particular area of practice. Equally, a difference in payment can lead to differing levels of status within a team. Status may play a major part in the decision-making process, and nurses may have to work proactively to ensure that their views on good practice are heard and evaluated.

Chapter 16

1a. Professional practice can be viewed from many different starting points depending on who it is that is defining it. The common elements arise, however, from expectations about a practitioner's behaviour as a professional that arise from the profession's code of conduct and from legal responsibilities.

1b. The responsibilities for professional practice are defined in the NMC *Code of Professional Conduct* (2002) and encapsulated by the following statement:

    As a registered nurse or midwife, you must:
    ● protect and support the health of individual patients and clients

- protect and support the health of the wider community
- act in such a way that justifies the trust and confidence the public have in you
- uphold and enhance the good reputation of the professions.

As a registered nurse or midwife, you are personally accountable for your practice.

Individual responsibilities are listed in Chart 16.1.

2a. The *Code of Professional Conduct* is the document produced by the UKCC that outlines the roles and responsibilities of a registered practitioner. It acts as a standard for professional practice, enabling the profession to judge practitioners in terms of misconduct.

2b. Students are given their own, amended, version of the *Code of Professional Conduct*. If you are not familiar with this, it is important that you read it before proceeding with your studies.

2c. You are accountable for your own actions as a citizen of this country and must therefore not undertake criminal activities. You are also accountable to your employer for your actions while working, and you are accountable under civil law for all of your actions, whether these occur at work or elsewhere.

2d. Students clearly cannot be professionally accountable because they are not entered on the professional register, but they are accountable in the other three ways listed in 1b above. This does not, however, mean that students are not responsible for their actions.

2e. Informed consent is a decision to agree to treatment based on a full explanation of the intervention involved, including information about the benefits and risks of the treatment proposed, and alternative treatments. It is needed for all nursing procedures. A competent adult or a child judged to be competent can give consent. A parent or nominated other may give consent for a child under 16. Any person delivering care can obtain consent, the person giving the care/treatment ideally doing this.

3. We all practise from a belief and value system that has arisen from our own personal experiences of life and what we have encountered in the way of experience, education and professional socialisation. In the same way that our own style of nursing is directed by our beliefs and values, so also will be the care delivered by a team of nurses working together.

4. The primary purpose of a model of care is to help nurses to understand nursing from a particular viewpoint and use that to direct their care. Formal models occur when the values, beliefs and ways of working are

made explicit and shared by the team of nurses in the clinical area. They enable groups of nurses to think about, and carry out, nursing in a fairly similar way, with clear objectives for the delivery of care because the model aims to represent the nursing care to be achieved by that team.

5a. Quality assessment measures the standard of care that is used as a judgement evaluating the services being delivered. It is used to evaluate services against the promises made to clients in the Patient's Charter and against targets set by purchasing agencies, as well as to provide information for improving nursing care.

5b. Clinical governance provides a framework for the continual improvement of services to patients so it requires participation from all nurses. It will require a change in the culture of nursing, away from the separatist practice that we have had in the past towards integration and collaboration between all professions involved in health-care delivery. Clinical governance places reponsibility on all of us to strive for high standards of care and ensure that the best quality is delivered.

6. The basic answer here is that this is required by the NMC and written into Clause 6.1 of the *Professional Code of Conduct*. Apart from that, however, you would consider it ethically wrong if you consulted, for example, a lawyer and he or she was not up to date with the pertinent laws relating to your case. Similarly, we must as professional nurses ensure that we provide the best possible care to our clients, and as professionals it is incumbent upon us continually to keep abreast of developments in our speciality and practise appropriately.

● Activity Answers

Chapter 4

Activity 6

The nurse needs to understand that, as the body is about 60 per cent water, it affects many physiological processes, including the circulation of the blood (Chapter 6) and elimination (Chapter 5). Fluid and electrolytes are gained from eating and drinking, and lost in urine and sweat. Intravenous therapy (Chapter 6) makes no sense without an understanding of fluid compartments.

Activity 7

The client's urine will be pale and plentiful, defaecation easy, the skin well hydrated and the eyes not sunken.

Activity 8

Look around the supermarket to identify whole-grain cereals, for example:

- wholemeal bread, flour, pasta and brown rice
- Weetabix, Shredded Wheat, muesli and porridge
- bran-enriched cereals such as All Bran and Bran Flakes.

A trip to the supermarket will also identify loaves fortified with folic acid, for example Mighty White.

Folic acid is needed in very early pregnancy, often before the woman realises that she is pregnant.

Activity 9

A lack of sunlight on the skin can deprive the person of this source of vitamin D. Vitamin B deficiency will lead to osteomalacia with muscle weakness and bone pain and tenderness.

Activity 10

Channel Islands' breakfast milk has 134 mg calcium per 100 ml, skimmed cow's milk has 124 mg/100 ml, semi-skimmed milk has 122 mg/100 ml and whole milk has 119 mg/100 ml.

Activity 12

Non-starch polysaccharides (NSP/fibre) are digested by colonic bacteria, with methane as a byproduct. Intestinal flora synthesise vitamin B6.

The products of bacterial metabolism vary according to the types of bacterium present, which are different in different people, and their number, which is also subject to a wide variation. If the volume of food residue from the small intestine increases, the number goes up. Thus, if the amount of NSP/fibre in the diet is increased, or the digestion of carbohydrate and protein in the small intestine is incomplete (for example because of enzyme deficiency), the bacterial population in the large intestine increases (Rutishauser, 1994, pp. 123–4).

The metabolic activities of colonic bacteria result in the protein products of ammonia, urea and nitrogen; the NSP products of short-chain fatty acids, carbon dioxide, methane and hydrogen; and primary bile salts producing secondary bile salts, stercobilin from bilirubin (Rutishauser, 1994, pp. 123–4).

Activity 13

Eggs are classified in the meat and alternatives section, and potatoes in the starchy foods section.

Activity 14

Anabolism is the building up of body substance, such as occurs during convalescence or body-building. There will be increased nutritional demands compared with the normal steady state.

Catabolism is the breakdown of body substance, the destructive phase of the acute stress response, as occurs, for example, after trauma or surgery. Muscle may be very much depleted, and nutritional support is directed towards minimising the impact of this process.

Activity 23

The pH of gastric juice ranges from 1.0 to 7.0, depending on the stomach contents. This is acid enough to dissolve razor blades, hence the rare 'sport' of eating cars and bicycles.

Activity 24

The eustachian (auditory) tube runs between the pharynx and the middle ear and can transmit infection introduced by nasogastric tube placement.

Index

Page numbers in **bold** type refer to figures; those in *italic* to tables and charts. Page numbers marked with an asterisk (*) indicate the presence of glossary points in the margin in addition to any material in the main text; those marked with (w) include a relevant website address.